SKIN BIOPSY – PERSPECTIVES

Edited by **Uday Khopkar**

Skin Biopsy – Perspectives
Edited by Uday Khopkar

Published by InTech

Janeza Trdine 9, 51000 Rijeka, Croatia

Publishing Process Manager Dragana Manestar

Technical Editor Teodora Smiljanic

Cover Designer InTech Design Team

Additional hard copies can be obtained from orders@intechopen.com

Skin Biopsy – Perspectives, Edited by Uday Khopkar
p. cm.
ISBN 978-953-307-290-6

For EU product safety concerns:
IN TECH d.o.o., Prolaz Marije Krucifikse Kozulić 3, 51000 Rijeka, Croatia,
info@intechopen.com or visit our website at intechopen.com.

Meet the editor

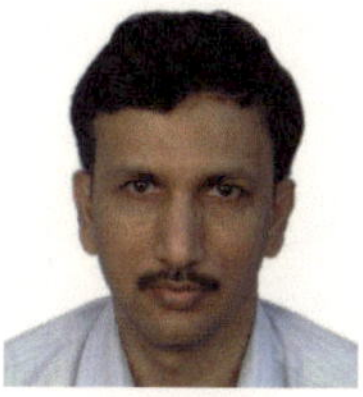

Dr. Uday Khopkar is a Consultant Dermatologist, Dermatopathologist, Professor and Head of Dermatology at the GS Medical College and KEM Hospital in Mumbai, India. After doing post-graduation in Dermatology at the Topiwala National Medical College and Nair Hospital, Mumbai, he did Fellowships in Dermatopathology in 1992 and 1994-95 with A. Bernard Ackerman in USA. He started the first countrywide dermatopathology referral system in India and currently gives opinion on about 6000 skin biopsy specimens per year. His other contributions to Indian Dermatology are giving a face-lift to the national journal, viz. Indian Journal of Dermatology, Venereology and Leprology during his 6 year tenure as the Chief Editor of IJDVL, getting it indexed, and authoring popular texts for medical undergraduates and postgraduates in India. Dr. Khopkar has wide research interests covering dermatopathology, dermoscopy, clinical trials, clinical trichology and management of autoimmune skin diseases.

Contents

Preface

I am pleased to present this book on the techniques and applications of skin biopsy.

The book is organized into four sections as per the applicability of the techniques described in each of the chapters.

Skin biopsy is the most frequent diagnostic investigation undertaken by a dermatologist. Large amount of information is available upon interpretation of skin biopsies. However, in clinical practice, difficulties in interpretation of skin biopsies are not uncommon. Many of these difficulties arise from variations in technique of performing or processing a skin biopsy. It is with this intent that we decided to focus on the methodology of performing skin biopsies in different clinical scenarios.

The first section of the book deals with common clinical applications of skin biopsy in humans. While it is focused largely on the nuances and pitfalls in technique of performing a skin biopsy, the second section is dedicated to specialized applications of skin biopsy in the diagnosis of uncommon diseases. These clinical situations, being uncommon, demand special attention to appropriate technique while taking the biopsy in the clinic as well as processing it in the laboratory. Some of these conditions are systemic diseases establishing diagnosis for which is dependent on the correct sampling and processing of skin biopsy.

Technology is moving at a rapid pace and finds applications in every field. Skin as a tissue is being increasingly used in research laboratories around the world. Many research methods have been developed based on skin tissue culture and these have been dealt with in some detail in the third section of this book.

Finally, the last section deals with the use of skin biopsy to monitor impact of environmental changes on animals, more specifically - marine life. This brings into focus the wider applications of skin biopsy in environmental sciences and biology in general.

I am thankful to the authors for contributing their excellent scientific material to this book, in spite of their busy schedules, which requires special appreciation. I am also indebted to the InTech team for coordinating all the correspondence and looking after the technical matters and following a strict publication protocol. Special thanks are due to Dragana Manestar of InTech for her patience and perseverance in correspondence that has led to this successful conclusion.

This book is basically aimed at improving outcomes of skin biopsies aimed at diagnosing skin diseases. I hope that this drop in the ocean of information around us improves this outcome for the final beneficiary of all medical literature - the patient.

Uday Khopkar
GS Medical College and KEM Hospital
Mumbai, India

Part 1

Skin Biopsy Procedure – Do's and Don'ts

1

Skin Biopsy Procedures: How and Where to Perform a Proper Biopsy

Z. Seia, L. Musso, Stefania Palazzini and M. Bertero
Ospedale S. Croce e Carle of Cuneo, SC Dermatologia
Italy

1. Introduction

1.1 Skin biopsy

The skin biopsy is a relatively simple, but essential procedure in the managment of skin disorders. As a diagnostic method, skin biopsy is most commonly used in dermatology rather than in other medical specializations. The most common indication is to diagnose or exclude cutaneous malignancies. Properly performed, it may confirm a diagnosis, remove cosmetically unacceptable lesions, and provide definitive treatment for a number of skin conditions yielding a sample of skin for histopathological or other investigation. Before performing a skin biopsy it is necessary to take prior arrangements with a laboratory for sending specimens, particularly for specialised investigations such as direct immunofluorescence or molecular biology. Otherwise it would be better to send the biopsy to selectioned centers even far away because a wrong diagnosis is worse than a lack of diagnosis. It is also necessary a foolproof system for sending specimens, receiving and filing reports, documenting and executing action plans. Patients must give a well drafted, written consent form for invasive procedures.

Skin biopsy techniques should ideally be quick and easy to perform, yielding specimens of high quality and adequate size while leaving the smallest possible tissue defect and a good cosmetic result. Skin biopsies can be performed with minimal risk in critically ill patients, and a timely skin biopsy may avoid other, more invasive procedures. Skin biopsies are infrequently performed by internist. This may involve lack of proficiency, or uncertainty regarding indications, choice of procedure, specimen handling, or subsequent wound care. Nevertheless, many dermatoses have nonspecific histopathology and biopsy cannot substitute for good clinical skills.

There are few absolute controindications to skin biopsy, but all patients should be told that biopsies leave scars. A biopsy should not be done at an infected site, although occasionally infection may be the indication for the procedure. Inquiry should be made regarding allergies to topical antibiotics, antiseptics, local anesthetics and reaction to tape. Patient should be asked about systemic diseases, bleeding disorders, bleeding with previous surgery, and use of drugs known to interfere with hemostasis.

There are several methods to perform biopsy: curettage, shave biopsy, punch biopsy, excisional biopsy.

1.1.1 Surgical safety

Performing skin biopsies places the operator at risk of blood-borne infections. Universal precautions should be observed by wearing gloves and eye-guards. Shave and punch biopsies are clean but not sterile procedures; mask, gown and sterile gloves are not always necessary. These are indicated for excisions, and are reasonable for any patient at increased risk of infection. Material that is contamined with blood or other body fluids should be disposed in special „contaminated-materials" plastic bags.

1.1.2 Preparing the site

To prepare the biopsy site common skin antiseptics can be used (such as isopropyl alcohol, providone-iodine, chlorhexidine gluconate). It is useful to mark the intended lesion with a surgical marker as the border may be temporarily obliterated by the anesthetic injection. For excision, a surgical fenestrated drape is placed over the biopsy site after cleansing and before anesthesia.

1.1.3 Anesthesia

The most commonly used anesthetic is 1% or 2% lidocaine. This is a vasodilator, and so small amounts of epinephrine are added to constrict blood vessels, decrease bleeding, and prolong anesthesia. It is better to avoid the use of epinephrine for acral lesions, tip of nose, or when large quantities are needed, especially in patients with cardiovascular disease. The onset of vasoconstriction is slower than that of anesthesia. The sting of injection can be minimized by mixing 1 mL of $NaHCO_3$ with 9 mL of lidocaine, using a 30-gauge needle, and by making the initial injection perpendicular to the skin. Deep injections sting less than superficial injection, but prolong the time to adequate anesthesia. For small lesions the anesthetic can be injected directly into, or immediately adjacent to the lesion. For larger lesions it is better to perform a field block by placing a ring of anesthetic around the surgical site.

2. Biopsy procedure

2.1 Curettage

The curette is a spoon-like blade attached to a pencil-like handle ranging in diameter from 2 to 10 mm (fig 1)

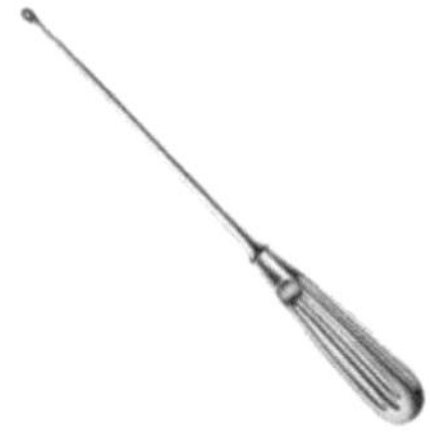

Fig. 1. This is a Volkmann curette. In commerce there are also disposable curettes with a circular cutting top.

Curettage is performed by scraping the lesion with a curette. It can also be used to treat superficial nonmelanocytic skin cancers. Four mm diameter curettes are usually used for small lesions (less than 1 cm in diameter). Bigger curettes can give more tissue to make histological evaluation possible. Haemostasis is achieved by compression, cauterisation or laser.

2.2 Shave biopsy

Shave biopsies are quick, require little training, and do not require sutures for closure. The shave biopsy can be facilitated by raising the lesion with a wheal of injected anesthetic, allowing it to be propped up and stabilized between the thumb and forefinger. To shave a lesion , a blade is held parallel to the skin surface. The depth of the biopsy is controlled by the angle of the blade. Care should be taken to keep the blade parallel to the skin surface, avoiding irregular, deep penetration. A double-edge razor blade cut longitudinally can also be used for shave biopsies. The razor technique has several advantages; it is sharper than most blades, the razor can be bent concave or convex with the thumb and forefinger to better conform to the surface being cut, and depth is easily controlled by increasing the convexity of the curve. Curved scissors are an efficient means of removing skin tags and other small, exophytic growths. The lesion to be removed is stabilized with toothed forceps, then cut at the base.

Lesions that are most suitable for shave biopsies are either elevated above the skin, or have pathology confined to the epidermis (Fig 2).

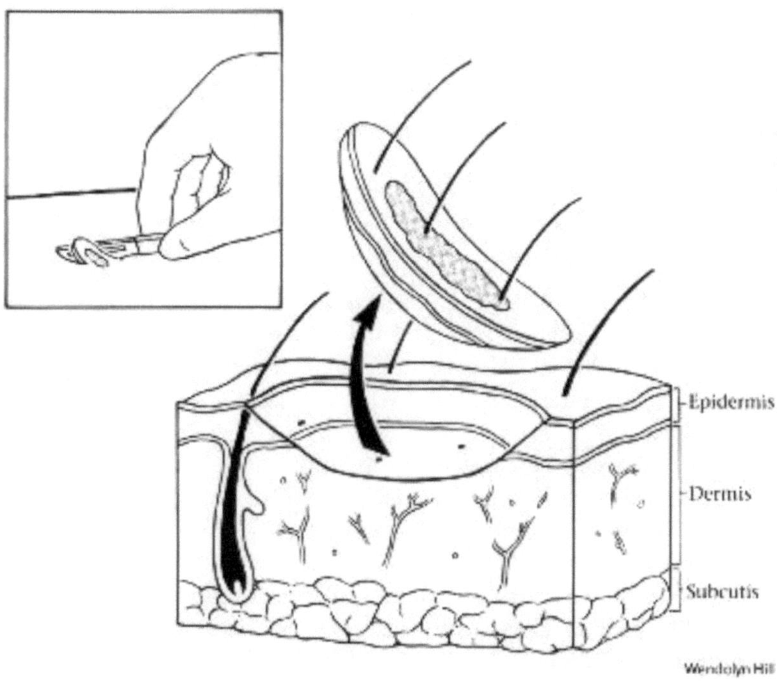

Fig. 2. An example of a shave biopsy. Note that the lesion depth was restricted only to the epidermis and the dermis.

It is acceptable if the lesion is small and the risk of malignancy is low. Common indications include seborrhoeic or actinic keratoses, skin tags, and warts. Shave biopsies should not be used for pigmented lesions. With shave biopsies, a small, depressed scar does occur.

2.3 Punch biopsy

Punch biopsy is considered the primary technique to obtain diagnostic, full-thickness skin specimen (Fig 3).

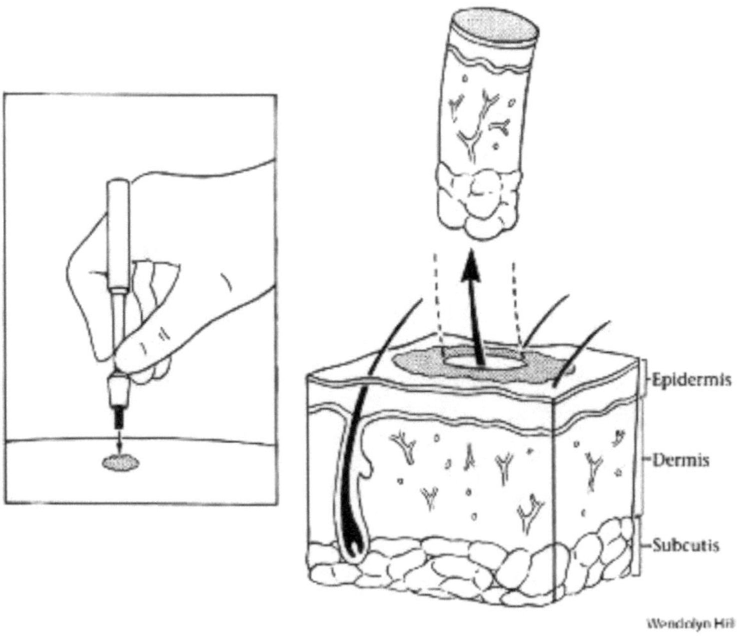

Fig. 3. An example of punch biopsy. The cylinder of tissue includes the epidermis, dermis and sometimes the subcutaneous fat.

It is performed using circular blade or trephine attached to a pencil-like handle ranging in diameter from 2 to 10 mm, but 3 mm is the smallest size likely to give sufficient tissue for consistent and accurate histologic diagnosis. The punch biopsy yields a cylindrical core of tissue that must be gently handled (usually with a needle) to prevent crush artifact at the pathological evaluation.

Large punch biopsy sites can be closed with a single suture and generally produce only minimal scarring. Because linear closure is performed on the circular-shaped defect, stretching the skin before performing the punch biopsy allows the relaxed skin defect to appear more elliptical and makes it easier to close. The skin is stretched perpendicular to the relaxed skin tension lines, so that the resulting elliptical-shaped wound and closure are parallel to these skin tension lines. The punch is then firmly introduced and rotated to obtain the specimen. This procedure is suitable when all skin layers are to be examined, or when the area of skin to be removed is unacceptably large for an excision.

Punch biopsy of inflammatory dermatoses can provide useful information when the differential diagnosis has been narrowed. The active edge of a dermatosis is usually chosen as the biopsy site. Cutaneous neoplasm can be evaluated by punch biopsy, and the discovery of malignancy may alter the planned surgical excision procedure (Fig 4).

A punch biopsy of a melanoma does not influence the prognosis of the neoplasm (Pflugfeldern A et al 2010; Bong Jl et al 2002), however it is currently recommended only for the histopathologic diagnosis of large tumors in facial, mucosal, and acral locations. Routine biopsy of skin rashes is not recommended because the commonly reported nonspecific pathology result rarely alters clinical managment.

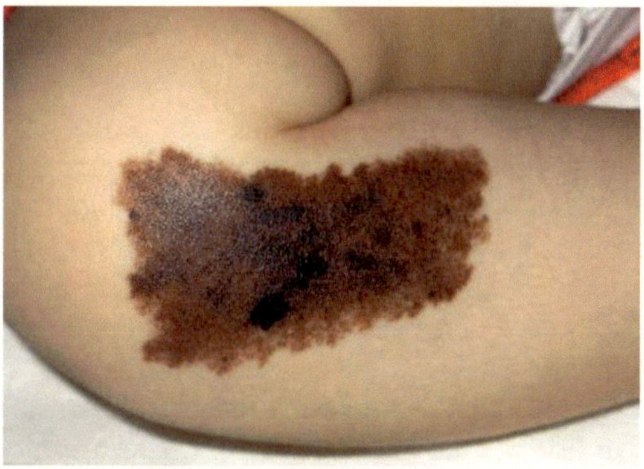

Fig. 4. In a case of giant congenital nevus a punch biopsy is useful to perform a histological evaluation of more atypical areas before deciding wheter to remove the entire lesion.

2.4 Excisional biopsy

In an excision biopsy, the entire skin lesion is removed with an elliptical excision. The classical fusiform excision has a 3 to 1 length-to-width ratio and a 2-to-5 mm margin of normal skin around the lesion. This tecnique produces an angle of 30 degrees or less at the end of the wound. The long axis of the wound should be oriented parallel to the lines of least skin tension to improve the final scar outcome. Holding the scalpel with a nuber 15 blade like a pencil, the incision begins at one apex with the blade perpendicular to the skin. As the incision progresses, it should be made using more of the belly of the blade, raising it to the perpendicular again at the next apex. A number 11 blade can be also used instead of the 15 one. The incision must be deep enough to see subcutaneous fat when the sample is removed. Once the ellipse has been incised, the sample edge should be carefully lifted with fine forceps and completely undermined at the level of subcutaneous fat with scalpel or scissors. A properly designed fusiform excision can be closed primarily and should nor result in the formation of raised tissue at the ends of the wound (known as „dog ears“). The skin should not be grasped with forceps, because the resulting skin damage can produce necrosis and scarring. Hematomas at the base of the excision inhibit wound healing, create excessive scarring and produce a depressed and more noticeable scar following normal scar retraction. Subcutaneous bleeding sites can be controlled with instrument clamps, electrocautery, or absorbable suture ligation. Interrupted, deep-buried absorbable sutures placed down to the level of the fascia eliminate dead space, provide excellent haemostasis, reduce tension on skin sutures and generally improve the cosmetic and functional result.

Excisions are reserved for lesions that cannot be removed with a punch owing to size, depth, or location. Their main advantage is the amount of tissue that can be excised, allowing for multiple studies (culture, histopathology, immunofluorescence, electron microscopy) from one biopsy site. Excisions are especially well suited for removal of large skin tumors or inflammatory disorders deep in the skin, involving the panniculus. Excision may be indicated for lipoma, dermatofibroma, keratoacanthoma, pyogenic granuloma, or epidermoid cysts. The wound is closed by suturing. This procedure can be curative for many lesions, but requires adequate time, expertise and suitable equipment. Excisional biopsy is also the procedure of choice for suspicious pigmented lesions (Tadiparthi S et al 2008) and for definitive treatment of skin cancer after diagnostic biopsy.

3. Choise of site

3.1 Introduction

Skin biopses are unique because the lesion can be visualized, allowing for proper selection of biopsy site and technique. It is a common fact that more errors are made from failing to biopsy promptly than from performing unnecessary biopsies. Nevertheless, many dermatoses have nonspecific histopathology, and biopsy cannot substitute for good clinical skills. Biopsy is indicated in all suspected neoplastic lesions, in all bullous disorders, and to clarify a diagnosis when a limited number of entities are under consideration.

One of the more difficult initial decisions is selecting the biopsy site. Whenever possible, avoid important cosmetic areas, such as the face, areas with poor healing characteristics and areas where a nerve or an artery damage is possible. Hypertrophic scarring tends to occur over the deltoid and chest areas, and delayed healing can be a problem over the tibia, expecially in diabetic patients or in patients with arterial or venous insufficiency. The incidence of secondary infection in the groin and axillae is high; therefore biopsy these areas only if other sites are unavailable.

3.2 Biopsy of the scalp

The biopsy of the scalp is usually performed to diagnose squamous carcinomas which are very frequent especially in an elderly patient. These tumors frequently derive from chronic actinic damage in a solar exposed area where the hair protection is lost. The scalp area is a highly vascular area and biopsy of the scalp should be performed in an aseptic surgical room by expert trained operators. The fusiform excision is to be preferred since in case of an artery damage (usually some branches of the superficial temporal artery) it is easier to stop bleeding with a suture of the artery. It is also important to not extend the incision deep to the galea capitis to lead a better and faster healing.

Considering inflammatory and cicatritial alopecias, it is nowadays considered more useful to have not just vertical but also horizontal histological sections in order to analyze the type of inflammatory infiltration and its localization around hair follicles. So in these cases, it is better to perform two punch biopsies of the scalp usually of 4-5 mm of diameter deep to the adipous layer. One tissue cylinder will then be cut vertically as usual leading to longitudinal sections, while the other will be cut horizontally leading to tangential sections Fig 5 and Fig 6).

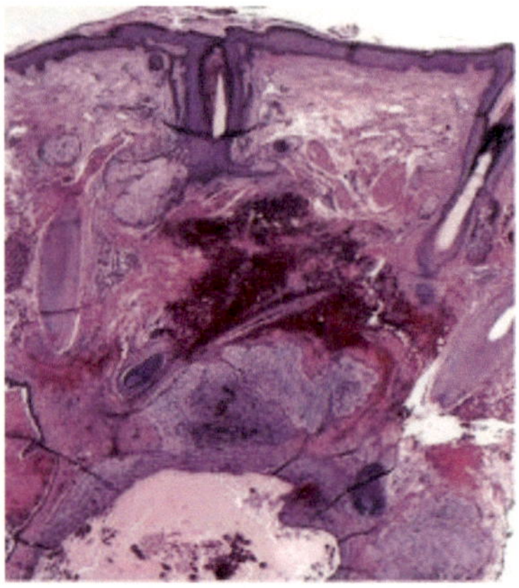

Fig. 5. Longitudinal classic histology of a biopsy of the scalp. It is possible to make a qualitative examination of the hair structures and it is possible to localize the inflammatory infiltrate.

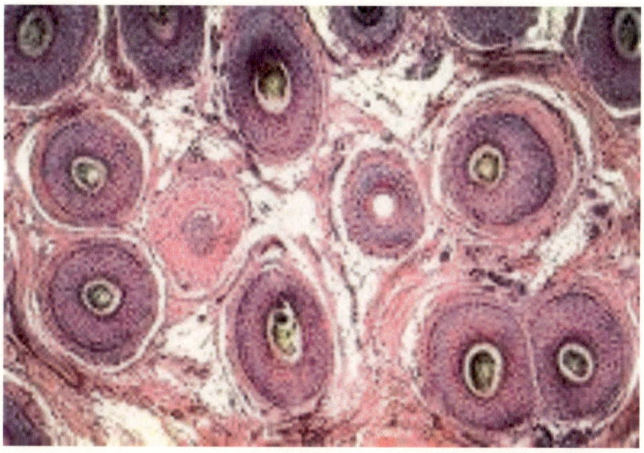

Fig. 6. A tangential histological evaluation of a scalp biopsy. With this section it is possible to localize the inflammatory infiltration, and to make a quantification of hair structures.

The timing of suture removal is usually 7-12 days.
A particular case of scalp biopsy is the biopsy of the Superficial Temporal Artery when there is a suspicion of Horton Temporal arteritis. Since the important risk is bleeding, this procedure must be done only by expert operators. For this particular biopsy it is better to obtain a sample of a Fronto-Temporal Artery branch. The artery can be recognized by the pulsations, but sometimes the vasculitic process could stop them. Before taking the biopsy it would be better to localize the exact biopsy site by Doppler marking with a skin-pen. Then the artery will be exposed with a scalpel cut paying attention not to damage it; with two hemostatic Klemmers the artery should be clamped proximally and distally in order to obtain the artery sample in the middle of the clamped area. Then both the edge of the cut artery must be accuratly sutured in order to avoid the risk of post-operatory bleeding(Fig 7).

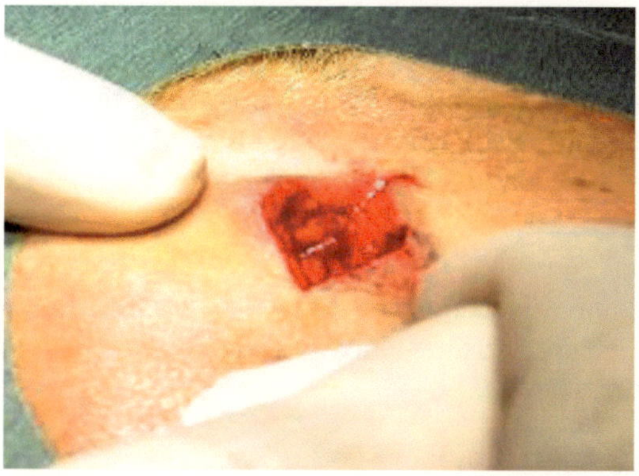

Fig. 7. The image shows the surgical preparation of the Temporal Artery before the biopsy.

3.3 Biopsy of the face

An incisional biopsy of the face can lead to a permanent cosmetic damage, so it should be performed only if necessary. The long axis of the wound should be oriented parallel to the lines of least skin tension lines (Kraissl lines in the living, Langers lines in anatomic studies) to improve the final scar outcome (Fig 8).

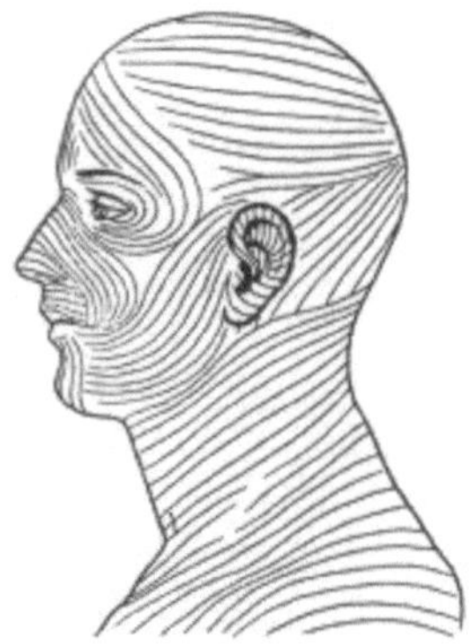

Fig. 8. The picture shows the orientation of Langers lines to follow while making an elliptical excision.

The face is a bleeding prone site and in some areas such as the nose, the anesthetic injection can be painful and difficult. The sting of injection can be minimized by using a 30-gauge needle with anesthetic cream applied two hours before. For cosmetic reason one should use the thinnest suture size (5-0 or 6-0) and suture in the face can be removed in 3 to 7 days eventually followed by the application of semipermanent adhesive strips to reduce wound tension. After the second or third day if there are some crusts on the suture, they should be washed away with wet gauze since they could cause depressed puntiform scars.
A particular attention has to be paid to the area above the zygomatic arch for the presence of the Fronto-Temporal Nerve and the preauricular area innervated by the Facial Nerve. A lesion of these two nerves can lead to a permanent functional and cosmetic damage. Placing a good volume of anesthetic beneath the lesion effectively increases the thickness of the skin and subcutaneous tissues, thereby keeping the incision more superficial.

3.4 Biopsy of the lip, of the tongue and of the oral mucosa

These sites are not particularly diffucult to biopsy but they are easily bleeding. The dermatological competence for the oral cavity is limited to the anterior one-third of the entire area, the other part is usually let to Otorinolaringoiatry specialists.

3.5 Biopsy of the breast

Usually a biopsy in this area is performed to analize a suspected naevus. In the areola is common Paget disease. The fusiform biopsy in this area should have a semilunar shape near or directly on the areola edge.

3.6 Biopsy of the finger

In the fingers it is better to use a ring block anesthesia in order to limit the pain. It has to be performed at the proximal lateral site of the finger with a 30 gauge needle, avoiding the use of epinephrine; the volume of anesthetic injected should be as less as possible in order to prevent compression ischemia.
Fingers are usually the site of pigmented lesions that are difficult to diagnose if they are located under the finger-nail. They require a biopsy of the nail matrix which has to be as small as possible in order to minimize aesthetic nail damage (Fig 9).

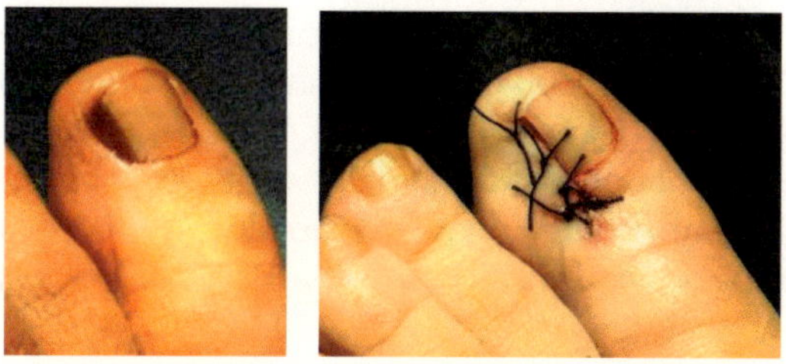

Fig. 9. Excisional biopsy of the medial edge of the thumb nail for the diagnosis of a suspected pigmented lesion.

3.7 Biopsy of the penis

A biopsy of the penis should be performed using anesthesia without epinephrine. If the lesion is on the shaft it is enough to make an injection under the lesion, while if the sample has to be taken on the glans it is better to perform a ring block anesthesia.

4. Choice of the lesion

A representative lesion at the height of its intensity, unmodified by trauma or treatment, will best show the more characteristic histological features; evolutionary changes may take several days and a too-early biopsy may reveal only nonspecific features. The major exceptions are blisters (and pustules), which should be preferably less than a day old when the specimen is taken. An old blister with secondary changes such as crusts, fissures, erosions, excoriations, infection and ulceration should be avoided since the primary pathological process may be obscured. For non bullous lesions, the biopsy should include maximal lesional skin and minimal normal skin. For lesions between 1 and 4 mm in diameter, biopsy the center or excise the entire lesion, for larger lesions, biopsy the edge, the thickest portion, or the area that is most abnormal in color, because these sites will most likely to contain the distinctive pathology. When the edge of the lesion is well demarcated it is usually best to take the specimen from the edge to include a small portion of normal skin. The edge is often the most active part of the lesion, and the normal skin serves as a built-in control. Whenever possible, remove vesicles intact, with adjacent normal-appearing skin, because disruption makes histological interpretation more difficult. Similarly, bullae should be biopsied at their edge, keeping the blister roof attached. If the differential diagnosis is broad, biopsy several sites to minimize sampling error or to assess the evolution of varied morphology of lesions.

4.1 Examples

- **Suspected melanoma.** A correctly performed biopsy is a crucial initial step in the management of malignant melanoma. Excision biopsy is the recommended method for suspected malignant melanoma as it enables diagnosis, staging of the tumour, and determines future investigation, treatment, and prognosis. The initial biopsy should be performed with a minimum lateral clearance of 2 mm and a cuff of subcutaneous fat deep to the tumour. This provides the pathologist with the maximum opportunity to diagnose a malignant melanoma in a given biopsy sample, as well as the depth of invasion. Breslow thickness, the most powerful prognostic parameter, together with the presence of ulceration and the mitosis number, subsequently provides a guide to the margin of clearance required for delayed wide excision and need for sentinel node assessment and/or adjuvant therapy (Tadiparthi S et al 2008; Swanson NA et al 2002). To assess the thickness of a neoplasm, the base must be visualised; this can be done with confidence only if excision is done with a scalpel and is complete. An incisional biopsy is considered suboptimal because it does not provide the entire lesion for analysis. Incision biopsy is only acceptable for large lesions in cosmetically sensitive areas (facial, mucosal or acral locations) (Newton Bishop JA et al 2002) or when the suspicion for melanoma is low (Fig 10).

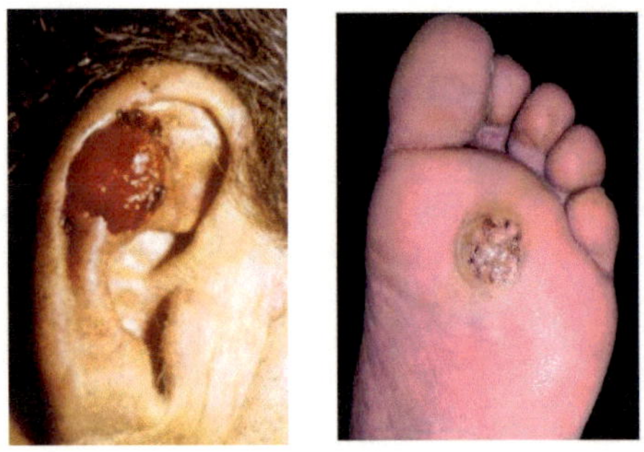

Fig. 10. An amelanotic melanoma is a lesion difficult to recognize. In this case a biopsy is required before making a complete excision.

Incision biopsy may also be warranted in an area of a recent change within a giant congenital naevus (Newton Bishop JA et al 2002). It is a controversial issue whether an incisional biosy is associated with an unfavorable patient prognosis in melanocytic lesions. Evidence of one of the larger, prospective randomized controlled trial is that incisional biopsies were not associated with an unfavorable prognosis for melanoma patients (Pflugfeldern A et al 2008). Other methods of biopsy, such as punch and shave, are not recommended as they do not allow complete histological staging (Newton Bishop JA et al 2002).

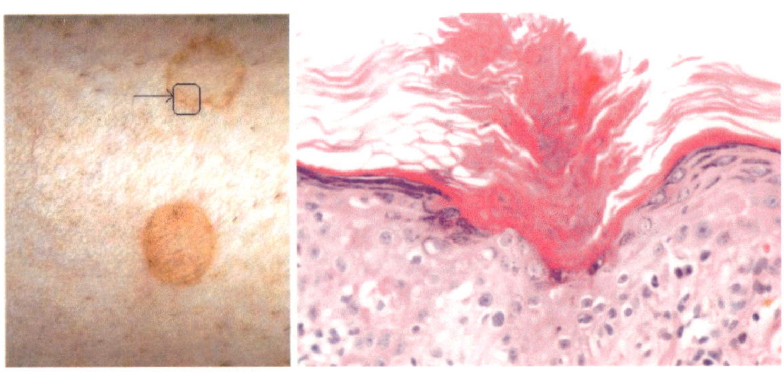

Fig. 11. In the clinical image on the left the arrow shows the exact area to be included in the biopsy. On the right a histological image of the cornoid lamella which arises from a small indentation in the epidermis while extends like a thin column through the entire stratum corneum, and the underlying granular cell layer is diminished.

- **Porokeratosis.** In porokeratosis the histopathologist can make a fast and correct diagnosis by recognozing in the histological slide the"cornoid lamella" which is the clue of this dermatitis. To obtain this clue in our sample it is necessary to biopsy one edge and a part of the internal area of the lesion (fig 11).

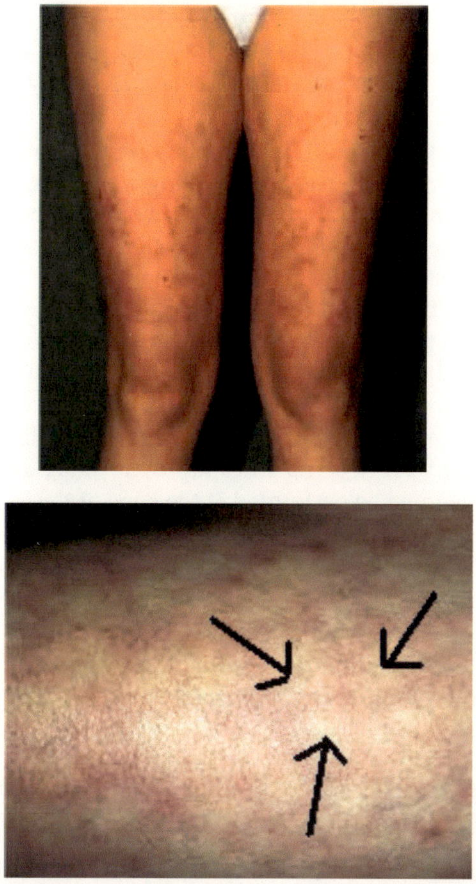

Fig. 12. A clinical example of reticulated dermatitis (livedo reticularis). The biopsy should be done on the center of the red ring in order to obtain evidence of the arteriolar damage.

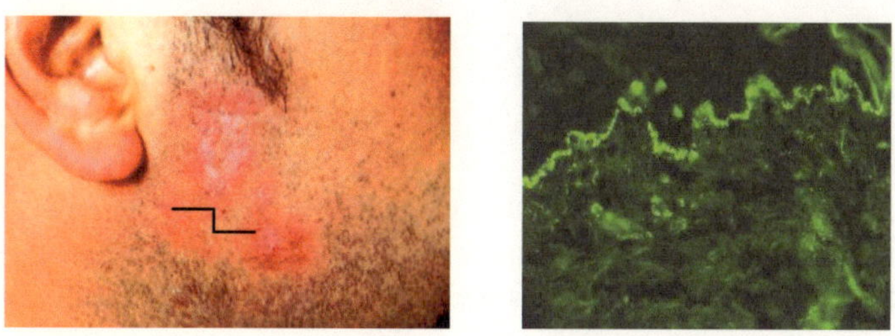

Fig. 13. In case of suspected lupus erythematosus the biopsy should be done in a non-scarring inflammatory area (see the arrow) in order to demonstrate at the direct immunofluorescence examination the specific lupus band.

- **Granuloma annulare.** Granuloma annulare should be biopsied on its elevated periferal edge where the biopsy sample should show the granulomatous infiltrate. Sampling a part of the center of the lesion or a part of the external normal skin would be useful to have a built-in negative control. A biopsy performed in the center of the lesion does not show the peculiar granulomatous infiltrate.
- **Reticulated dermatitis.** Livedo reticularis, erythema ab igne, livedo racemosa and other reticulated dermatitides should be biopsied in the center of a „red ring". In fact only the white center of the vascular lesion can show the real arteriolar damage that leads to the reticular skin pattern (Fig 12).
- **Bullous dermatitis.** Blisters should be preferably less than a day old when the specimen is taken. An old blister with secondary changes such as crusts, fissures, erosions, excoriations, infection and ulceration should be avoided since the primary pathological process may be obscured. Perilesional skin is the best site for immunofluorescence, and should form the greater proportion of the specimen.
- **Lupus.** it is necessary to select early and mature lesions, avoiding those too recent or too late for finding the basal layer damage and still find immunofluorescence alterations (lupus band and perivascular deposits) (Fig 13).
- **Non-scarring alopecia** (androgenethic alopecia, telogen effluvium, alopecia areata, traction alopecia). The biopsy must be performed where the disease is mostly expressed.
- **Scarring alopecia** (peripilar lichen planus, lupus erythematosus, folliculitis decalvans). In this case the biopsy must be performed at the edge of the scarring area.
- **Pyoderma gangrenosum.** The biopsy should be done on a small early pustule and moreover it should be deep enough to reveal the suppurative folliculitis which is the main clue of the disease.
- **Lymphomas and erythrodermic diseases.** Since in these dermatitides there are usually different lesions in different clinical stages a good histological diagnosis is easily reached if more biopsies are performed in different areas from different lesions (Fig 14).

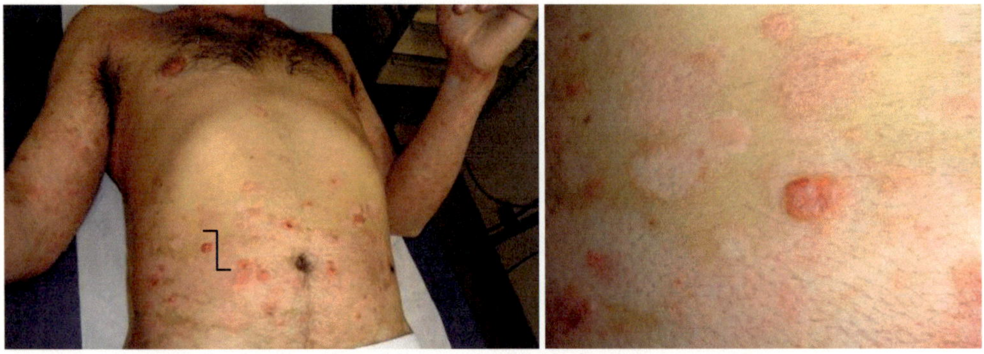

Fig. 14. A case of nodular mycosis fungoides. On the right a higher magnification of the clinical image where it is possible to see a nodular lesion and other flat lesions. In order to have a complete diagnosis, it is necessary to biopsy all the different lesions.

- **Vasculitis.** In suspecyted vasculitis a biopsy should be performed within 24 hours of appearance of the lesion, otherwise fibrinogen and immunoglobulin deposits may be difficult to find.

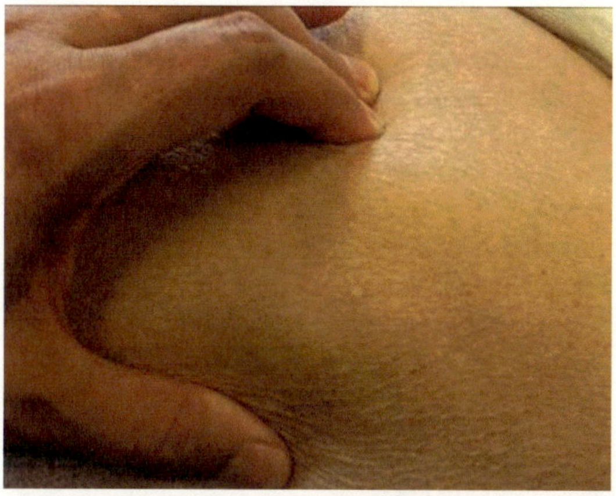

Fig. 15. A case of nephrogenic sclerosis (on the left). Since the dermatitis is a deep inflammatory process a deep biopsy is necessary to demonstrate the diagnostic clue.

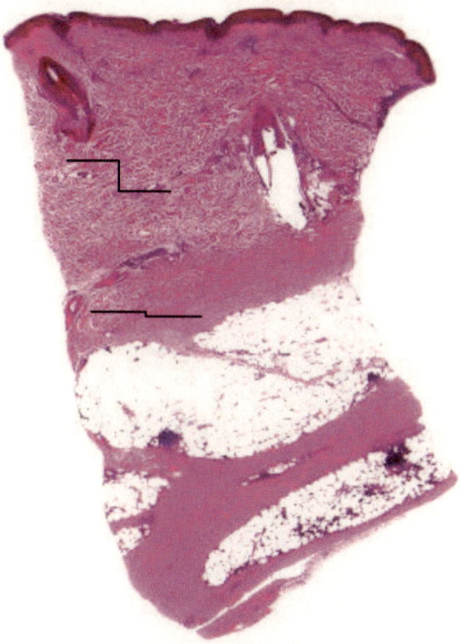

Fig. 16. The rows show the deep sclerosingprocess with fibrotic strands in the fat layer. A superficial biopsy would have given a false negative result.

- **Deep dermatitis.** In order to make an exact diagnosis of deep dermatitis such as panniculitis, necrobiosis lipoidica, cellulitis,…it is necessary to perform a deep biopsy which includes a thick layer of adipous tissue. This could help to differentiate different forms of cutaneous panniculitis that usually do not show peculiar alteration of superficial skin layers. The deep biopsy would lead to the differentiation between lobular or septal panniculitis and should demonstrate the type of inflammatory infiltrate (Fig 15 and Fig 16).

- **Dermatomyositis.** While performing a biopsy in a muscle, a second anesthetic injection should be done when the muscle is reached to reduce pain.
- Scabies (**Acariasis).** Even if is not always possible to isolate the „Sarcoptes" from the skin sample, it should be known that the acarus can not be found in the site of a cutaneous lesion (such as a crust or an excoriated lesion); it usually lies at a few millimeter distance away from the lesion.
- **Keratoacantoma.** The specimen should include a segment of the shoulder of the lesion extending into the central crater, along with adjacent normal skin and subcutaneous fat Fig 17).

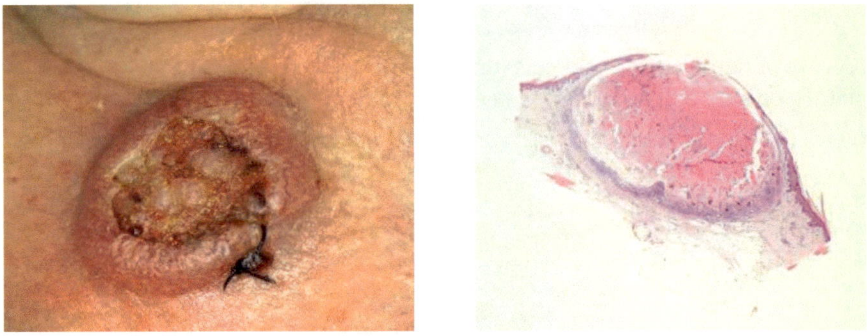

Fig. 17. A clinical image of a biopsied keratoacanthoma (image on the left). The biopsy of the elevated edge permits demonstration of the typical histologiacl architecture of a depressed cup limited by two cutaneous collarettes (image on the right).

5. Procedure pitfalls/complications

Complications are usually related to inadequate operator experience or an insufficent knowledge of the anatomy or to undrerlying clinical conditions of the patient. Most frequent complications are:

Excessive bleeding during or after the procedure. A particular attention to patient in therapy with aspirin or coumarin and to special site such as the nose or the scalp.

If the wound only closes in the center with hard tugging on the tissue, it will be prone to **gaping**. It is a frequent complication in a lesion of the back especially if a patient does not respect a period of rest.

Wound infection. It is uncommon if proper aseptic technique is followed. The operative time should be as short as possible. Antibiotic ointment should be applied to the wound immediately following the surgery and then daily until the sutures are removed or the wound heals. Wound-edge redness not associated with pus or drainage is not infection but instead it represents reparative or inflammatory changes associated with healing. Care must be taken when performing procedures in certain areas at higher risk for infection such as the groins or lower legs. Particular attention must be paid to an immunodepressed patient.

„Dog ears“ at the ends. "Dog ears" are mounds of elevated tissue that occur at the ends of some linear wound after closure. Dog ears can occur with excisions on convex surfaces such as the arms and legs and most commonly develop from an improperly designed fusiform excision. The wound should be long enough to have at least a 3 to 1 length-to-width ratio. Dog ears can be removed by excising a fusiform island of skin in the direction of the original wound or by removing a lateral piece of redundant skin and extending the wound laterally.

Damage to nerves or arteries. Incisions that extend deep into tissues have the potential to cause permanent nerve and artery damage. An increased quantity of anesthetic beneath it can keep the lesion more superficial avoiding the deep structures damage.

Discomfort during the procedure. It is usually related to inadequate anesthetization before starting the procedure. Five to ten mL of anesthetic should be administered before most procedures.

The final scar is thick and unsightly. Properly designed incisions that follow the lines of least skin tension usally result in cosmetically acceptable scars. Wounds that cross flexion creases or perpendicular to the lines of least tension can thicken into hypertrophic scars. **Keloids** are frequent on chest, chin, or ear lobules. African or asian patients are mostly involved in **keloids formation**.

6. Conclusions

Skin biopsy is an essential technique in the management of skin diseases, but it cannot replace clinical knowledge. Shave biopsy requires the least experience and time, but its use is limited to superficial lesions and should not be used for pigmented lesions. Punch biopsy is the primary diagnostic procedure in dermatology, is simple to perform, has few complications, and small biopsies can heal without suturing. Although closing with sutures improves the cosmetic result, it requires more expertise and time. Excisions are ideal for removing large or deep lesions, provide abundant tissue for multiple studies, and can be curative for a number conditions including cancer. However, excisions require the greatest amount of expertise, time, and office resources, and are associated with more complications, including bleeding and infection. Because of its complexity and complication potential, clinical training is highly recommended prior to attempting an excisional biopsy.

7. References

Bong Jl, Herd RM, Hunter JA. (2002). Incisional biopsy and melanoma prognosis. *J Am Acad Dermatol*, 46 (5):690-4.

Newton Bishop JA, Corrie PG, Evans J, Gore ME, Hall PN, Kirsham N et al. (2002). UK guidelines fort he manegement of cutaneous melanoma. *Br J Plastic Surg*, 55:46-54.

Pflugfeldern A, Weide B, Eigentler TK, Forschner A, Leiter U, Held L, Meier F, Garbe C. (2010). Incisional biopsy and melanoma prognosis: facts and controversies. *Clin Dermatol*, 28(3):316-8.

Swanson NA, Lee KK, Gorman A, Lee HN. (2002). Biopsy techniques: diagnosis of melanoma. *Dermatol Clin*, 20:667-80.

Tadiparthi S, Panchani S, Iqbal A. (2008). Biopsy for malignant melanoma-are we following the guidelines? *Ann R Coll Surg Engl*,90:322-325.

2

General Methods in Preparation of Skin Biopsies for Haematoxylin & Eosin Stain and Immunohistochemistry

Khitam Al-Refu
Mutah University,
Jordan

1. Introduction

Cutaneous Pathology (dermatopathology) is the microscopic examination of skin biopsies in order to determine a specific diagnosis or a list of differential diagnoses. Usually the diagnosis can be determined by the routine stain for tissue sections (Hematoxylin and Eosin).

Hematoxylin is a basic stain that stains basophilic structures such as chromatin and ribosome's a deep purple or blue. Eosin is an acidic stain that stains acidophilic structures red. The advantage of this stain is that it provides a clear stain of the cell nuclei; it provides a good stain for the cell membrane. These stains are not as specific for the tissue it stains. Nonetheless, this stain aided pathologists in diagnoses.

In addition to hematoxylin and eosin, the pathologist may use additional special stains to narrow a differential diagnosis or confirm an initial impression and one of these is immunohistochemistry. Immunohistochemistry has become an important technique and widely used in many medical research laboratories and is dependent on the localization of antigens in tissue sections by the use of labeled antibody as specific reagents through antigen-antibody interactions that are visualized by a marker such as peroxidase.

2. Skin lesion selection

For assessment of the skin biopsies by immunohistochemistry and usual haematoxylin satin, the skin lesions which developed recently according to the patient history should be selected for that purpose. Detailed clinical information (age, sex and site of skin biopsy) of the investigated patients should be provided. Biopsies from healthy donors may be analyzed for control purposes in some cases.

3. Types of skin biopsy

There are four main types of skin biopsies: shave biopsy, punch biopsy, excisional biopsy, and incisional biopsy. The choice of the different skin biopsies is dependent on the suspected diagnosis of the skin lesion. Shave biopsy is done for shaving a thin layer from the top of a lesion. The punch biopsy includes the full thickness skin and subcutaneous fat and is done by using round shaped knife ranging in size from 1mm to 8 mm. In Excisional

biopsy procedure, the doctor uses a scalpel to take off the entire lesion. Incisional biopsy is essentially the same as excisional one, except that part of lesion or tumor is included.
The skin is swabbed with an antiseptic and then injected with a local anaesthetic. In some patients, the biopsies are taken from the affected site in such a way as to include the three zones of the activity of the disease (scarred, active and apparently normal skin). Shave biopsies do not usually need stitches, while punch, excisional, and incisional biopsies will sometimes be closed with sutures.
A request form should accompany specimens that includes patient details including age, sex, site of the biopsy, brief clinical history with suspected and differential diagnosis and if there if any treatment applied prior to the biopsy.
The skin biopsies are either frozen samples or paraffin embedded. Some of the antibodies (in case of immunohistochemistry) work on frozen sections as is the case for the majority of the antibodies against the basement membrane antigens, while other antibodies such as granzyme and cutaneous lymphocytic antigen work better on paraffin sections.

4. Preparation of paraffin embedded biopsies

The purpose of fixation is to preserve the skin specimen indefinitely in a life-like state. For normal histological sections, the sample should be transported in fixative (usually 10% neutral buffered formalin); the volume should be at least ten times that of the tissue and should be labeled with the patient's full name, date of birth, the site of the biopsy and the date of taking the biopsy. It remains in this preservative for a minimum of 24 hours prior to processing. Formalin is a good fixative media by forming cross-links between lysine residues in the proteins of the tissues without alterations to their structure.
The biopsies are processed in the tissue processing machine for 24 hours; this machine automatically processed the tissues in graded alcohols and xylene. This involved first replacing the 70% (v/v) ethanol with 90% (v/v) ethanol, before placing in absolute ethanol. This is then repeated with xylene and liquid paraffin. The biopsies should not be kept in the machine for more than one week as this may affect the process of the antigen retrieval.
Skin biopsies are embedded in metal moulds filled with paraffin wax with particular attention to the position of the biopsies to ensure orientation of the tissues from the epidermis down to the subcutaneous tissues, using ice to hold the tissue in place. The cassette is positioned and the blocks are left in the ice to set. The mould is removed whilst cold and the excess wax is trimmed manually using a dissecting blade.
The wax blocks are cooled in ice and sectioned at a thickness of 4 µm using a microtome. The sections are floated on a 40 °C water bath and collected on adhesive slides to minimize section loss during heat-mediated retrieval. They are then incubated at 37 °C overnight for 24 hours on slide racks, and kept in special slides container at room temperature, to be used later on for immunohistochemistry and H&E staining.
If the paraffin sections are not processed carefully, various artifacts may be present on the slide. Fine black spots may be seen if the formalin used is too acidic (unbuffered). In addition, holes within the sections due to tearing by microtome because of insufficient tissue dehydration or the presence of hard material such as calcium or sutures.

5. Frozen samples preparation

Orientation of the tissue to the knife is is an extremely important aspect of the frozen section preparation so that the knife meets the tissue in a specific orientation. Fat should be the last thing to hit the blade or should hit the blade by itself whenever possible. When fat hits the blade before the more manageable tissues it may smear the rest of the section.

The biopsies for frozen sections are snap frozen in liquid nitrogen, and are used directly for mounting and cutting or stored for later processing in liquid nitrogen at -196°C. Each biopsy is placed on a sample block within a cryostat cabinet set at a -25ºC and embedded in especial mounting medium, one drop is placed on the mounting plate and the biopsy is placed centrally on top. The embedding medium used for frozen tissue to ensure optimal cutting temperature; it is used to embed tissue before sectioning on a cryostat. Whilst freezing, additional drops of mounting medium fluid are added in order to completely embed the biopsy.

The frozen block (containing the biopsy) is sectioned at a thickness of 6µm and sections mounted on superfrost slides. The slides are soaked in 100% acetone for five minutes, drained and left to air dry for 12-24 hours at room temperature. The slides are wrapped in aluminium foil, labelled and stored at -70ºC in liquid nitrogen. When required, the slides are removed from the freezer and allowed to stand for thirty minutes for any condensation to evaporate.

6. Haematoxylin & Eosin staining (H &E)

6.1 Principles of H & E staining

H&E stain, or hematoxylin and eosin stain, is a popular staining method in histology. It is the most widely used stain in medical diagnosis. The stain works well with a variety of fixatives and displays a broad range of cytoplasmic, nuclear, and extracellular matrix features (figure 1).

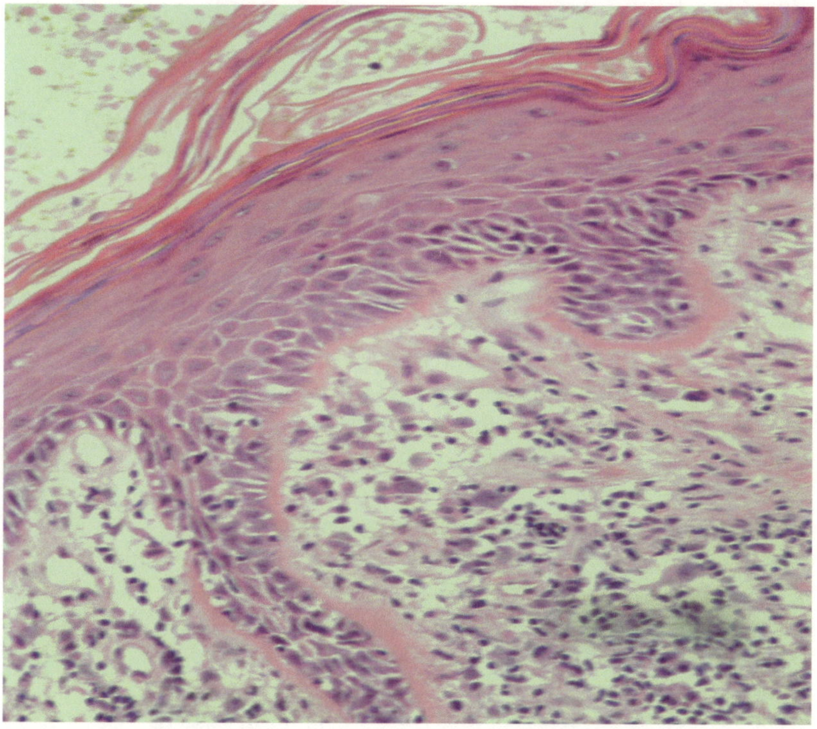

Fig. 1. Hematoxylin and eosin stain for a skin biopsy from a discoid lupus erythematosus skin lesion.

The staining method involves application of hematoxylin, which is a complex formed from aluminium ions and oxidized hematoxylin. This colors nucleus of cells (and a few other objects, such as keratohyalin granules) blue. The nuclear staining is followed by counterstaining with eosin, which colors eosinophilic other structures in various shades of red and pink.
Optimization may be necessary to achieve staining (hematoxylin may be diluted in H2O and eosin may be diluted in ethanol as needed).

6.2 H & E staining of paraffin and frozen sections

Paraffin sections are prepared for H&E staining by mounting on superfrost slides, drying on a hot plate, and then immersing into three sets of xylene for 10 minutes each followed by three sets of absolute ethanol for 10 minutes and finally rinsed with tap water. The purpose is to remove the wax and dehydrate the sections. Frozen sections are stained directly without using hot plates for drying or dehydration in sets of xylene and alcohol.
Slides (frozen and paraffin) are placed into haematoxylin for 5 minutes and rinsed thoroughly under tap water for approximately 4-5 minutes. Excess haematoxylin is removed by adding 1% acid alcohol (1% HCl in 70% (v/v) alcohol) for 5 seconds followed by a tap water wash.
The pink haematoxylin stain is converted to blue by adding Scott's tap water, for approximately 10 seconds until the sections turned blue. The slides are rinsed in tap water before being stained in eosin (1% (w/v)) for 15 seconds with a subsequent wash in running tap water for 1-5 minutes. The sections are then dehydrated in two washes of absolute alcohol and in two washes of xylene for 10 minutes each before being mounted in DPX mountant and covered with glass cover slips.

7. Immunohistochemistry by Immunoperoxidase Labelling (IHC)

7.1 Principles of immunohistochemistry

Antigen-antibody interactions in tissues sections can be visualized in a number of ways. In the most common technique, an antibody is conjugated to an enzyme, such as peroxidase (immunoperoxidase staining) (figure 2), that can catalyze a color-producing reaction (see immunoperoxidase staining). Alternatively, the antibody can also be tagged to a fluorophore, such as fluorescein or rhodamine (immunofluorescence).
Immunohistochemistry or IHC refers to the process of localizing antigens in a tissue section by binding specifically with antibodies. Immunohistochemical staining is widely used in basic research to understand the distribution and localization of antigens in different parts of tissue sections.

7.2 Retrieval of antigens from paraffin and frozen sections

Tissues fixed in formalin (wax embedded) generally require some form of antigen unmasking for immunohistochemistry to be successful; formalin fixation and paraffin processing leads to inter and intra molecular cross linking, which mask or destroys antigenic sites in tissue specimens. Antibodies are then unable to bind them. Antigen retrieval sometimes makes the tissue act like a frozen tissue.
The most common method involves routinely heating paraffin sections in a retrieval solution, then cooling, rinsing, and proceeding with routing immunohistochemistry staining. Microwave oven, pressure cooker and steamer are the most commonly used heating methods.

The main pitfall when performing heating methods is that extreme care must be taken not to allow the sections to dry out or overheat as this can destroy antigens and produce section artifacts. Where possible the antigen retrieval solutions were flushed from the container with cold running water, the sections could then be removed when the fluid was cool.

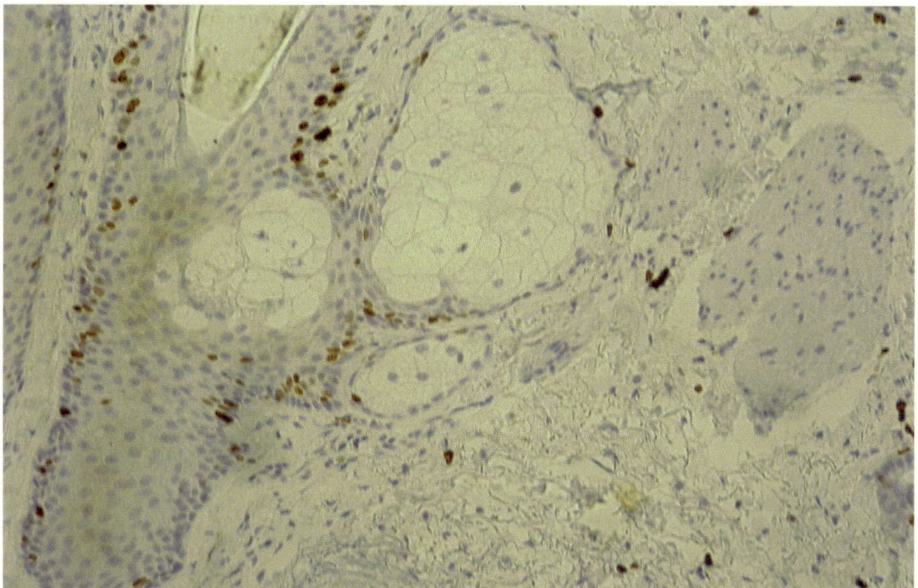

Fig. 2. Staining of skin biopsy from normal control by immunoperoxidase technique.

The type of antigen retrieval solution is different according to the primary antibody being used. The followings are commonly used Tris EDTA buffer (X10 concentrate), this solution is prepared as follows: Tris (12.0 g), EDTA (1.0 g), 1M HCl (10 ml) and 500 ml of distilled water. This solution is kept refrigerated and is diluted 1/10 with distilled water, and adjusted to pH 9.0 using NaOH before use. Citrate buffer, this solution is prepared as follows: 2.94 g sodium citrate with 1000 ml distilled water. The pH is adjusted to either 2.6 or 6.0 using HCl. The pH of solutions is measured using a pH meter. The pH meter is calibrated using solutions of pH 4,7 and 10 made from buffer tablets dissolved in deionised water. The pH of the solutions is adjusted using 1 M HCl, or 1 M NaOH which is added drop-wise with stirring.

8. Immunohistochemistry techniques

8.1 Sample preparation for immunohistochemistry

A prerequisite for good immunohistochemistry is that sections (paraffin and frozen) are of the highest quality and cut from adequately fixed tissue blocks. This is critical to maintain cell morphology, tissue architecture and the antigenicity of target epitopes. Sections (frozen and paraffin-embedded) are picked up on superfrost slides to minimize section loss during heat-mediated retrieval.

De-paraffinization and rehydration of paraffin sections is required only for paraffin sections. The paraffin sections are deparaffinized in three sets of xylene for 10 minutes, each followed by three sets of absolute ethanol for 10 minutes and finally rinsed with tap water. The purpose is to remove the wax and rehydrate the sections. Because of the method of fixation and tissue preservation, the sample may require additional step to make the epitopes available for antibody binding, including antigen retrieval; this step often makes the difference between staining and no staining.

Additionally, depending on the tissue type and the method of antigen detection, endogenous biotin or enzymes may need to be blocked or quenched, respectively, prior to antibody staining. Endogenous peroxidase activity is found in a wide variety of mammalian tissues in red blood cells, granulocytes, monocytes, macrophages and myoglobin. The most frequently used method of blocking this endogenous enzyme activity is to use its substrate (hydrogen peroxide). Two drops of Peroxide Block (3% Hydrogen peroxide) is used for all sections (frozen and paraffin) for 5 minutes, which are then washed twice in distilled water for 10 minutes.

Although antibodies show preferential avidity for specific epitopes, they may partially or weakly bind to sites on nonspecific proteins that are similar to the the target antigen. The nonspecific binding causes high background staining that can mask the detection of the target antigen. To reduce background staining in IHC, , the samples are incubated with a protein block that reduce the non-specific binding of primary antibodies and polymers and this done by adding two drops (100 µl) of the blocking serum to the section.

The sequential steps of staining were interposed with (PBS) washing for 10 minutes.

Due to the high volume usage; PBS was made in large quantities as follows; 74 g sodium dihydrogen orthophosphate and 286.5g disodium hydrogen orthophosphate in 25 litters of distilled water. The pH of this solution was 7.4.

8.2 Antibodies types

The antibodies (or antisera) used for specific detection can be polyclonal or monoclonal. Polyclonal antibodies are antibodies that are obtained from different B cell resources. By contrast, monoclonal antibodies are derived from a single cell line. Monoclonal antibodies show specificity for a single epitope and are therefore considered more specific to the target antigen than polyclonal antibodies. Polyclonal antibodies are a combination of immunoglobulin molecules secreted against a specific antigen, each identifying a different epitope. These antibodies are typically produced by immunization of a suitable mammal, such as a mouse, rabbit or goat and then purified from the mammal's serum. Thus, polyclonal antibodies are a heterogeneous mix of antibodies that recognize several epitopes.

8.3 Sample labeling by immunohistochemistry

Each section, except for the negative control, is then incubated with optimally diluted primary antibody (as recommended for each one). The optimum dilution of the primary antibody is the concentration of the primary antibody, which give the optimal specific staining with the least amount of background staining. This is determined by experiments using control sections at different concentrations and for different times. The optimal dilution is dependent upon the type and duration of fixation.

The incubation with post primary block increases penetration of the secondary reagents, the biotinylated secondary antibody was added for the slides for 30 minutes. The final incubation step involved the addition of a peroxidase conjugated avidin/biotin complex for 30 minutes. This incubation was for detection of any tissue-bound primary antibody.

Additional of DAB working solution is required for visualization of the primary antibodies. The primary antibodies are visualized by the addition of the substrate/chromogen, 3, 3'-diaminobenzidine (DAB). This working solution isprepared by adding 50 µl of DAB chromogen to 1 ml of DAB substrate buffer and is used within 6 hours of preparation. Reaction with the peroxidase produces a brown insoluble precipitate at the antigen site. The colour development is monitored by light microscopy.

After immunohistochemical staining of the target antigen, a second stain is often applied to provide contrast that helps the primary stain stand out. Many of these stains show specificity for discrete cellular compartments or antigens, while others will stain the whole cell. A vast array of reagents to fit every experimental design, hematoxylin is commonly used. So the sections are counterstained with Haematoxylin for 5 minutes followed by rinsing in water for 5 minutes before dehydration in two sets of absolute alcohol for 10 minutes, clearing in two sets of xylene for another 10 minutes, and mounting the sections with DPX mountant and covered with glass cover slips.

9. Development of optimal immunohistochemical methods

There are various protocols available. Antibodies may react differently, when using antigen retrieval solutions with a different pH. Unfortunately, there is not one method which can be applied to all antigens; some methods work with some and not others (Figure 3).

The specific staining may be too light and this may due to using too low concentration of the primary antibody (Figure 4). Or it may be too dark and this is may be due to using the primary antibody at high concentration or the incubation times may be too long (Figure 5).

10. The controls in immunohistochemistry

Controls validate immunohistochemistry results. Inclusion of a known positive control demonstrates the correct performance of reagents. Omission of primary antibody on one test preparation is essential. This provides information on any non-specific reactions intrinsic to the labelling system. A negative control is used on every test in which the primary antibody was omitted to test for non-specific reactions of the secondary reagents to the tissue.

11. Double labelling protocol in immunohistochemistry

11.1 Principle of double labelling technique in immunohistochemistry

In this technique, two primaries, raised in different species, are applied to the section. Two primaries visualized by different satins. Usually brown satin (DAB) for one and another satin which may be red, blue or others for the second primary. This double immune staining should not be carried out for co-stain of antigens located on the same structure (nucleus, membrane cytoplasm) as the brown stain of the DAB (the stain of the first primary antibody) combining with the blue stain (the stain of the second antibody) would give a third colour which would be difficult to differentiate from the other two colours.

Pre-request for this double immunostaing is that the secondary antibodies for both primary antibodies should be different and the antigen retrieval method in case of paraffin sections should be similar.

In peroxidase staining, the same procedure described is employed for the first antibody but without haematoxylin counterstaining.

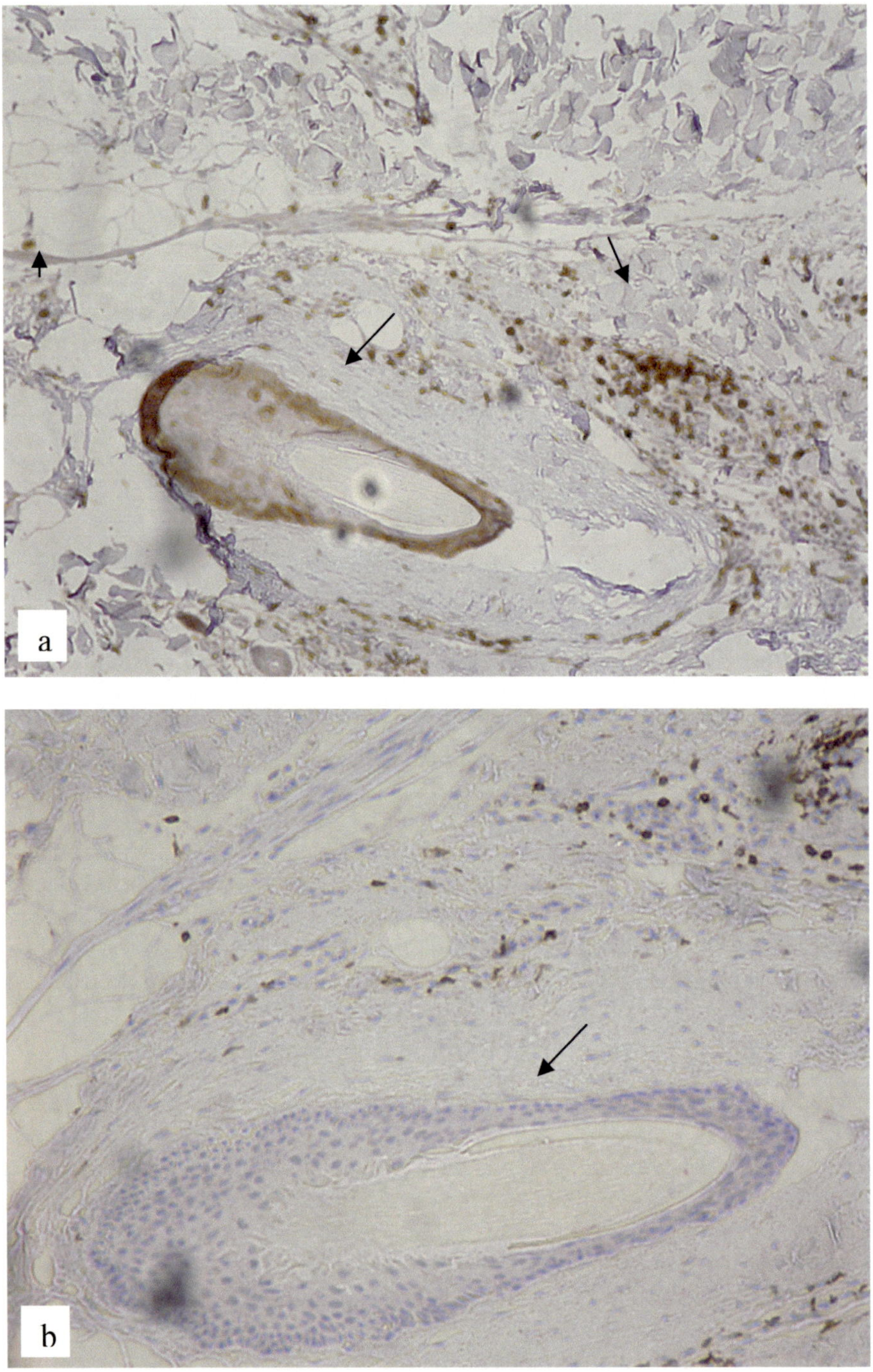

Fig. 3. This is an immunohistochemistry stain using C8/144B as a primary antibody, this can satin part of the external sheath of hair follicle and cytotoxic cells (CD8+) as demonstrated in (a) by arrows, but changing the method of antigen retrieving; the satin was very weak for the CD8 cells and without staining of the hair follicle.

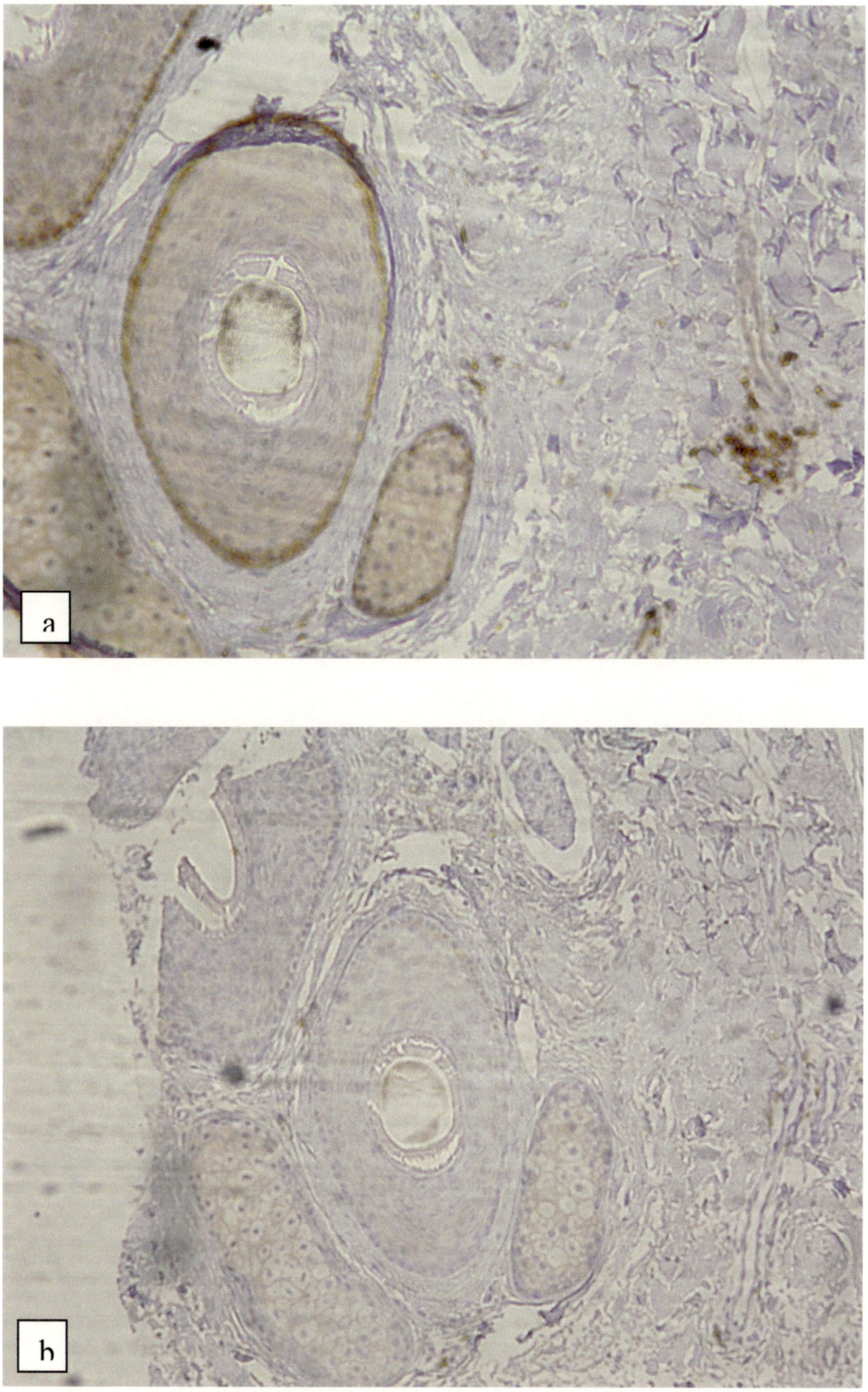

Fig. 4. This demonstrates the optimal dilution of CK-15 in (a) compared to very low concentration of this antibody in (b).

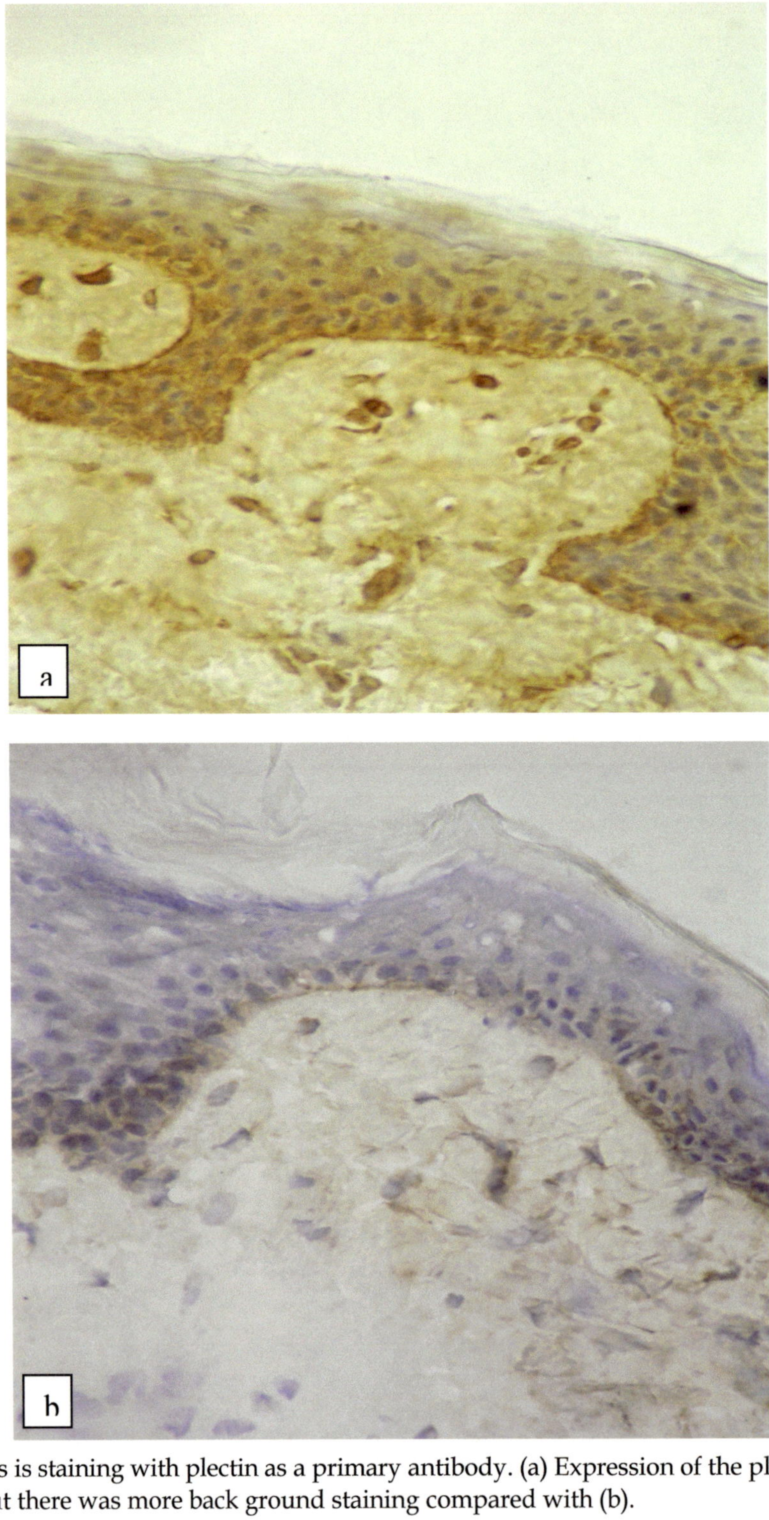

Fig. 5. This is staining with plectin as a primary antibody. (a) Expression of the plectin was normal but there was more back ground staining compared with (b).

11.2 Double labelling technique in immunohistochemestry

The paraffin-embedded samples are sectioned and mounted on super adhesive slides and then de-paraffinized and rehydrated in two sets of xylene and two sets of absolute alcohol for 10 minutes. The antigen retrieval process is performed as required for both of the tested antigens. At this stage, the antigen retrieval method is similar for both of the antigens to be visualized. The endogenous peroxidase is neutralized by using peroxidase block for 5 minutes. The sections are then incubated with protein block as required for the first primary antibody followed with incubation with the optimally diluted primary antibody. This is followed by addition of the post primary block and secondary antibody as required for the tested first primary antibody. The visualization of the first antibody is carried out by DAB working solution. At this stage, there is no counterstaining with haematoxylin. The slides are then washed with BPS as usual.

Staining with the second primary antibody as described below.

11.3 Primary staining with the second antibody

The slides are incubated with the protein block as required for the second primary. The second antibody is added to the slides after dilution with BPS. This is followed by addition of the secondary antibody as required for the second primary antibody. After washing of slides with BPS as usual, the specific reagent for visualization of the second primary antibody is added to the sections. The blue colour is the best to be combined with the brown stain of the DAB stain. The sections are mounted with DPX mountant and covered with glass cover slides without haematoxylin staining. Using of haematoxylin staining may mask the required satin of the second antibody (which will be stained with blue colour).

12. References

[1] Kiernan JA (2008). Histological and Histochemical Methods: Theory and Practice. 4th ed. Bloxham, UK: Scion.

[2] Lillie RD, Pizzolato P, Donaldson PT (1976). Nuclear stains with soluble metachrome mordant lake dyes. The effect of chemical endgroup blocking reactions and the artificial introduction of acid groups into tissues. Histochemistry 49: 23-35.

[3] Ramos-Vara, JA (2005). "Technical Aspects of Immunohistochemistry". Vet Pathol 42 (4): 405–426. doi:10.1354/vp.42-4-405.

[4] Al-Refu K, Goodfield M (2009). Hair follicle stem cells in the pathogenesis of the scarring process in cutaneous lupus erythematosus. Autoimmun Rev. 8 (6):474-7.

[5] Al-Refu K, Edward S, Ingham E, Goodfield M. Br J Dermatol (2009). Expression of hair follicle stem cells detected by cytokeratin 15 stain: implications for pathogenesis of the scarring process in cutaneous lupus erythematosus 160 (6):1188-96.

[6] Al-Refu K, Goodfield M. Immunohistochemistry of ultrastructural changes in scarring lupus erythematosus (2011). Clin Exp Dermatol 36(1):63-8.

[7] Shi S - R, Cote RJ, Taylor CR (1999). Standardization and further development of antigen retrieval immunohistochemistry: strategies and future goals. J. Histotechnol 22: 177 - 192.

[8] O' Leary TJ (2001). Standardization in immunohistochemistry. Appl. Immunohistochem. Mol. Morphol 9: 3 – 8.

[9] Scanziani E (1998). "Immunohistochemical staining of fixed tissues". Methods Mol Biol 104: 133–40.

3

Types and Selection Criteria for Various Skin Biopsy Procedures

Divey Manocha, Nidhi Bansal and Ramsay S. Farah
SUNY Upstate Medical University, New York, USA

1. Introduction

The skin biopsy is a simple procedure that can assist with the diagnosis of cutaneous disorders. More errors are made from failing to biopsy promptly than from performing unnecessary biopsies. Properly performed, it may confirm a diagnosis, remove cosmetically unacceptable lesions, and provide definitive treatment for a number of skin conditions. Skin biopsies are unique because the lesion can be visualized, allowing for proper selection of biopsy site and technique. Skin biopsies can be performed with minimal risk in critically ill patients, and a timely skin biopsy may avoid other, more invasive procedures.[1] Skin biopsies may be performed with shave, punch, excisional or incisional techniques.

There are few absolute contraindications to skin biopsy, but all patients should be made aware that biopsies leave scars. In most cases, a biopsy should be avoided at an infected site, although occasionally ruling out infection may be the indication for the procedure. Inquiry should be made regarding allergies to topical antibiotics, antiseptics, local anesthetics, and to tape. Patients should be asked about bleeding disorders and use of drugs known to interfere with hemostasis (anticoagulants and antiplatelet agents). Generally, lesions with the most advanced inflammatory changes should be chosen; evolutionary changes may take several days and a too-early biopsy may reveal only nonspecific features.[2,3, 5, 6] However for blistering diseases, the earliest lesions reveal the more specific histopathology. Consequently, only the newest vesicles and blisters should be biopsied, usually within 48 hours of their appearance.[2, 3, 4] Older lesions with secondary changes such as crusts, fissures, erosions, excoriations, and ulcerations should be avoided since the primary pathological process may be obscured. For nonbullous lesions, the biopsy should include maximal lesional skin and minimal normal skin. For lesions between < 4 mm in diameter, the central region should be biopsied or the entire lesion be excised. For larger lesions, the edge, the thickest portion, or the area with abnormal coloration should be biopsied, because these sites will most likely contain the distinctive pathology. Vesicles should preferably be biopsied intact with adjacent normal-appearing skin, because disruption makes histological interpretation more difficult. Similarly, bullae should be biopsied at their edge, keeping the blister roof attached. If the differential diagnosis is broad, taking biopsy from several sites can minimize sampling error. Important cosmetic areas, such as the face should be approached with caution, and areas with poor healing characteristics should be avoided if other sites are available for biopsy.[4, 6] Hypertrophic scarring tends to occur over the deltoid and chest areas, and delayed healing can be a problem over the tibia, especially in diabetic patients or in patients with arterial or venous insufficiency.[6] The incidence of secondary infection in the groin and axillae is high; therefore, these areas should only be biopsied if others are unavailable.[3]

2. Surgical safety

Performing skin biopsies places the operator at risk of blood-borne infections. Accordingly, vaccination for hepatitis B is indicated, and universal precautions should be observed by wearing gloves and eye-guards.[7] Shave and punch biopsies are clean but not sterile procedures so mask, gown and *sterile* gloves are not necessary.[5] A mask is recommended for operators or assistants known to be respiratory carriers of *Staphylococcus* or *Streptococcus* organisms. Mask, gown, and sterile gloves are indicated for excisions, and are reasonable for any patient at increased risk of infection.[5] Recapping used needles increases the risk of needle sticks, and should never be attempted. Use of forceps during handling of surgical needles is highly recommended to minimize chances of injury. (Fig. 1) Materials that are contaminated with blood or other body fluids should be disposed appropriately in contaminated-materials plastic bags.

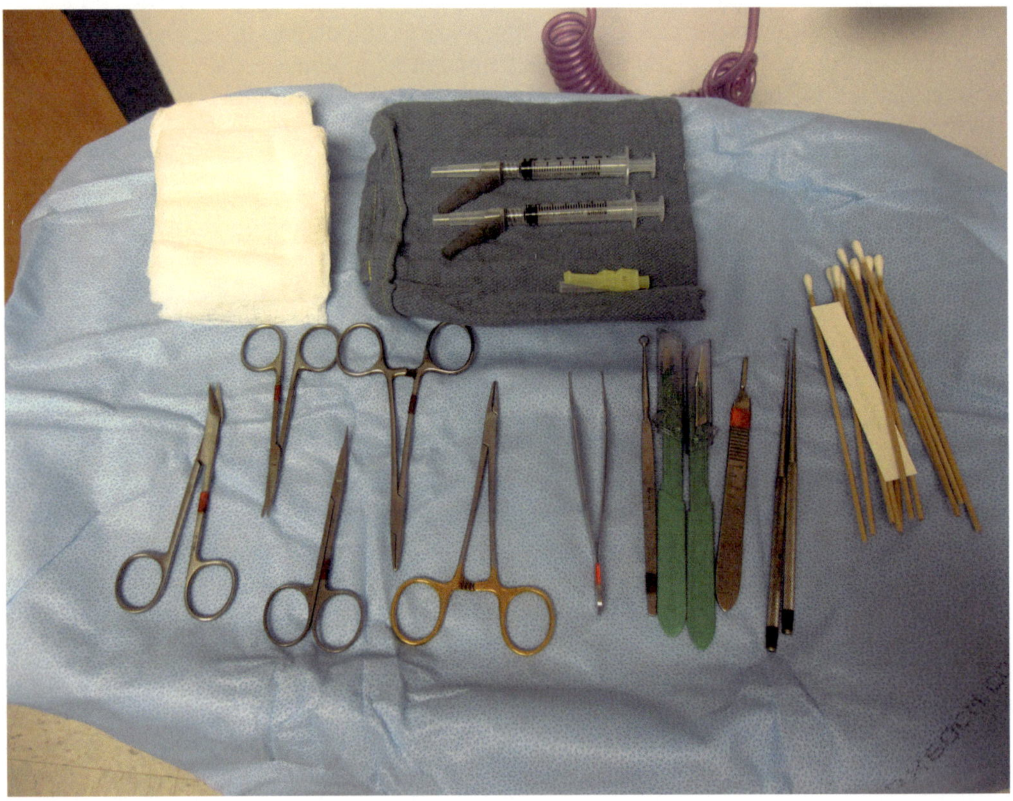

Fig. 1. Instruments used in skin biopsy procedures

3. Preparing the site

Common skin antiseptics such as isopropyl alcohol, providone-iodine, or chlorhexidine gluconate can be used to prepare the biopsy site. [3, 5] Mark the intended lesion with a surgical marker as it may be temporarily obliterated following injection of the anesthetic. (Fig. 2) Marking the outlines for excisional biopsies can be very helpful. For excisions, place a fenestrated surgical drape over the biopsy site after cleansing, but before anesthesia. Round wounds tend to be pulled open in the direction of skin tension lines known as Langer's lines, which are generally parallel to the direction of collagen in the dermis. Tension lines can be demonstrated by gently compressing relaxed skin with the thumb and index finger, and wrinkle lines on the face are another good indicator. Surgical incisions placed parallel to tension lines will close more easily and cosmetically than those placed at right angles. [7, 8, 9]

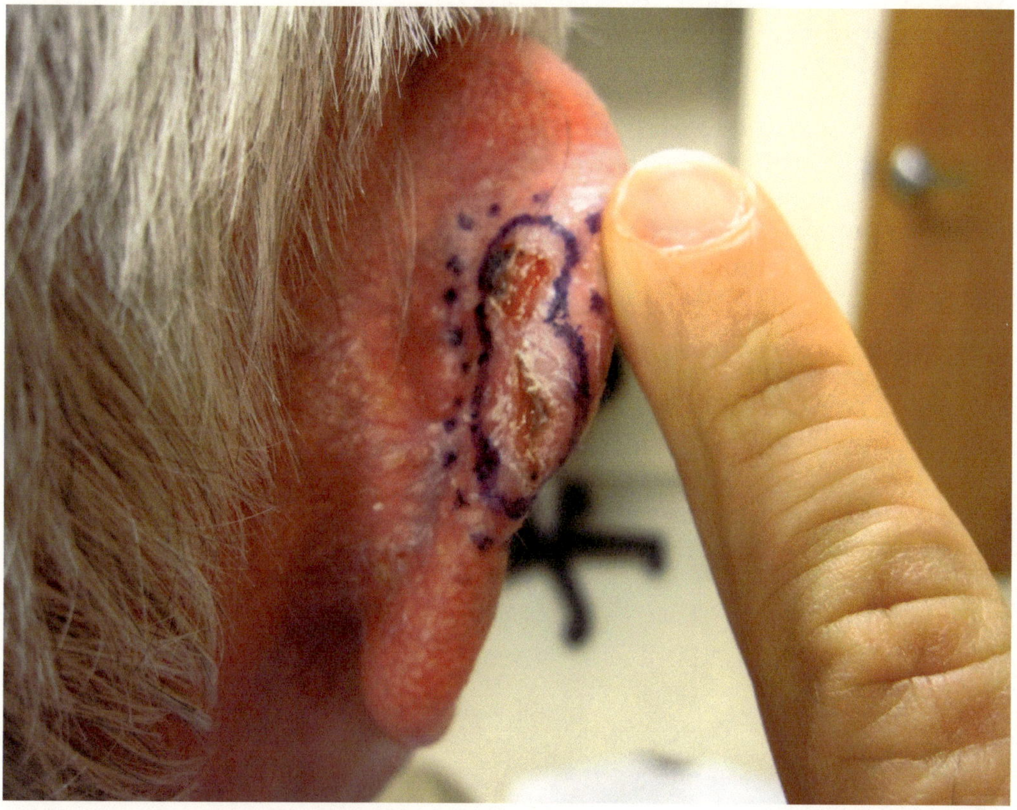

Fig. 2. Lesion on the back of right ear marked for biopsy

4. Anesthesia

The most commonly used local anesthetic is 1% or 2% lidocaine. Allergy to lidocaine is rare and is often secondary to the preservative. [10] An allergy to procaine (Novocain) is not a contraindication to the use of lidocaine, since they are chemically different, and cross reaction is rare. [11] Because lidocaine is a vasodilator, small amounts of epinephrine(1: 100,000) are added to constrict blood vessels, provide some degree of hemostasis, prolong anesthesia, and limit lidocaine toxicity.[12, 13] Avoid the use of epinephrine for acral lesions or when large quantities are needed, especially in patients with cardiovascular disease. [8, 14] However, epinephrine is absolutely contra indicated in digital and penile blocks because it may compromise the blood flow in a confined space. [11, 15] The onset of vasoconstriction is slower than that of anesthesia; plan to use this time efficiently by injecting the biopsy site first, then use the subsequent waiting period to select instruments, fill out forms, and explain follow-up care to the patient. (Fig. 3) Adjunctive techniques utilizing topical anesthetics, cryotherapy (ice or liquid nitrogen) or psychologic distraction may compliment routine use of lidocaine. Sterile saline or diphenhydramine (Benadryl) may be substituted in the rare patient allergic to lidocaine. The anesthetic effect of these two agents is primarily attributed to increased turgor pressure. [10, 16]

The sting of injection can be minimized (presumably by raising the pH) by mixing 1 mL of $NaHCO_3$with 9 mL of lidocaine, using a 30-gauge needle, and by making the initial injection perpendicular to the skin.[3, 7, 12] Deep injections sting less than superficial injections, but prolong the time to adequate anesthesia.[3] Small syringes (1 and 3 cc) permit easier injection and are less cumbersome to handle. For small lesions the anesthetic can be injected directly into, or immediately adjacent to, the lesion. Some schools of thought recommend not injecting directly into lesions in which a malignancy is being considered highly among the differential diagnoses. This practice protects against the small potential of seeding the area during the procedure. For larger lesions, perform a field block by placing a ring of anesthesia around the surgical site, always advancing and injecting through a site that has been previously anesthetized.[7, 1]

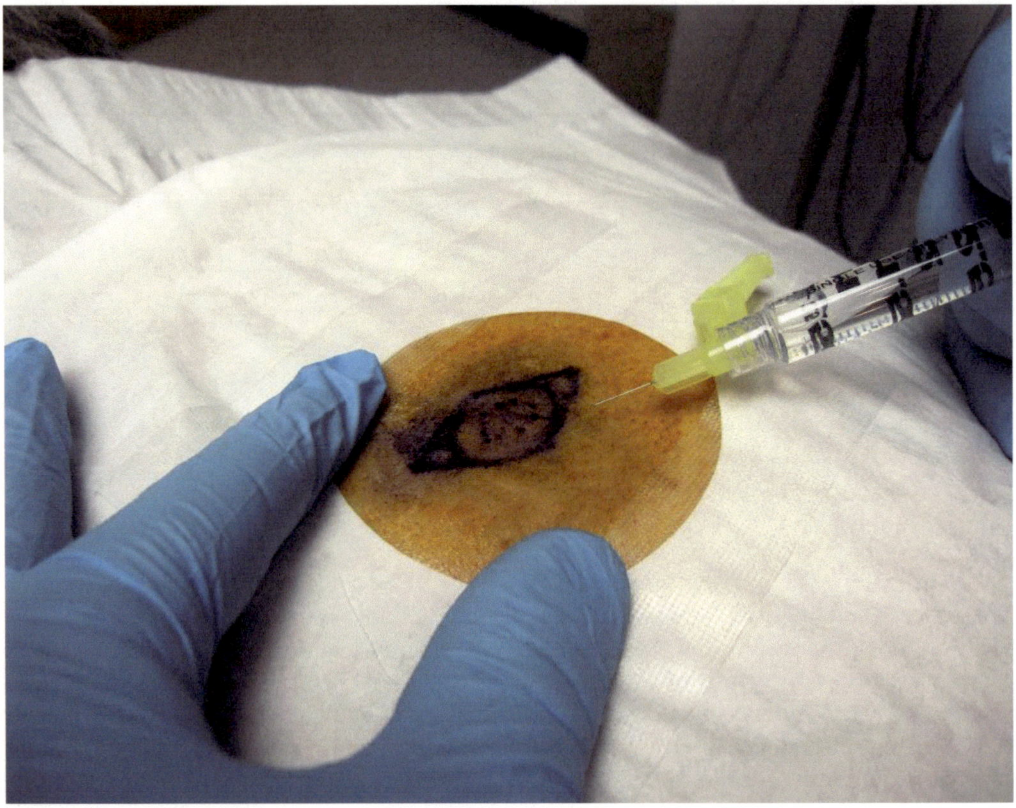

Fig. 3. Administration of local anesthetic agent at the site of skin biopsy

Technique	Advantages	Disadvantages
Shave Biopsy	• Rapid removal of protruding portion of superficial, raised or pedunculated lesions (e.g., milia, warts, seborrheic keratosis, molluscum contagiosum, benign-appearing nevi).	• Potential bisection of melanoma, • disrupting staging evaluation. • False-negative reports whenpathology lies in deeper tissues.
Excisional	• Improved diagnostic sensitivity for tumors of uncertain diagnosis or lesions suspicious for melanoma. Evaluation of deep pathology in toto removal of lesions larger than 6 mm; useful for multiple studies from a single biopsy. (e.g., culture, routine histology, immunofluoroescence).	• Increased time needed forprocedure. Occasionally creates a large skin defect that necessitates layered closure with sutures.
Punch Biopsy	• Rapid, simple and safe technique • Easy removal of small tumors • Useful when multiple biopsies are needed for diagnosis of systemic skin disorders (e.g., psoriasis,erythema multiforme, connective tissue disorders, sarcoidosis and bulous skin diseases').	• May be inadequate for diagnosisof melanoma.
Incisional	• Conservative biopsy of deep subcutaneous disorders (e.g., panniculitis, fibrous tumors) • Diagnosis of large lesions without in toto removal.	• May be inadequate for diagnosisof melanoma.

Table 1. Comparison of Four Common Biopsy Techniques

5. Shave biopsy

Shave biopsies are quick, require little training, and do not require sutures for closure. Lesions that are most suitable for shave biopsies are either elevated above the skin, or have pathology confined to the epidermis. Examples include seborrheic or actinic keratoses, skin tags, warts, and superficial basal or squamous cell carcinomas. Shave biopsies should not be used for pigmented lesions; if an unsuspected melanoma is partially removed, it cannot be properly staged. (Table 1) [5, 12, 18]

5.1 Performing a shave biopsy

Shave biopsies are classified into superficial and deep. Superficial shave biopsies are done across or nearly parallel to the skin surface and extend into the epidermis only or epidermis and limited superficial dermis. The shave biopsy can be facilitated by raising the lesion with a wheal of injected anesthetic, allowing the lesion to be propped up and stabilized between the thumb and forefinger.[8, 14] To shave a lesion, a number 15 blade is held parallel to the skin surface, and the biopsy is performed by using a smooth sweeping stroke rather than a sawing motion. (Fig. 4) Near the end of the shave maneuver, place the index finger on top of the lesion to stabilize and prevent tearing with the exit of the blade. The depth of the biopsy is controlled by the angle of the blade. Care should be taken to keep the blade parallel to the skin surface, avoiding irregular, deep penetration.

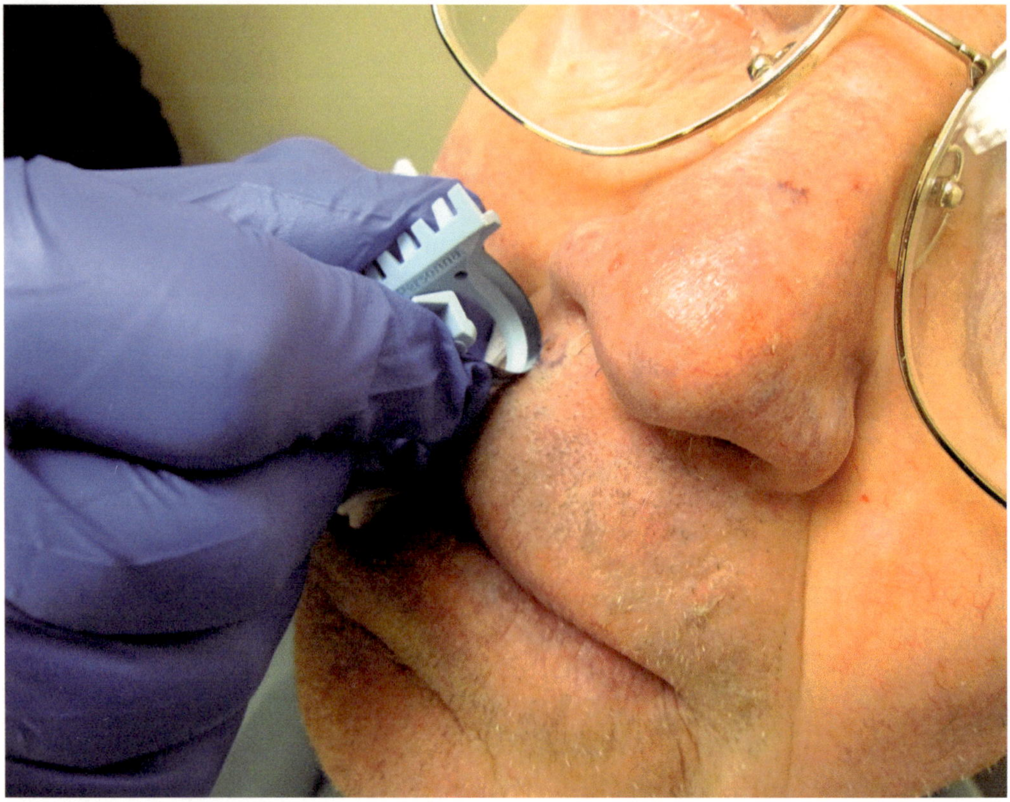

Fig. 4. Performing shave biopsy

A double-edge razor blade cut longitudinally can also be used for shave biopsies. The razor technique has several advantages; it is sharper than most blades, the razor can be bent concave or convex with the thumb and forefinger to better conform to the surface being cut, and width is easily controlled by increasing or decreasing the convexity of the curve. The depth of the shave biopsy can be controlled by varying the angle of contact between razor blade and the skin surface. Curved scissors can be used to perform shave biopsies. Curved scissors are an efficient means of removing skin tags and other small, exophytic growths.[12] The lesion to be removed is stabilized with toothed forceps, and then cut at the base.

The deeper shave biopsy (also known as "saucerization" biopsy) facilitates sampling of dermis and epidermis which is important for assessing basal cell and squamous cell carcinomas. The scalpel is held like a pen to make a small vertical incision into the skin with the beveled tip. The scalpel is then turned and blade is moved forward in a horizontal sawing motion, turning it up towards the surface to finish the excision. [19] This procedure can also be accomplished with the same amount of ease using a double edged razor blade as an alternative. The defect created is that of a saucer.

5.2 Hemostasis

Shave biopsies are quick and do not require sutures for closure. Bleeding following small shave biopsies can often be controlled with pressure alone. Persistent oozing can be stopped with 20% aluminum chloride in absolute alcohol, which is the most commonly used haemostatic agent. (Fig. 5) It is very efficacious and causes minimum tissue destruction. Other hemostatic agents, in order of increasing corrosiveness, are Monsel's solution (ferric sub sulfate), trichloroacetic acid, and silver nitrate. Although Monsel's solution is more effective than aluminum chloride, it also causes more tissue destruction and, like silver nitrate, can result in skin pigmentation.[3, 7]

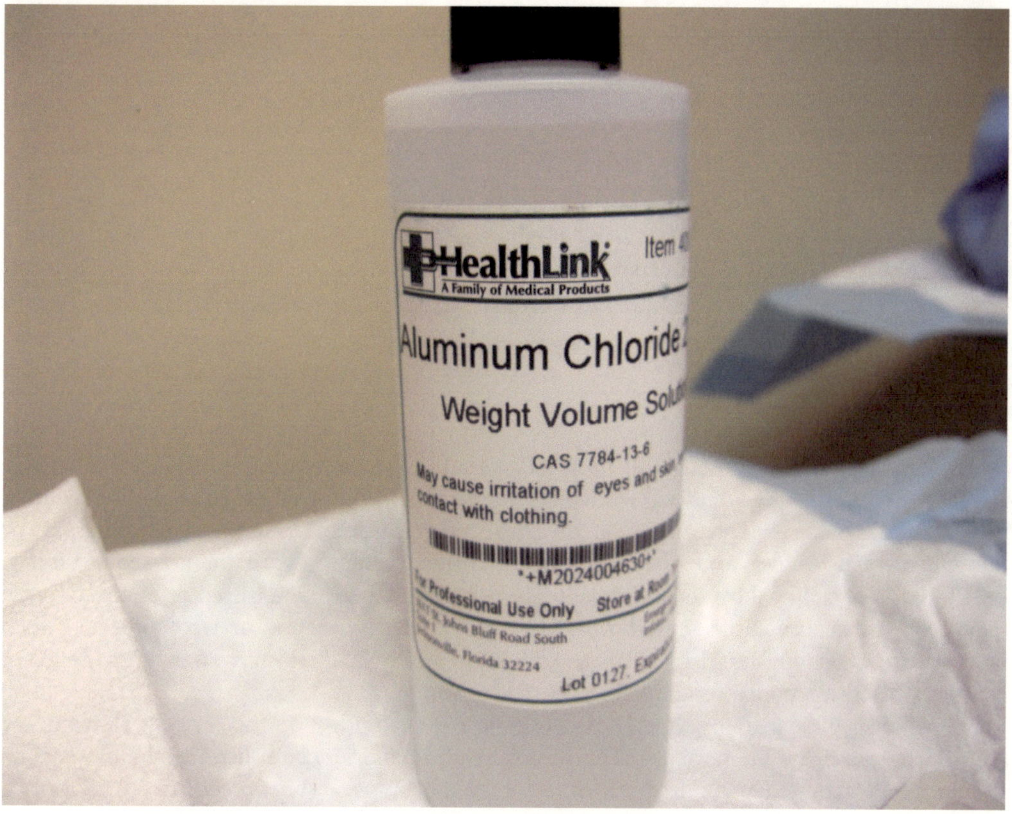

Fig. 5. Aluminum chloride: Most commonly used hemostatic agent

For hemostatic agents to be effective; the wound must be as dry as possible, following which the agent is applied with a cotton applicator using firm pressure with a twisting motion. (Fig. 6) In general, excellent hemostasis following shave biopsies can be achieved in patients with bleeding disorders or in those taking warfarin or aspirin with the combined use of aluminum chloride and several minutes of direct pressure over the wound.

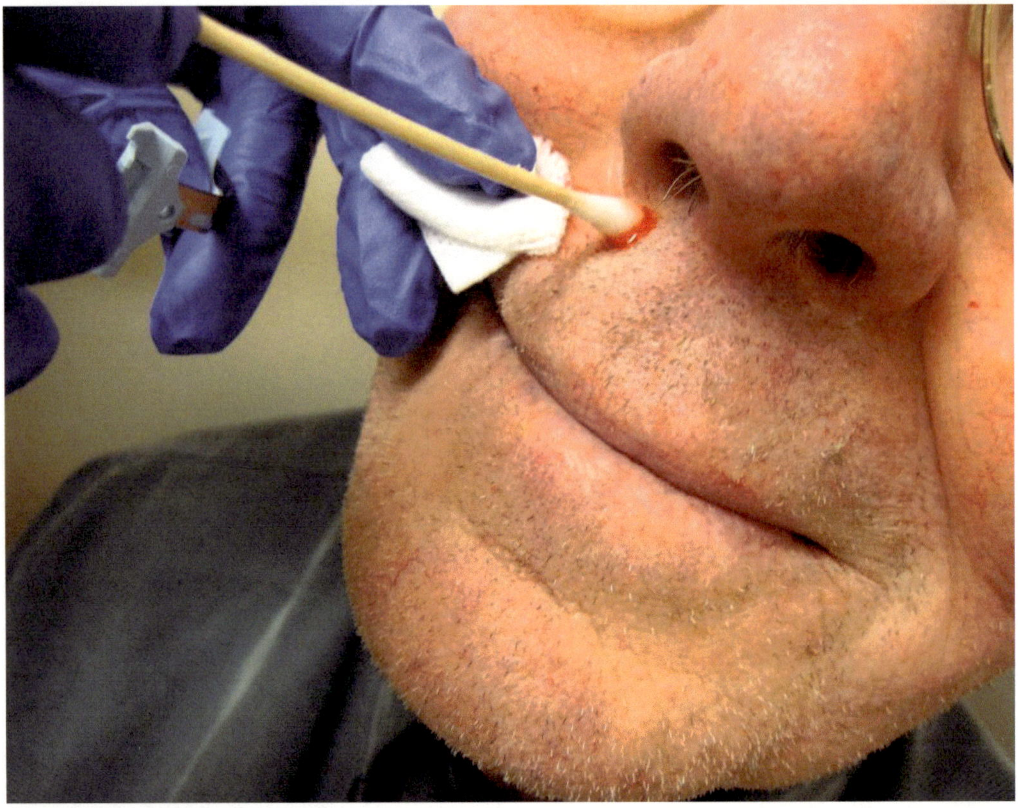

Fig. 6. Application of local haemostatic agent

6. Punch biopsy

Punch biopsies are performed with round, disposable knives ranging in diameter from 2 to 10 mm, but 3 mm is the smallest size likely to give sufficient tissue for consistently accurate histologic diagnosis.[20] The punch is an ideal procedure for diagnostic skin biopsy or removing small lesions, and often provides a better cosmetic result than a shave biopsy. Punch biopsies can heal by secondary intention, but punches greater than or equal to 3 mm may produce unacceptable scarring and are best closed with one or two sutures. Punch biopsies are easily mastered by most practitioners, are quick, and have a low incidence of infection, bleeding, nonhealing, or significant scarring.[3, 5]

Punch biopsies yield a cone shaped core of tissue with its widest diameter at the skin surface and narrowest at the biopsy base. The direction of the skin tension lines at the biopsy site should be determined prior to performing a punch biopsy. The procedure to perform a punch biopsy is as following:

Raise an intradermal wheal with anesthetic agent. Stabilize the skin with the thumb and forefinger, stretching it slightly perpendicular to the normal skin tension lines; this will produce an oval rather than round defect, facilitating closure. (Fig. 7) [4] Place the punch perpendicular to the skin and apply firm and constant downward pressure with a circular twisting motion. Removal of the punch to "check the progress" should be avoided as this may result in a ragged wound and a shredded biopsy sample. [21]

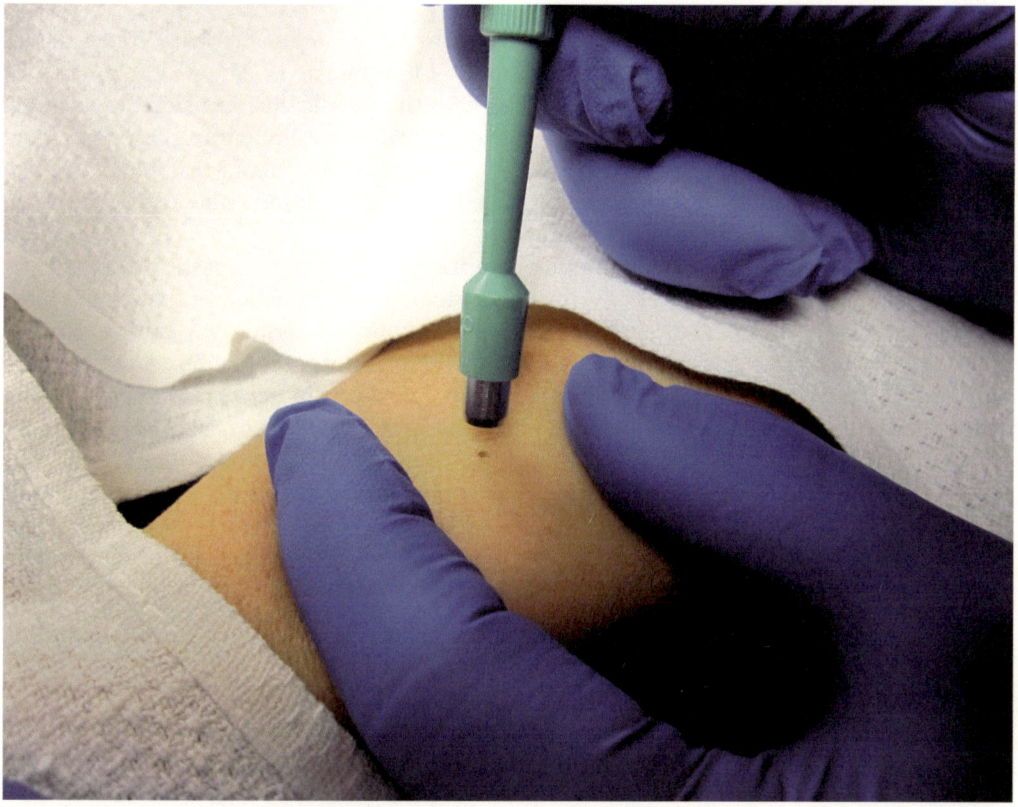

Fig. 7. Performing punch biopsy procedure

A definite "give" occurs when the punch reaches the subcutaneous fat, indicating that a full-thickness cut has been made. Remove the punch and apply downward finger pressure at the sides of the wound to pop up the core. Completely elevate the core with gentle use of forceps or a needle tip and excise it at its base with small tissue scissors. The pressure applied through forceps to elevate the core should be gentle to minimize the destruction and distortion of tissue in the biopsy sample. After finishing the harvest of the tissue, prepare the biopsy site for closure.

Punch biopsies of the scalp for diagnosis of hair disorders are best accomplished using a 4 mm punch and holding it at 20° to the surface of the scalp, roughly along the axis of the hair follicle. [5] Biopsies of scalp lesions suspected of being malignant are performed in the same manner as other punch biopsies, with the punch perpendicular to the skin surface.

Punch biopsies can be closed with one or two sutures or allowed to heal by secondary intention. Wounds that are allowed to heal by secondary intention may be treated with a hemostatic agent such as aluminum chloride or absorbable gelatin. These agents are not needed if sutures are to be used. Contraindications to suturing include biopsies in infected or poorly healing skin; these wounds heal better by secondary intention. The punch is an ideal procedure for diagnostic skin biopsy or removing small lesions. It often provides a better cosmetic result than a shave biopsy. [5]

7. Excisional biopsy

Excisions are reserved for lesions that cannot be removed with a punch owing to size, depth, or location. Excisions are especially well suited for removal of large skin tumors or inflammatory disorders deep in the skin, involving the panniculus. Excisions require the greatest amount of expertise and time; they almost always require sutures, and are more easily performed with an assistant.[3, 5] It is strongly recommended that practitioners receive clinical training before attempting an excisional biopsy, or refer patients requiring an excision to a qualified dermatologist or surgeon.

These are performed for lesions that require complete removal for diagnostic or therapeutic purposes. An excisional biopsy allows for histopathologic examination of an entire lesion. Another advantage of an excisional biopsy is the amount of tissue that can be excised, allowing for multiple studies (culture, histopathology, immunofluorescence, electron microscopy) from one biopsy site.[5] The direction of the skin tension lines should be determined in preparation for an excision. Align the long axis of the excision parallel to the skin tension lines. Using a surgical marking pen, draw an ellipse around the lesion to be excised, including a 2 to 5 mm margin of normal skin around the lesion, with 30° angles at each apex, and the length three times the width. (Fig. 8) Holding the scalpel with a number 15 blade like a pen, begin the incision at one apex with the blade perpendicular to the skin. As the incision progresses, use more of the belly of the blade, raising it to the perpendicular again at the next apex.[14]

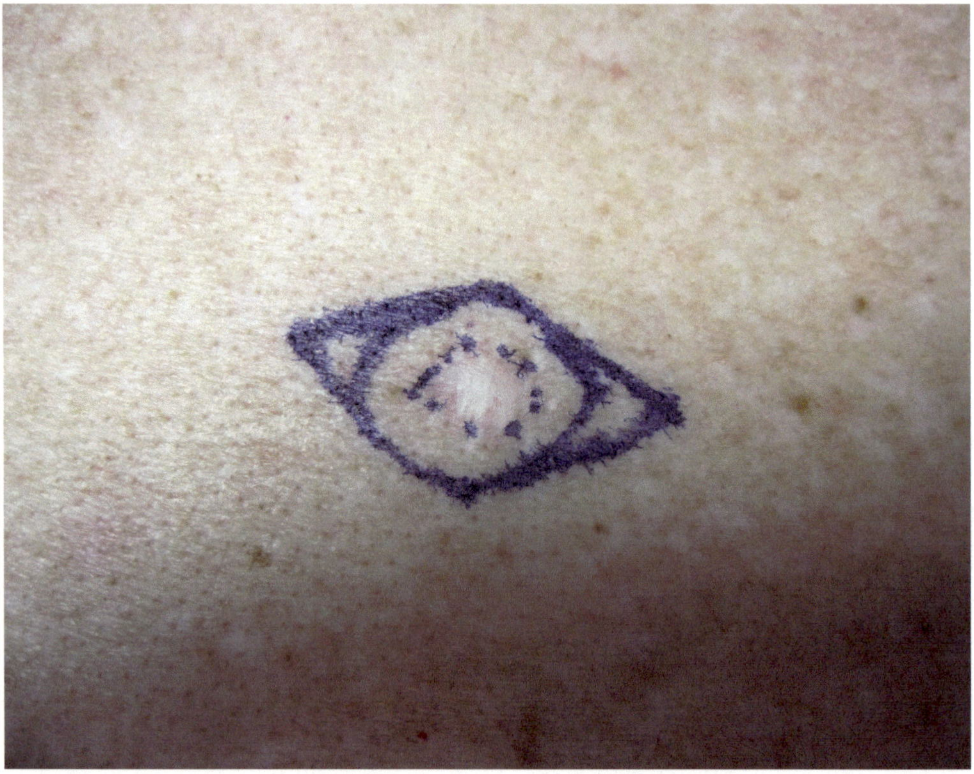

Fig. 8. Lesion marked in elliptical fashion prior to excisional biopsy

The blade should be angled away from the lesion, slightly undermining the wound edge. This will allow for easier eversion of the wound edge during closure, improving the cosmetic result and decreasing the risk of dehiscence. (Fig. 9) Carefully lift the sample edge with fine forceps once the ellipse has been incised and completely undermine the sample at the level of the subcutaneous fat with scalpel or scissors. Apply pressure to the wound with gauze in preparation for closing.

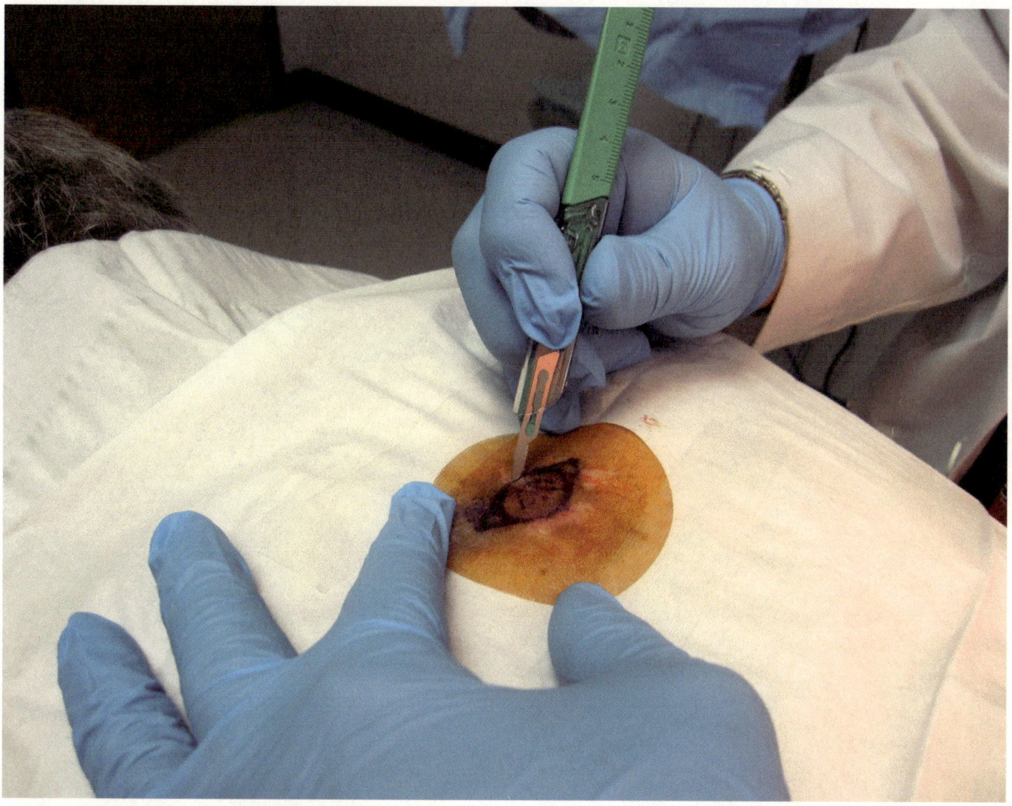

Fig. 9. Performing excisional biopsy

For some physicians, it will be technically easier to perform a diamond-shaped excision for small lesions, and a hexagonal-shaped excision for larger lesions.[4] The lines of the excision can be marked with a surgical marker prior to anesthesia. For diamond excisions, the blade is inserted vertically into the skin to make the four straight-line incisions of the diamond. For the hexagon, two straight and parallel lines are incised on either side of the lesion and then connected at each end by two more straight incisions to form the hexagon.[4]
Excisions require the greatest amount of expertise and time; they almost always require sutures, and are more easily performed with an assistant.[5]

8. Processing the biopsy sample

For light microscopy, the specimen should be placed in a 10% buffered formalin solution provided by pathology; each specimen should be placed into a separate bottle and identified. Specimens less than 1 cm in greatest dimension can be fixed in 30 mL of formalin, but larger specimens will require more formalin for adequate fixation. (Fig. 10) If a large complicated specimen needs to be sectioned, clue the pathologist to the location of the lesion by sectioning through its center and marking the normal skin borders with surgical marker. Careful attention must be paid to labeling the specimen. Include patient and physician name, date, and location of the lesion. The latter is especially critical if more than one lesion is removed. The specimen label must match the pathology request form and the description in the medical record. On the request form, list the clinical diagnoses and give a short clinical history and description of the lesion or rash.[10, 12] Focused clinical history and differential diagnoses are of immense help to the pathologist to arrive at a correct histological diagnosis. If a tumor has been removed, request that the margins be checked for tumor. Whenever possible, the specimen should be submitted to a dermatopathologist.[3]

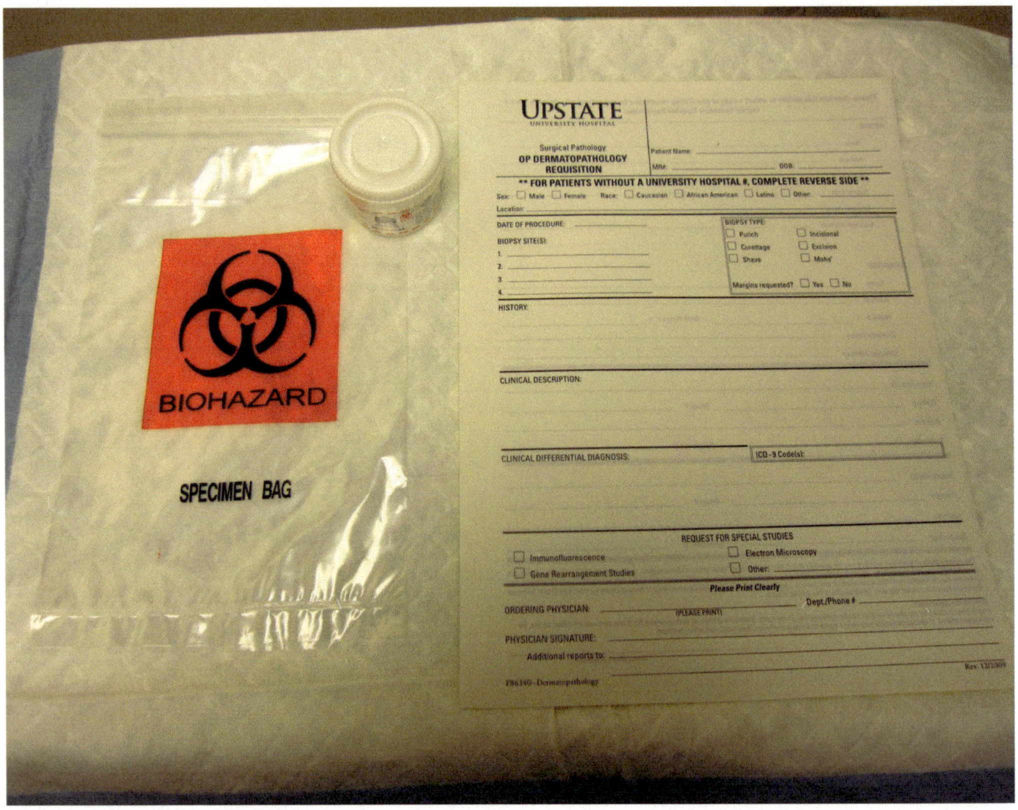

Fig. 10. 10% buffered formalin solution and Pathology request form

9. Preparing the wound for suturing

Prior to closing excisional wounds, the edges of the wound may need to be undermined either sharply with a scalpel or bluntly with scissors. Blunt dissection is performed by advancing the closed scissors under the wound edge, and quickly spreading them open. The width of undermining varies with the size of the wound, but for most wounds, 5 to 10 mm is sufficient. Undermining allows the skin edges to evert more easily and reduces tension on the sutures. (Fig. 11) It is a very useful technique; however care should be taken not to overdo it to minimize tissue destruction, risk of bleeding and post procedure pain. [3, 5, 16]

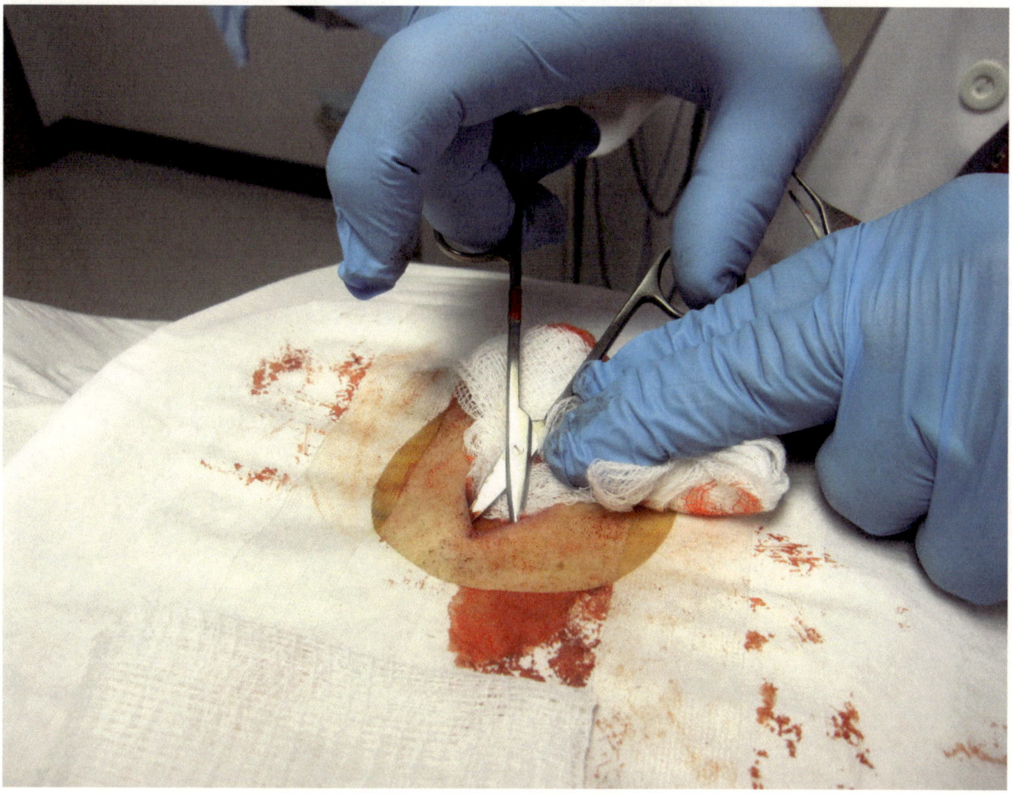

Fig. 11. Undermining the excision site prior to suturing

10. Choice of suture and needle

The qualities most important in suture are flexibility, strength, secure knotting, and infection potential.[22] The two major categories of suture are absorbable and nonabsorbable. Absorbable suture is made from synthetic polymer or mammalian-derived collagen (gut). Common synthetic absorbables include polyglactic acid (Vicryl), polyglycolic acid (Dexon), and polydixanone (PDS). Absorbable sutures are usually placed deep in larger wounds to reduce skin tension for the final closure.

Nonabsorbable sutures are used for skin closure and permanent internal placement. Common nonabsorbable sutures include silk, nylon (Ethi-lon), and polypropylene (Prolene). Silk and nylon suture can be braided, adding strength and improving knotting potential, but are more likely to harbor infection. Polypropylene and unbraided nylon are monofilaments, and are less likely to harbor infection, but knots are less secure and more difficult to tie. Silk and gut, as natural materials, cause considerable tissue inflammation and have been largely replaced by synthetic suture material. [8, 22]

Generally, 4-0 or 5-0 monofilament nylon can be used on the body and scalp, and 6-0 nylon on the face.[7, 16] Polypropylene can be considered for the scalp, primarily because it is blue and easy to see.

Suture needles are made of noncorrosive stainless steel, especially forged to achieve maximum strength and ductility, the ability to bend under pressure without breaking.[22] Suture needles have an eye, body, and point. Most needles have a swaged eye where the metal of the needle is molded around the end of the suture. This part of the needle is soft and likely to bend or break if mishandled. The body of the needle is designed for great strength and secure grasping; it is usually flattened with slight convex or concave sides to avoid rotation in the holder while suturing. Three types of needle points are common: cutting, tapered, and blunt. Cutting needles allow for easy passage through tough tissue and are ideal for skin. The size of the needle is ranked by a number, with higher numbers identifying larger needles. Needle curvature is measured in terms of proportion of a circle, with one-quarter, one-half, and three-eight curves available. When wound closing seems more difficult than expected, reassess the appropriateness of the instruments. Needle selection is often a prime factor in the ease of suturing and final cosmetic result.[17]

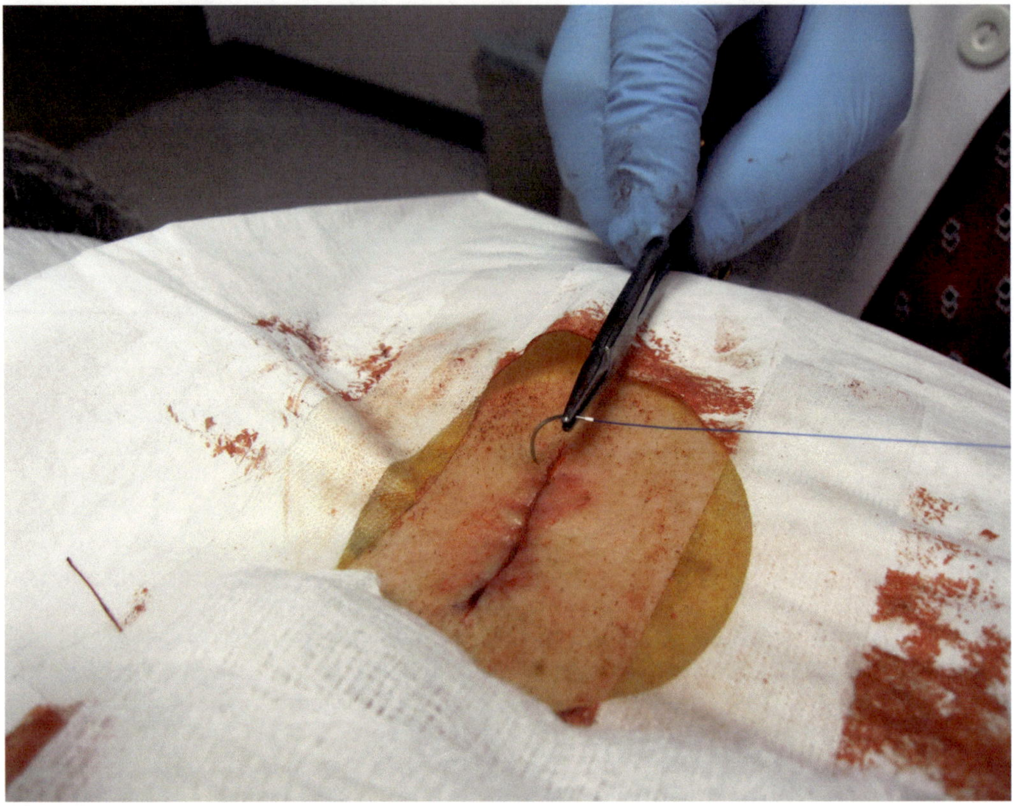

Fig. 12. Handling technique for suture needles

11. Closing

Primary closure of a punch wound can be accomplished with one or two, single-layer, interrupted sutures. Excisions can be closed in one or two layers, with two-layer closures giving better cosmetic results in the larger wounds. The most common closure technique is a simple, interrupted suture.[7] To begin, grasp the needle with the needle-holder at midpoint or about one third the distance from the eye. (Fig. 12) This will provide maximum driving force and diminish the likelihood of bending or breaking the needle. A palm grip is recommended to increase the driving force of the needle through the skin. Place the handle of the holder in the palm, wrap the thumb and fingers around the handles, and extend the index finger down over the tip of the holder near the needle. The needle point is placed perpendicular to the skin surface about 2 mm away from the wound edge, and is driven down, then up into the center of the wound. A second insertion begins in the center of the wound, and exits the skin on the opposite side, 2 mm from the wound edge, perpendicular to the surface. If done properly, the suture will make a flask-shaped loop; the loop beneath the skin surface is farther apart than the entry and exit points on the surface. For small excisional wounds, and for most punch wounds, a needle exit in the middle of the wound is not necessary, but depends on the size of the needle and the ease that the wound edges can be approximated and everted.

The instrument tie is fast and efficient. To begin, hold the needle holder parallel to the long axis of the wound with the free end and needle end of the suture on either side of the holder. Wrap the needle end of the suture twice around the holder, then grasp the free end of the suture with the holder and pull through, tightening the knot. (Fig. 13) At this point the needle end and free end of the suture should have switched sides relative to the beginning. The process is repeated as needed, reversing the position of the free end and needle end of the suture with each knot. "Approximate, don't strangulate" acknowledges the importance of proper tension on the suture. Excessive tension can be recognized by blanching of the wound edges, and may indicate the need for subcutaneous sutures or simply less tension on each suture.

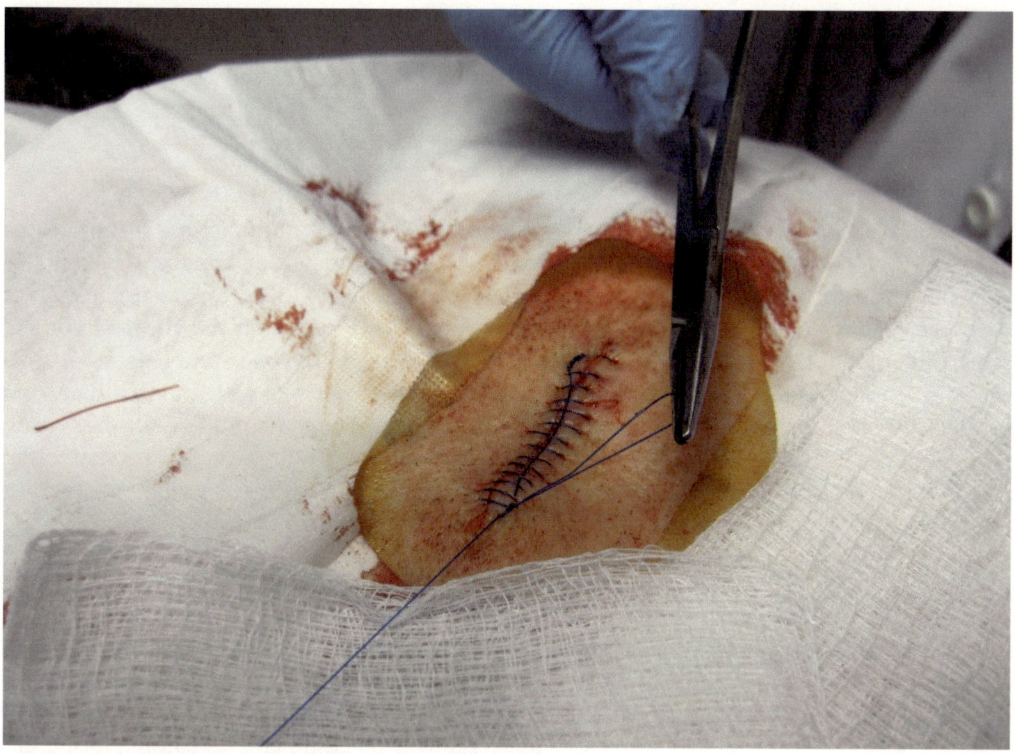

Fig. 13. Placement of sutures at excisional biopsy site

Placement of sutures for elliptical excisions can be facilitated by following the "rule of halves."[7] The wound is divided in half by the initial suture placement, and each half is itself halved by the subsequent placement of sutures. Similar halving continues until all wound edges are approximated. Starting the initial suture at an apex rather than the middle runs the risk of "dog ears" at the opposite apex owing to the creation of uneven wound edges.
In large wounds, the skin tension can be reduced by placing a temporary initial suture at the midpoint of the wound, but farther from the edge than usual. At a later time, this suture can be removed as the wound is approximated with the permanent sutures. Diamond and hexagonal excisions are easily closed by placing the initial sutures at the two opposing points of the diamond or four opposing points of the hexagon, then adding other sutures as necessary to completely approximate the wound. The straight lines of the diamond and hexagon provide better approximation of edges for the beginner than do the curved surfaces of the ellipse.[10]

12. Wound dressing

Wounds heal faster when moist, and under an occlusive or semi occlusive dressing. All biopsy wounds can be dressed with a thin film of an antibiotic ointment (bacitracin, polysprin, mupirocin) or plain petrolatum to prevent crust formation, then covered with a Band-Aid or other nonadherent covering, and topped with a gauze dressing and tape.[7, 23] The dressing should be removed in 12 to 24 hours and thereafter cleaned with soap and water twice daily. After cleaning, the wound should be covered with an antibiotic ointment or petrolatum. Wounds healing by secondary intention need to be redressed after each cleaning until healed over, or for at least 5 days, whereas this is optional for sutured wounds. For sutured wounds, showering is permitted after 24 hours, but use of hot tubs is prohibited until the sutures are removed.[24]

13. Suture removal

There is a balance between the tendency for wound dehiscence or stretching if the sutures are removed too early, and the production of suture marks if they remain too long.[8, 22] Generally, sutures on the face can be removed in 3 to 5 days, followed by the application of semi permeable adhesive strips to reduce wound tension. Sutures on the chest, abdomen, arms, and scalp can be removed in 7 to 10 days, and those on the back and legs in 12 to 20 days.[7, 22, 23] Physicians should remove sutures from their patients to learn first-hand the results of their suturing technique and wound healing. Any crust should be washed away with wet gauze, then the suture is gently lifted near the knot, and one side cut close to the skin surface. The suture is removed by pulling *across* the wound surface; pulling away from the wound puts tension on the wound and may cause dehiscence.[7]

14. Complications

The major complications include bleeding, infection, and allergic reactions. Most bleeding can be controlled with simple pressure on the wound.[10] If this is not successful after 5 minutes, a single suture may be sufficient. If bleeding remains uncontrolled, remove the suture, find and tie off the bleeding vessel, then resuture. Bleeding and hematoma formation can be minimized by using a pressure dressing directly over the wound. Tape a folded 4 × 4

gauze pad tightly over the wound, or secure it with an elastic bandage or self-adhering wrap. An ice pack applied for 3 to 5 minutes several times during the first 24 hours will also help decrease bleeding, hematoma formation, pain, and edema.[23]
Infection, though relatively uncommon, is usually the result of *Staphylococcus*, *Streptococcus*, or *Candida*. If the wound is frankly purulent, or has an associated cellulitis, culture the discharge and begin oral antibiotics. Infected wounds in the hands, feet, and intertriginous areas are often infected with *Candida* and can respond to topical antifungal ointments. [25] Occasionally patients will develop reactions to topical antibiotics.[26] The wound will be red, itchy, and may have vesicles. If this occurs, stop the antibiotic and apply a topical corticosteroid ointment. Tape reactions are usually irritant rather than allergic and improve simply by not taping, or sometimes by changing the direction of the tape on the skin.[27]

15. Documentation

All procedures must be documented in the medical record. Minimal content includes location and nature of the lesion, indications for procedure, what was done, and how it was performed, specimen disposition, and instructions to and follow-up plans for the patient. Documentation of location with diagrams, pictures and accurate measurements with a ruler using nearby anatomical landmarks as reference points should be done. This is especially important if there is the possibility of further excision at the original biopsy site in future. Often the original biopsy defect may heal so well as to completely conceal the original site.[1]

16. Snip biopsy

Snip biopsies are especially indicated for very superficial or pedunculated lesions such as acrochordons (skin tags), filliform warts, or seborrheic keratosis. The lesion is secured with a forceps and raised. This enables one to expose the base of the lesion and provide traction. A sharp scissors is then placed at the base of the lesion and it is cut (or snipped off). (Fig. 14)

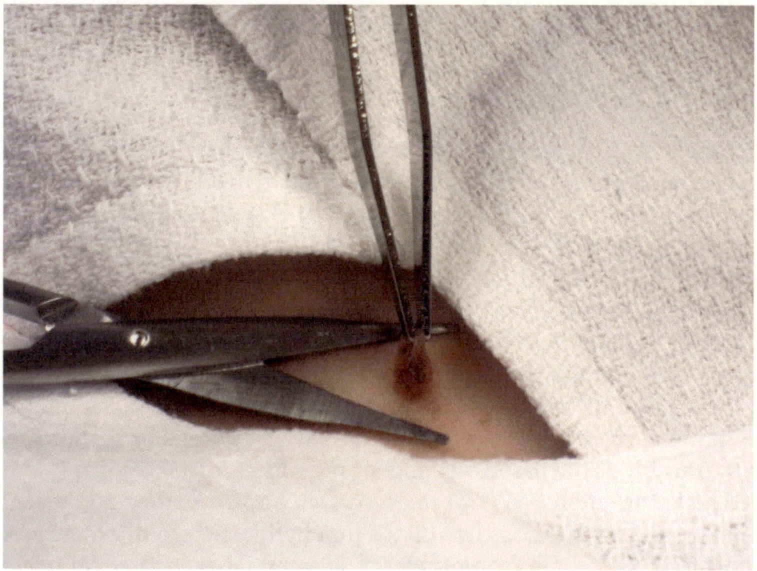

Fig. 14. Snip Biopsy

17. Incisional biopsies

Incisional biopsies usually include a part of a lesion, or part of the affected skin plus part of the normal skin to show the interface between the two. These are usually performed for inflammatory processes involving the subcutaneous tissue or fascia, or well demarcated conditions where the specimen needs to include normal and abnormal skin. The location within the lesion should be chosen to include the most raised or pigmented part of the lesion. The depth of the incision is through the entire dermis down to the subcutaneous fat. Incisional biopsies have particular uses when the subcutaneous tissues must be examined (i.e., panniculitis, fibrous tumors).
Long and thin deep incisional biopsies are excellent on the lower extremities as they allow a large amount of tissue to be harvested with minimal tension on the surgical wound. Advantage of the incisional biopsy over the punch method is that hemostasis can be done more easily due to better visualization. [18]
The technique of the incisional biopsy closely resembles that of the excisional biopsy. They are also a practical aid in planning definitive treatment of large lesions. The disadvantages of incisional biopsy include risk of bleeding and scarring, and limited tissue for histology in pigmented lesions, the incisional biopsy, like the punch biopsy, is only used where the excision is undesirable because of functional or cosmetic considerations.[15]

18. Oral biopsies

The same techniques that are used in the skin are also utilized in the oral cavity. Oral mucous membrane is histologically similar to the skin except for the absence of a stratum corneum. Hemostasis is difficult to achieve after the procedure because of the vascular nature of the oral cavity and limited access into an enclosed space. Special devices are used such as a Chalazion clamp greatly aids in performing these procedures. The physician should also be aware that oral biopsies may produce esthetic compromise as a result of scarring or residual deformity. The esthetic outcome is of particular concern when a lesion on the lip is near the vermilion border.[28]

19. Pigmented lesions (Melanoma)

An important caveat regarding removal of pigmented lesions is the possibility of malignant melanoma. The incidence of melanoma has almost tripled in the past three decades, growing faster than that of any other cancer. Because melanoma is notorious for its poor prognosis, accuracy and speed of diagnosis are essential. A high clinical suspicion for melanoma should be entertained for any pigmented lesion characterized by the ABCDs of malignant melanoma: asymmetry, /border irregularity, color variegation and (diameter more than 6 mm, or rapid growth over a period of weeks to months. [16]
Excisional biopsy can optimize the sampling of tissue suspicious for melanoma. The excision should be at the level of the subcutaneous tissue, where the Breslow depth of invasion and therefore the grade of melanoma can be determined. An elliptic or fusiform excision may span the entire breadth of the tissue, yet allow for good cosmetic results. [29] Early diagnosis of melanoma has led to improved cure rates. In fact, approximately 50 percent of patients with melanoma present with lesions less than 1 mm in thickness, a thickness associated with a cure rate of 90 to 95 percent.[30] Prompt referral is essential even after complete excision so further evaluation and therapy can be planned. Shave biopsy is never used for a pigmented

lesion that may be melanoma. Shave biopsy of a malignant melanoma may destroy valuable information by transecting the lesion, making accurate measurement of depth and prognosis difficult.[16] Punch biopsy should only be used with discretion for lesions suspicious for melanoma. Small lesions indicative of melanoma can be removed by a punch technique, provided that the lesion can be completely removed. In one study, only 32 percent of punch biopsies provided sufficient material for both definitive and complete evaluation of melanoma. Many of these biopsies were performed in lesions where suspicion of melanoma was minimal.[30] However, the problem of sampling error is a critical factor in pathologic interpretation of pigmented nevi. The lack of invasive melanoma in one punch biopsy specimen within a large lesion does not prove the lack of cancer in another portion of the lesion. It is advisable to refer patients with large or awkwardly located suspicious lesions to dermatologist, rather than attempt a biopsy that may carry a high risk of either disfigurement or inadequate sampling.

20. Summary

Skin biopsy is an essential technique in the management of skin diseases. It can enhance dermatologic care but is not a substitute for clinical knowledge and decision making. Shave biopsy requires the least experience and time, but its use is limited to superficial lesions and should not be used for pigmented lesions. Punch biopsy is the primary diagnostic procedure in dermatology, is simple to perform, has few complications, and very small biopsies can heal without suturing. Although closing with sutures improves the cosmetic result, it requires more expertise and time. Excisions are ideal for removing large or deep lesions, provide abundant tissue for multiple studies, and can be curative for a number conditions including cancer. However, excisions require the greatest amount of expertise, time, and office resources, and are associated with more complications, including bleeding, infection and possibly scarring. Because of its complexity and complication potential, clinical training is highly recommended prior to attempting an excisional biopsy.[7, 9]

21. References

[1] Patrick CA, Barbara MM. Skin Biopsy Techniques for the Internist. J Gen Intern Med. 1998 January; 13(1): 46–54.

[2] Fitzpatrick TB, Bernhard JD. The structure of skin lesions and fundamental of diagnosis. In: Fitzpatrick TB, Eisen AZ, Wolff K, Freedburg IM, Austen KF, editors. *Dermatology in General Medicine.* 3rd Ed. New York, NY: McGraw-Hill; 1987. p. 47. In. Ed.

[3] Pariser RJ. Skin biopsy: lesion selection and optimal technique. *Mod Med.* 1989; 57:82–90.

[4] Pinkus H. Skin biopsy: a field of interaction between clinician and pathologist. *Cutis.* 1977; 20:609–14.

[5] Peters MS, Winkelman RK. The biopsy. *Dermatol Clin.* 1984;2:209–17.

[6] Krull EA, Babel DE. Diagnostic procedures of the skin, part two: skin biopsy and other tests. *J Fam Pract.* 1976; 3:427–31.

[7] Dinehart SM, Hanke CW, Geronemus RG. *Dermatologic Surgery for Medical Students.* Schaumburg: Association of Academic Dermatologic Surgeons; 1993.

[8] Harrison PV. A guide to skin biopsies and excisions. *Clin Exp Dermatol.* 1980; 5:235–43.

[9] Snell G. Skin biopsy. In: Pfenninger JL, Fowler GC, editors. *Procedures for Primary Care Physicians.* St. Louis, Mo: Mosby-Year Book; 1994. pp. 20–6. In: Eds.
[10] Grekin RC, Auletta MJ. Local anesthesia in dermatologic surgery. J Am Acad Dermatol 1988; 19:599- 614.
[11] Fewkes JL, Sober AJ. Skin biopsy: the four types and how best to do them. Primary Care and Cancer, 1993:13:35-9.
[12] Arca MJ, Bierman JS, Johnson TM, Chang AE. Biopsy techniques for skin, soft-tissue, and bone neoplasms. *Surg Oncol Clin North Am.* 1995; 4:157–74.
[13] Ritchie JM, Greene NM. Local anesthetics. In: Gilman AG, Rall TW, Nies AS, Taylor P, editors. *The Pharmacological Basis of Therapeutics.* 8th ed. New York, NY: Pergamon Press; 1990. pp. 311–31. In. eds.
[14] Bart RS, Kopf AW. Techniques of biopsy of cutaneous neoplasms. *J Dermatol Surg Oncol.* 1979; 5:979–87.
[15] Area M, Biermatin JS, Johnson TM, Chang AE. Biopsy techniques for skin, soft-tissue, and bone neoplasms. Surg Oncol Clin North Am 1995; 1:157- 74.
[16] Koh HK. Cutaneous melanoma. N Engl J Med 199I; 3Z'i: 17l-S2.
[17] Epperson WJ. Laceration and incision repair. In: Pfenninger JL, Fowler GC, editors. *Procedures for Primary Care Physicians.* St. Louis, Mo: Mosby-Year Book; 1994. pp. 7–11. In: eds.
[18] Achar S. Principles of skin biopsies for the family physician. Am Fam Physician. 1996 Dec; 54(8):2411-8.
[19] Olbricht, S. Biopsy Techniques and Basic Excisions. In: Dermatology, 1st edition,Bolognia, JL, Rapini, RP, et al (Eds), Mosby, London 2003. p.2269.
[20] Todd P, Garioch JJ, Humphreys S, Seywright M, Thompson J, du Vivier AWP. Evaluation of the 2-mm punch biopsy in dermatological diagnosis. *Clin Exp Dermatol.* 1996; 21:11–3.
[21] Grekin, RC. Simple dermatological surgical procedures. Res Staff Phys 1989; 35:61.
[22] Moy RL, Waldman B, Hein DW. A review of sutures and suturing technique. *J Dermatol Surg Oncol.* 1992; 18:785–95.
[23] Telfer NR, Moy RL. Wound care after office procedures. *J Dermatol Surg Oncol.* 1993; 19:722–31.
[24] Noe JM, Keller M. Can stitches get wet? *Plast Reconstr Surg.* 1988; 81:82–4.
[25] Bennett RG. Microbiological considerations in cutaneous surgery. In: Bennett RG, editor. *Fundamentals of Cutaneous Surgery.* St. Louis, Mo: CV Mosby Company; 1988. pp. 136–78. In: ed.
[26] Gette MT, Marks JG, Maloney ME. Frequency of postoperative allergic contact dermatitis to topical antibiotics. *Arch Dermatol.* 1992; 128:365–7.
[27] Grolnick M. Factors involved in the production of adhesive plaster irritation. *Am J Surg.* 1940; 50:63–78?
[28] Drore E. The Oral Mucosal Punch Biopsy. A Report of 140 Cases. *Arch Dermatol.* 1992; 128(6):815-817.
[29] Zuber TJ, Dewitt DE. The fusiform excision. Am Fam Physician 1994; 49:371-6,379-80.
[30] Devereux DF. Diagnosis and management of dysplastic nevus syndrome and early melanoma. Oncology 1990; 4:73-8l.

Part 2

Skin Biopsy Applications in Skin Diseases

4

New Diagnostic Applications in Sporotrichosis

Rosely Maria Zancope-Oliveira,
Rodrigo de Almeida-Paes, Manoel Marques Evangelista de Oliveira,
Dayvison Francis Saraiva Freitas and Maria Clara Gutierrez Galhardo
Instituto de Pesquisa Clínica Evandro Chagas – Fundação Oswaldo Cruz
Brazil

1. Introduction

Sporotrichosis is a subcutaneous mycosis that is globally distributed. Areas of high endemicity are Latin America, South Africa, India and Japan (Lopez-Romero et al., 2011; Queiroz-Telles et al., 2011). This infection is caused by the dimorphic fungus, previously described as the single species *Sporothrix schenckii* (Coura, 2005), that is now named the *S. schenckii* species complex (Marimon et al., 2006, 2007, 2008), which is associated with plants and soil (Ramos e Silva et al., 2007). In humans, sporotrichosis has been regarded as a job-related disease that usually occurs in the form of isolated cases or small outbreaks and affects only people exposed to plants or soil rich in organic matter and occasionally laboratory technicians (Copper et al., 1992; Hajjeh et al., 1997).

The fungus *S. schenckii* was isolated for the first time in 1896 by Benjamin Schenck from a 36-year-old male patient who presented with lesions on his right hand and arm. This isolate was classified into the genus *Sporotrichum* (Schenck, 1898). Hekton and Perkins described the second sporotrichosis case in 1900. These investigators isolated the fungus and created the current denomination, *Sporothrix schenckii* (Hekton & Perkins, 1900, as cited in Coura, 2005).

In the early 1900s, sporotrichosis was a common disease in France, and many features of the fungus and the less-common clinical manifestations were described. At the same time, potassium iodide began to be used to treat sporotrichosis (Kwon-Chung & Bennett, 1992) and is a satisfactory therapy for treatment of sporotrichosis, until now.

The first reported case of natural animal infection was described in 1907 by Lutz and Splendore in rats from Brazil (Lutz & Splendore, 1907, as cited in Coura, 2005). In 1908, in Brazil, Splendore described the asteroid bodies around *Sporothrix* yeast cells, which are used to diagnose sporotrichosis during histological examinations (Kwon-Chung & Bennett, 1992).

Classically, subcutaneous mycosis is usually associated with puncture injuries in farmers, florists, leisure gardeners, landscapers and greenhouse workers. However, in the zoonotic sporotrichosis endemic area of Rio de Janeiro, Brazil, transmission of the disease has been occurring broadly in the populace through the scratches or bites of *S. schenckii* infected cats (Schubach et al., 2008). Less commonly, other form of acquisition of the infection is inhalation of fungus conidia from soil (Rohatgi, 1980) and from infected animals, being cats the most involved. Sporotrichosis is primarily a cutaneous disease. After inoculation, a papule develops at the site of inoculation and generally ulcerates, forms into nodules and then develops proximal to the primary lesion followed by lymphatic distribution and often ulceration. This is the lymphocutaneous form and is followed in frequency by the fixed form, which is characterised by a localised lesion without lymphatic involvement (Schubach et al., 2008). Disseminated forms are unusual and frequently occur in immunosuppressed hosts (Schechtman, 2010). Disseminated cutaneous sporotrichosis is primarily characterised by multiple lesions scattered over several parts of the body or the spread of haematogenous lesions. Osteoarticular (Campos-Macías et al., 2006) and pulmonary lesions (Losman & Cavanaugh, 2004; Callens et al., 2005) are the most common extracutaneous forms. All forms are rare in normal hosts. Mucosal involvement is sporadic, and the conjunctiva is the most commonly affected mucosa (Schubach, et al., 2005). Meningitis is one of the worst complications of *S. schenckii* infection, and several recently reported cases describe AIDS as an underlying risk factor (Galhardo et al., 2010).

Pathogenic fungi of the genus *Sporothrix* are dimorphic in the environment or when cultured in the laboratory at 25-30°C. In the filamentous form, they present as hyaline, septate, branched hyphae with single-celled conidia of two types: hyaline and brown (dematiaceous). Hyaline conidia are small, ovoid and usually occur in the apical portion of conidiophores. Dematiaceous conidia are large and ovoid with a thick cell wall and are present along the entire length of the hyphae (Siegler et al., 1990). Macroscopically, filamentous *S. schenckii* colonies are initially white and gradually become brown to dark black as the fungus produces the conidia, which are unable to form chains. In contrast, the parasitic phase and the yeast phase of *S. schenckii* that develops when the fungus is cultured in appropriate culture media at 35°-37°C, resembles cigar-shaped oval yeast cells, which may have one or more buds (Ramos e Silva et al., 2007). Macroscopically, colonies of *S. schenckii* grown at 37°C have a yellowish-beige colour and a creamy texture.

Sporothrix schenckii belongs to the Fungi Kingdom. After the substantial fungal taxonomy revision by Guarro and co-workers, this fungus was placed in the *Ascomycota* Division, *Pyrenomycetes* Class, *Ophiostomatales* Order, *Ophiostomataceae* Family (Guarro et al., 1999). Recently, it was suggested that *S. schenckii* should not be considered the only taxon, which causes sporotrichosis in human and animals because four new species have been identified (Marimon et al., 2006, 2007, 2008).

Mycoses can be challenging to diagnose, and accurate interpretation of laboratory data is important to ensure appropriate treatment. Although the clinical manifestations of sporotrichosis are well described, the diagnosis of this mycosis cannot be based on clinical information alone because the symptoms of sporotrichosis overlap of with those of other diseases. Also, a definitive diagnosis requires isolation of *Sporothrix* spp. on specific culture media or visualisation of the yeast form during direct examination of clinical specimens using specific fungal staining techniques. However, these procedures are time consuming, usually taking a minimum of 15 days, and lack sensitivity. Furthermore, *Sporothrix* spp. structures can be confused with those of other fungal pathogens when visualised microscopically. Given these difficulties, other techniques have been developed to supplement culture and microscopic examination. These laboratory tests have a rapid turnaround time and reasonable specificity and sensitivity.

In this chapter, some of the well-established clinical and laboratorial diagnoses will be discussed and current conventional diagnostic tools will be reviewed. Additionally, we will outline of the development of novel diagnostic methods and discuss their relative merits and disadvantages.

2. Diagnosis

Sporotrichosis is classically diagnosed by correlation of clinical, epidemiological and laboratorial data. Erythematous, ulcerated, or verrucous lesions that appear at the site of a skin injury that are caused by trauma with material from vegetal origin or by a scratch or bite from an animal, such as a cat, with subsequent nodular lymphangitic spread, are strong clinical and epidemiological indicators of mycotic infection (Coura, 2005). To confirm the diagnosis, laboratorial examinations must be performed. Typical laboratory analyses involved in sporotrichosis diagnosis include microscopic examination and culture of clinical specimens, such as skin biopsies or pus, from the patient's lesions. Although, in cases of disseminated or extracutaneous sporotrichosis other specimens such as sputum, urine, blood, synovial and cerebrospinal fluids can be analysed depending on the affected organs or systems (Kwon-Chung & Bennet, 1992).

Currently, there are additional diagnostic tools available for the diagnosis of sporotrichosis. For instance, serological techniques involving antibody detection against *S. schenckii* antigens have been developed using different enzyme linked immunosorbent assays (ELISA) formats and antigenic preparations (Almeida-Paes et al., 2007a; Bernardes-Engemman et al., 2005). Molecular methods to detect *S. schenckii* DNA in clinical specimens, including tissue fragments, are also being studied in several laboratories to facilitate quick diagnosis of infection (Hu et al., 2003; Kano et al., 2003). The next sections will focus on these diagnostic applications for diagnosis sporotrichosis.

2.1 Clinical types and differential diagnosis

2.1.1 Clinical types

Sporotrichosis affects both sexes and can occur at any age. In most cases, sporotrichosis is a benign infection that is restricted to the skin, subcutaneous tissue and adjacent lymph vessels (Kwon-Chung & Bennett, 1992; Rippon, 1988).

The disease can be divided into four clinical forms (Sampaio et al., 1954, as cited in Ramos-e-Silva et al., 2007):

The **lymphocutaneous** form is the most common presentation and accounts for up to 75% of cases and is the easiest sporotrichosis to diagnose. The lesions are usually located on the upper extremities and are characterised by the appearance of a primary lesion at the site of inoculation after two or three weeks. This lesion can be ulcerated with an infiltrated base or a papular, nodular, nodular-ulcerative, ulcerative-gummy or vegetative plaque. From the initial injury, it forms a chain of painless nodules along the path of the lymph vessels, which may soften and ulcerate with little exudates that can be classified as sporotrichoid (Figure 1). Usually, the regional lymph nodes are not involved, and no skin changes are observed between the nodes. Erythema can be present, but the pain is usually mild. A secondary infection may occur and is associated with increased erythema and suppuration.

The **fixed cutaneous** form is the second most common and accounts for approximately 20% of cases. The lesion remains confined to the inoculation site and the lymph vessels are not involved. The lesions are ulcers (Figure 2), verrucous, or infiltrated plaques. Small satellite lesions are common and are frequently observed in children. The upper and low extremities are the most common sites of lesions, and children present with a high index of lesions on the face. Unlike the lymphocutaneous form, patients with the fixed cutaneous form do not present systemic symptoms. However, if left untreated, the lesions may evolve into a chronic course, and a spontaneous involution of the lesion can occur.

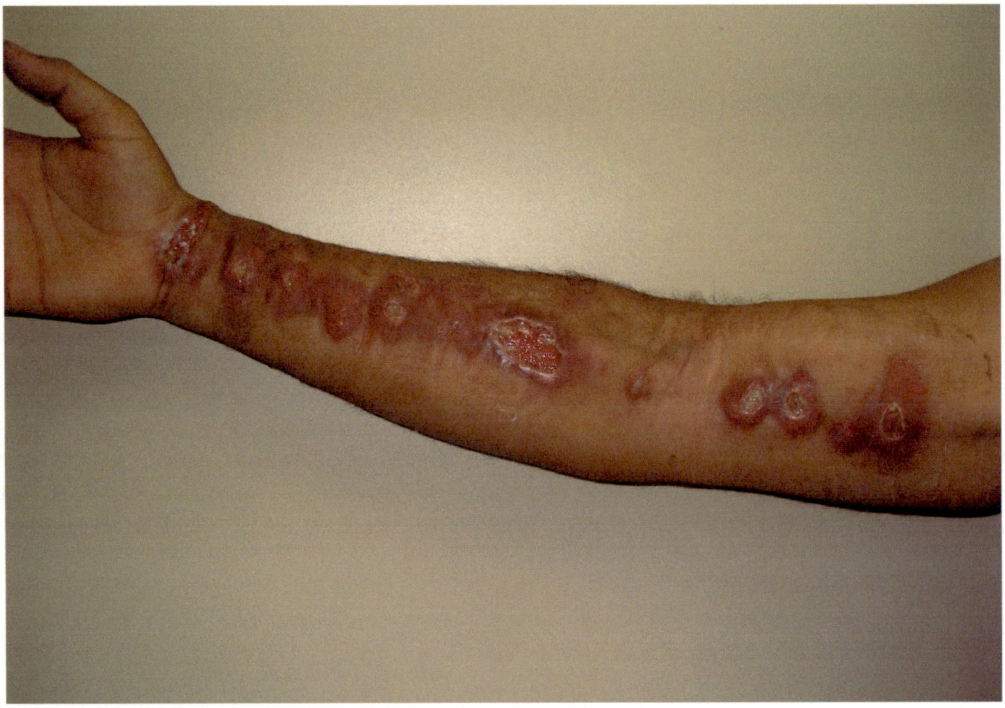

Fig. 1. Lymphocutaneous sporotrichosis.

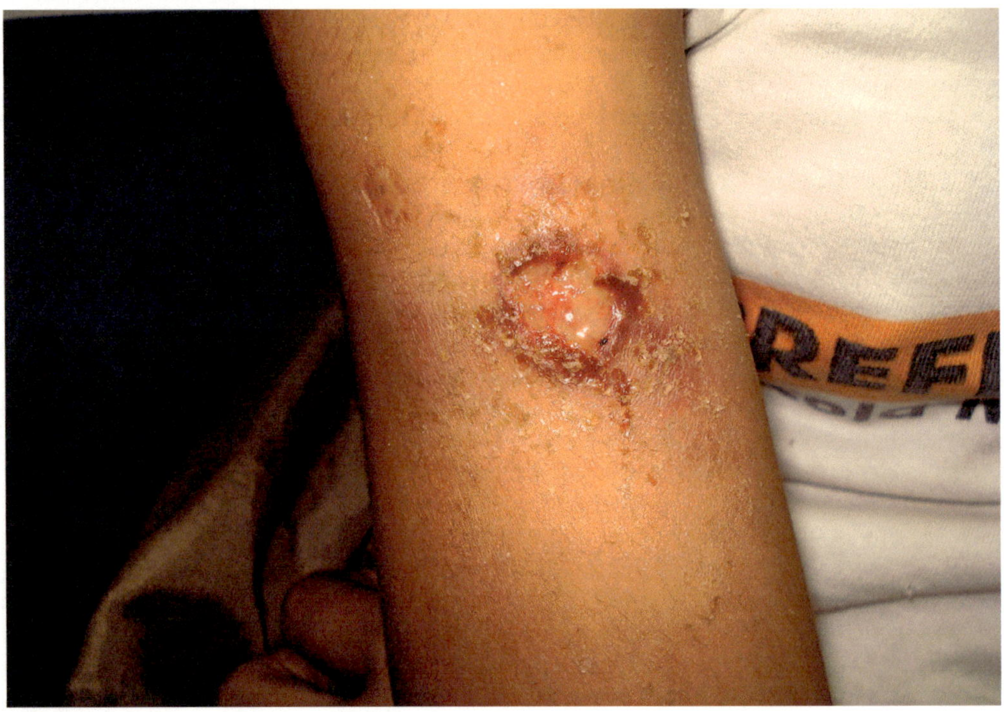

Fig. 2. Fixed cutaneous sporotrichosis.

The **disseminated cutaneous form** presents with nodular, gummy, or ulcerated disseminated lesions (Figure 3). Following inoculation of the skin, there is a haematogenous dissemination, which initially presents as softened subcutaneous lesions that can ulcerate after weeks or months. Although quite rare, it has been reported in AIDS patients and in patients submitted to a long course of steroid therapy as the first manifestation of this syndrome. Disseminated cutaneous sporotrichosis is more frequently observed (up to 16% of cases) during endemic zoonotic sporotrichosis in non-immunosuppressed patients infected by cat zoonotic transmission of the fungus (Barros et al., 2004; Freitas et al., 2010), which is attributed to multiple inoculations.

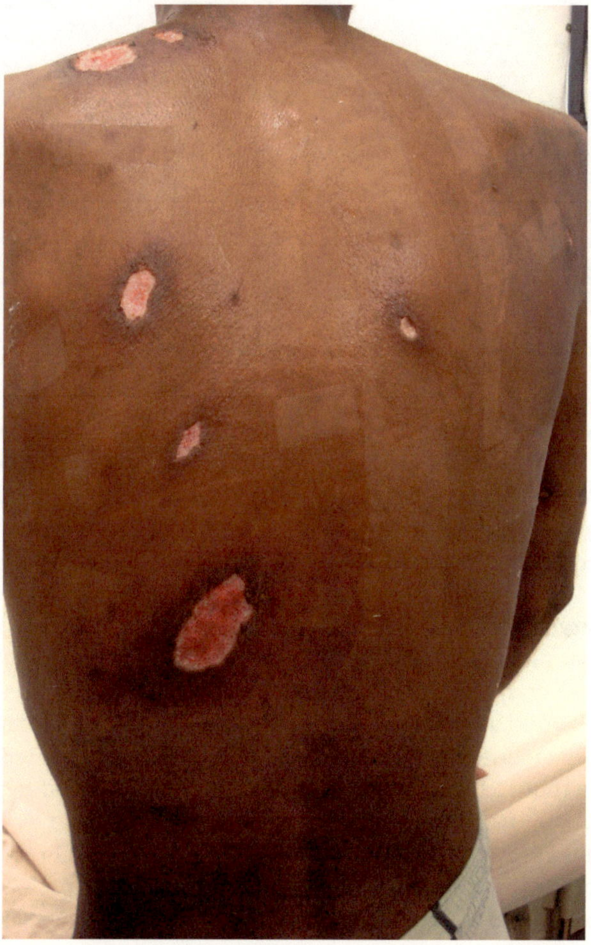

Fig. 3. Disseminated cutaneous sporotrichosis.

The **extracutaneous form** appears in less than 5% of cases and is difficult to diagnose. It arises after haematogenous spread of the fungus, conidial inhalation, contact with a skin lesion or direct inoculation of a mucosal site. Any organ or tissue can be affected by sporotrichosis, and the symptoms are specific to the organ involved and are then followed by fever and general commitment in some cases. Involvement can be unifocal or multifocal. Immunosuppression, caused by conditions such as diabetes, alcoholism, malignancy, steroid therapy, chronic obstructive pulmonary disease (COPD) and AIDS, is common in the pulmonary and nervous forms (Kwon-Chung & Bennett, 1992; Rippon, 1988). Some points of emphasis are:

- Bones and joints are the most commonly affected sites after the skin. The most commonly affected bones are the tibia, small bones of hands, radius, ulna, skull and face. Additionally, the joints of the hands, elbow, wrist, knee and ankle are also commonly affected. Most patients have infection of a single joint, which presents as a solitary granuloma. Destructive arthritis (Figure 4) or tenosynovitis may occur.

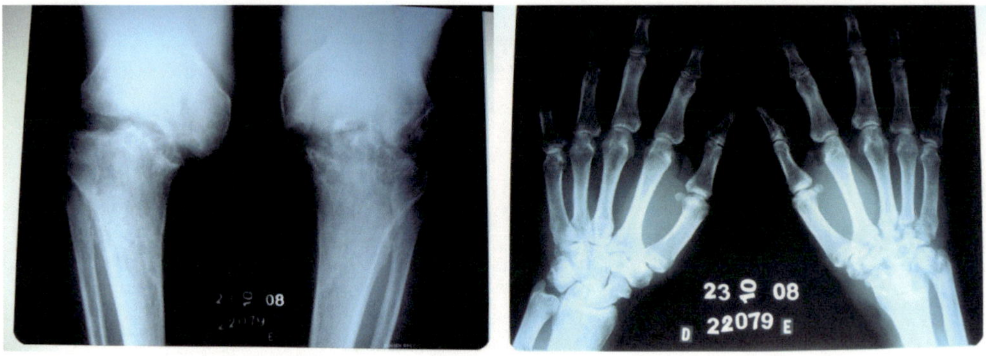

Fig. 4. Bilateral destructive lesions on the knees and on the left wrist in a patient with osteoarticular sporotrichosis.

- Pulmonary infection is frequently caused by inhalation of conidia and is not caused by dissemination of the fungus. Clinically, pulmonary sporotrichosis manifests as a chronic pulmonary disease with cavitation or hilar massive lymphadenopathy, the later has a certain frequency of spontaneous resolution.
- Ocular infection can result from an exogenous infection or haematogenous dissemination. It may manifest as conjunctivitis with characteristic visible granulomas, episcleritis, dacryocystitis, corneal ulceration, uveitis, nodular iritis, retrobulbar lesion, panophthalmitis, ulceration or ectropia and can lead to total blindness in rare cases. Cases of isolated granulomatous conjunctivitis have been reported in Brazil without cutaneous disease and are related to cat zoonotic transmission (Barros et al., 2004).
- The mucosa in the mouth, pharynx, larynx and nose can be infected by both direct and haematogenous routes. Exanthema, ulceration, suppuration and vegetation are clinical manifestations.
- Infection of the nervous system presents as brain abscesses or chronic meningitis, which is indolent and is associated with hypoglycorrhachia, hyperproteinorrhachia and low mononuclear cell counts. A common and potentially serious complication in these cases is hydrocephalus.

The first-choice for treatment of the cutaneous forms is oral itraconazole. Oral terbinafine is an alternative medication. Potassium iodide, despite being a classical and inexpensive drug, is difficult to tolerate and does not have sufficient scientific background to be recommended for sporotrichosis. Treatment with venous amphotericin B is reserved for severe patients and is also an option for the disseminated forms involving internal organs. Immunosuppressed patients often need higher doses of itraconazole and longer courses of treatment (Kauffman et al., 2007).

2.1.2 Differential diagnosis

Lymphocutaneous sporotrichosis is fairly common and can be confidently diagnosed. However pyoderma, atypical *Mycobacterium* and *Nocardia* infection as well as leishmaniasis must also be considered (Coura, 2005).

The clinical symptoms of the fixed form can be similar to pyoderma, paracoccidioidomycosis, chromoblastomycosis, cutaneous tuberculosis, atypical mycobacteria, tertiary syphilis, leishmaniasis, and even skin cancer.

Lesions of the disseminated cutaneous form can be confused with other deep mycosis, such as paracoccidioidomycosis or histoplasmosis, or with atypical mycobacteria and non-infectious granulomatous diseases.

The disseminated extracutaneous forms are diagnosed differently according to the affected organ. Other fungal conjunctivitis, bacterial osteomyelitis, pulmonary fungal infections, tuberculosis and sarcoidosis should also be considered.

2.2 Conventional diagnosis

Depending on which clinical specimen is sent to the mycology laboratory for diagnosis, some procedures must be performed before microscopic and culture analyses. Skin biopsies should be sent to the laboratory in a sterile physiological saline solution. Water and formaldehyde are not suitable as transporter because they interfere with the microbiological tests. In the laboratory, skin/mucosa fragments have to be triturated using surgical scissors (Figure 5). Grinding the clinical specimen with a mortar and pestle should be avoided because it can destroy fungal structures present on the material. Pus from ulcerated lesions does not require special treatment and can be analysed directly after sample collection (Molinaro et al., 2010).

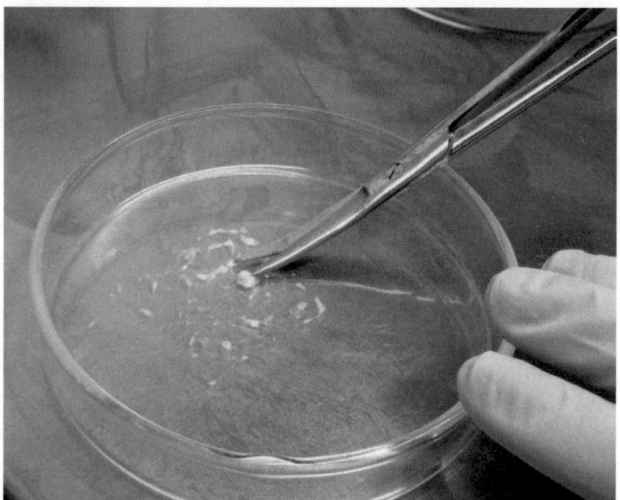

Fig. 5. Skin fragment being triturated for mycological examination.

Direct microscopic examination of the specimens is typically performed on specimens in 10% potassium hydroxide or 4% sodium hydroxide to detect parasitic cigar shaped-budding yeast-like cells using a light microscope with a magnification of 400X to 1000X. These fungal cells are small (2-6μm in diameter), rare and hard to detect during direct examination of the

specimens obtained from human patients (Kwon-Chung & Bennett, 1992) or from domestic animals, such as dogs (Schubach et al., 2006). On the other hand, when this test is performed on skin biopsies collected from cats infected with *S. schenckii* yeast cells are easily observable (Figure 6A) because cats have a high fungal burden on their lesions (Schubach et al., 2004). Although yeast-like cells can be observed during microscopic examination in a few cases, they do not provide a definitive diagnosis of sporotrichosis. *Histoplasma capsulatum* var. *capsulatum* and *Candida glabrata,* two other pathogenic fungi that may cause skin infections, can also appear as small, round or oval yeast cells similar to *S. schenckii* (Larone, 2002).
To identify the fungus, fluorescent methods using calcofluor white dye or fluorescent-antibody staining can be performed. However, these techniques are expensive and are not available in most laboratories, especially in underdeveloped countries. Staining methods, including the Gram and Giemsa preparations, also aid in the microscopic identification of clinical specimens from patients with sporotrichosis. When the Gram stain is performed on the clinical specimens, the yeast cells are positively stained and occasionally surrounded by giant or polymorphonuclear cells (Figure 6B). Although both fluorescent and staining methodologies facilitate the identification of fungal cells when compared to the clarification by hydroxide solutions, both procedures lack sensitivity (Lacaz et al., 2002).

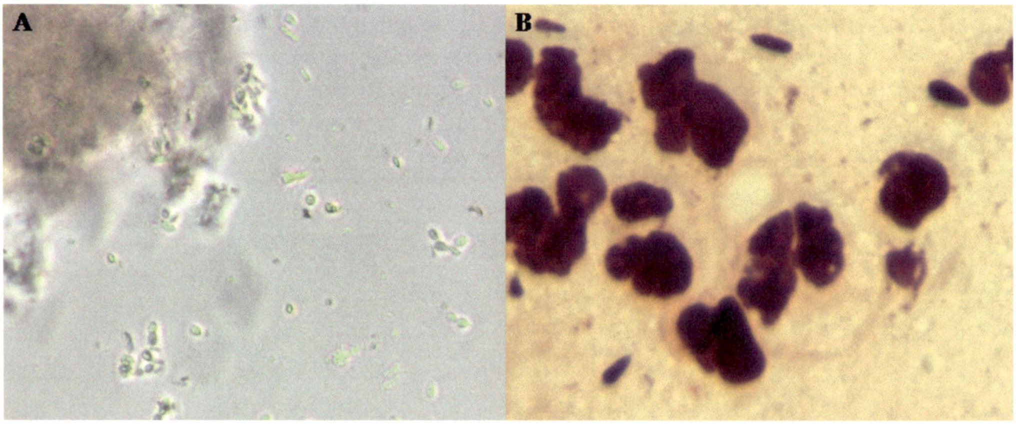

Fig. 6. Direct examination of clinical specimens from patients with sporotrichosis. (A) Skin biopsy of a cat with sporotrichosis showing several yeast-like budding cells. Magnification 400X. (B) Gram stain of pus from a human patient with sporotrichosis showing cigar shaped yeast-like cells. Magnification 1000X.

Histopathological examination using a tissue fragment in formaldehyde is important for the diagnosis of sporotrichosis. Although *S. schenckii* yeast-like cells may be seen in skin biopsies with the routinely used hematoxylin and eosin (H&E) stains, other stains such as Gomori methenamine silver (GMS) or periodic acid-Schiff (PAS) can be used to confirm identification of fungal elements (Figure 7A). Parasitic cells of *S. schenckii,* which can be found within phagocitic cells or in the extracellular space, are difficult to see due to the paucity of these cells in lesions from human patients (Larone, 2002; Quintella et al., 2011).
The reaction of the tissue is another important characteristic that should be evaluated during histopathologic examination of skin biopsies during diagnosis of sporotrichosis. *S. schenckii* usually causes a mixed suppurative and granulomatous inflammatory response in the dermis and adjacent subcutaneous tissue (Figure 7B). Cases of disseminated disease also present a

mixed inflammatory reaction. Fibrosis and micro abscess are frequently observed on cutaneous infections. Moreover, hyperkeratosis, parakeratosis and pseudoepitheliomatous hyperplasia may also occur (Larone, 2002). In addition to intact polymorphonuclear cells, the granuloma formed during sporotrichosis may also contain cellular debris, caseous material, lymphocytes, plasmocytes, giant and epithelioid cells, fibroblasts and yeasts (Quintella et al., 2011). Some authors also report that foreign material of vegetal origin related to the traumatic inoculation of the agent may be found in rare cases (Orellana et al., 2009).

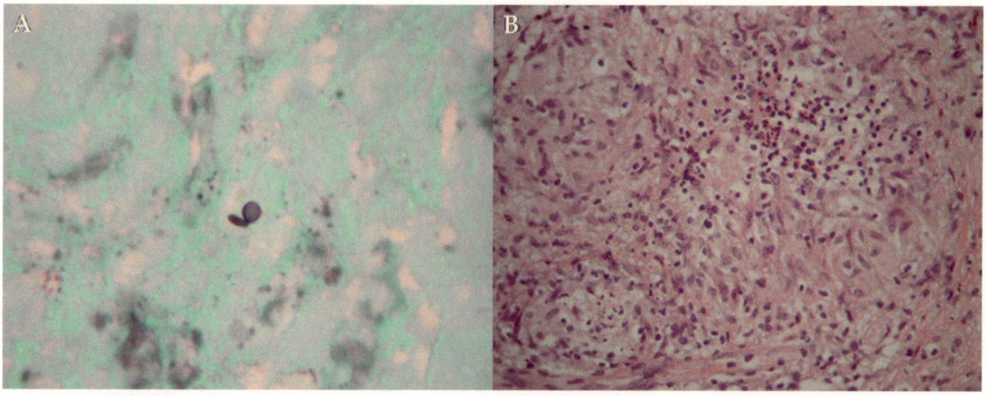

Fig. 7. Histological examination of skin biopsies from patients with sporotrichosis. (A) Gomori methenamine silver stain presenting a yeast-like cell with a cigar-shaped bud, suggestive of *S. schenckii*. Magnification 400X. (B) Hematoxylin and eosin stain presenting a suppurative and granulomatous reaction with neutrophils. Magnification 400X. (Courtesy of Leonardo P. Quintella.)

Some histopathologic changes on analysed tissues may be also related to the observation of the etiologic agent on tissue sections. The presence or predominance of epithelioid granulomas, caseous/fibrinoid necrosis and fibrosis as well as the occurrence of foreign body granulomas with predominance of lymphocytes is related to a lack of fungal observation. Suppurative granulomas, neutrophils and liquefaction are more common when *S. schenckii* yeast-like cells are encountered (Quintella et al., 2011).

Several authors observed the Splendore-Hoeppli reaction on histopathologic tissue sections from sporotrichosis patients. This reaction indicates a localised immunologic response to antigens of several infectious organisms, such as fungi, bacteria and parasites (Hussein, 2008), and appears as a radiating homogenous, refractile, eosinophilic, club-like material surrounding a central eosinophilic focus (Larone, 2002). Splendore first observed this structure in 1908 on tissue sections from patients with sporotrichosis and afterwards by Hoeppli in 1932 around schistosome larvae (Kwon-Chung & Bennett, 1992). Positive identification of this structure in tissue sections from patients with sporotrichosis ranges from 20% to 66% (Gezuele & Rosa, 2005); although other authors reported that this structure was not observed in several analysed samples (Quintella et al., 2011).

These histopathologic findings help to differentiate sporotrichosis from other diseases. For instance, during histoplasmosis infection, the neutrophilic inflammatory response is a mixed of suppurative and granulomatous reactions, and in sporotrichosis are not observed. Suppurative tissue reactions are observed in candidiasis, especially when it is caused by *C. glabrata,* where the absence of hyphae and pseudohyphae elements can mimic

sporotrichosis; however, granulomas are not usually formed (Larone, 2002). On dogs with sporotrichosis, lesions present well-formed granulomas with marked neutrophil infiltration. Frequently, lymphocytes and macrophages are absent on peripheral infiltrate, which facilitates the differentiation between sporotrichosis and leishmaniasis (Miranda et al., 2010).
Definitive diagnosis of sporotrichosis is based on the isolation and identification of its etiological agent in culture (Kwon-Chung & Bennett, 1992). Isolation of *S. schenckii* can be easily attained after spreading the clinical specimens on Sabouraud Dextrose Agar supplemented with 400mg/L chloramphenicol to avoid bacterial contamination and on culture media containing cycloheximide, such as Mycosel or Mycobiotic agar. Cycloheximide inhibits the growth of several anemophilous fungi that can contaminate cultures from clinical specimens obtained from non-sterile sites; however, this drug does not inhibit the mycelial form of *S. schenckii*, which grows well on this culture medium (Molinaro et al., 2010).
Traditional identification of *S. Schenckii* is based on the macro and micromorphologies of the mycelial and yeast forms (Figure 8). These analyses, however, do not differentiate the newly described species in the *S. schenckii* complex (Marimon et al., 2007). To differentiate the species within this complex, other tests such as carbohydrate assimilation (especially sucrose and raffinose), growth rates at 30°C and 37°C and the production of dematiaceous conidia are necessary. Moreover, molecular methods, which will be discussed below, are also important for the differentiation of these new species of *Sporothrix*.
Although *S. schenckii* can grow around body temperature, this is not the optimal temperature for this fungus growth. Therefore, to enhance the chance of fungal isolation, cultures must be incubated at 25 to 30°C after removing the fungus from stress condition and allowing it to grow, even if the patient fungal burden is low. After five to ten days of incubation at 25°C, filamentous hyaline colonies often start to develop. Only a few strains require extended incubation for growth. These colonies, after some time, may develop a dark colour, which is usually located in the centre or sectors of the colony (Kwon-Chung & Bennett, 1992). If there is no growth of *S. schenckii* after four weeks of incubation, cultures can be considered negative.
To identify a fungal isolate as *S. schenckii,* one needs to determinate if it can undergo *in vitro* dimorphism. Thus, it is necessary to make subcultures of the fungus at 35 to 37°C on enriched media such as brain heart infusion (BHI) agar, blood or chocolate agar, for five to seven days. Colonies with a creamy texture and with a yellow to tan colour will grow. Microscopically, they are composed of round to oval hyaline yeast-like cells that often have cigar-shaped narrow base buds (Larone, 2002; McGinnis, 1980).
Because environmental fungi of the genus *Sporothrix* can also form yeast-like cells when grown on the appropriate medium at temperatures around 35°C, a micromorphologic study of the filamentous form of the isolated fungus is necessary to correctly identify *S. schenckii* because environmental *Sporothrix* strains are not able to produce the virulence-related dematiaceous conidia of *S. schenckii* (Dixon et al., 1991). Slide culture preparations using potato dextrose agar (PDA) or corn meal agar incubated at 30°C are ideal to study *S. schenckii* conidiogenesis (Marimon et al., 2007). For this test, *S. schenckii* strains present hyaline hyphae usually less than 3 µm in diameter with regular septation and branching produced in strands. Hyaline conidia are produced in a flower-like arrangement at the tip of the sympodial conidiophores that arises at right angles from the sides of the hyphae. Dematiaceous conidia are produced mainly along the hyphae on extremely short denticles (Dixon et al., 1991; Kwon-Chung & Bennett, 1992; Larone, 2002).

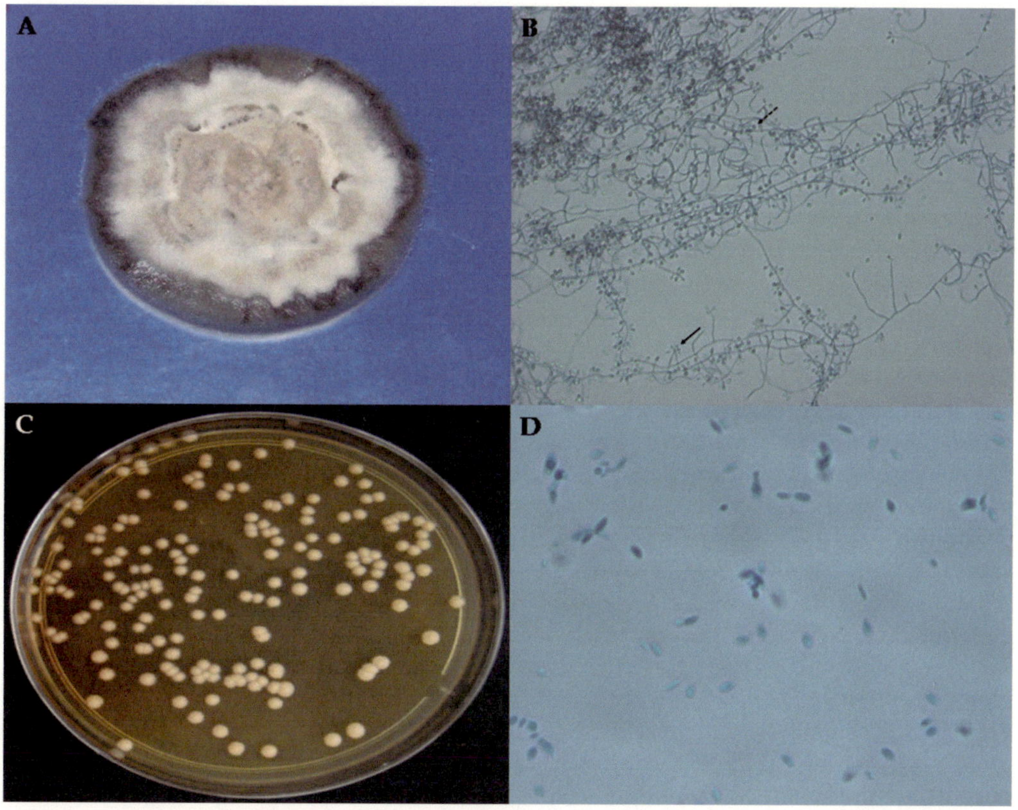

Fig. 8. *S. schenckii* identification: (A) Mycelial colony on Potato Dextrose Agar (PDA) after 21 days of incubation at 25°C. (B) Slide culture of the mycelial form on PDA, incubated at 30°C for 15 days and stained with lactophenol cotton blue. The continuous arrow indicates hyaline conidia on a sympodial conidiophore. The dashed arrow indicates dematiaceous conidia on a short denticle arising from the hypha. Magnification 400X. (C) Several white, smooth yeast colonies on a Brain Heart Infusion (BHI) agar plate after 10 days of incubation at 36°C. (D) Lactophenol cotton blue stain of oval yeast-like cells with cigar-shaped buds after growth on BHI agar. Magnification 400X.

2.3 New diagnostic approaches

Positive cultures provide the strongest evidence for sporotrichosis, but culture diagnosis has significant limitations. In particular, in some manifestations of the disease, such as *S. schenckii*-induced arthritis, the collection of material for culture is difficult (Morris-Jones, 2002.). Also, sporotrichosis may be mistaken for other infections, such as tuberculosis, leishmaniasis, paracoccidioidomycosis, gummatous syphilis, and chromoblastomycosis (Rippon, 1988; Sharma et al., 2005). Non-culture methods have been developed to improve the rate and speed of diagnosis. These tests include antibody detection as well as newer molecular techniques that have been developed to improve the diagnosis and identification of *Sporothrix* spp. in clinical specimens, as well for taxonomic purposes. The results from the described tests can provide a presumptive diagnosis of sporotrichosis and require clinical correlation for the correct evaluation and determination of the final diagnosis.

2.3.1 Serology

Several methodologies have been described for the immunological diagnosis of sporotrichosis based on antibody detection in sera from infected patients. Precipitation and agglutination techniques were first used (Albornoz et al, 1984; Blumer et al., 1973; Casserone et al., 1983; Karlin & Nielsen, 1970). Double immunodiffusion for sporotrichosis usually does not cross-react with sera from patients with chromoblastomycosis or leishmaniasis, which are infectious diseases with similar clinical manifestations. Immunoelectrophoresis has also been used, and in all positive cases, an anodic arc, called an S arc, is observed (Albornoz et al., 1984). Both methodologies that use an antigenic complex from fungal culture filtrate are highly sensitive. Tube and latex agglutination both have high sensitivity and specificity and have been used for sporotrichosis serodiagnosis since the 1970s (Blummer et al., 1973; Casserone, et al., 1983; Karlin & Nielsen, 1970). However, these tests lack sensitivity in cases of cutaneous sporotrichosis (Albornoz et.al., 1984; Rippon, 1988) and do not permit the determination of the immunoglobulin isotype involved.

Immunoenzymatic assays are increasingly used for the serodiagnosis of this mycosis. The first immunoblot assay used for serodiagnosis of sporotrichosis dates back to 1989, when exoantigen preparations from a *S. schenckii* yeast form presented 100% sensitivity and 95% specificity for the detection of antibodies (Scott & Muchmore, 1989). Later, another immunoassay (ELISA) was developed, using the concanavalin A binding peptide-rhamnomanan from the *S. schenckii* yeast cell wall, and antibodies were detected in 35 serum samples from patients with culture proven sporotrichosis, resulting in 100% sensitivity. However, the specificity was lower than previous tests because the sera from patients with cutaneous leishmaniasis cross-reacted (Loureiro Y Penha & Lopes Bezerra, 2000). The same group reported an ELISA test using the same antigenic preparation against sera from 92 patients with different clinical forms of sporotrichosis in Rio de Janeiro and reported 90% sensitivity, 80% specificity, and a global efficiency of 86% (Bernardes-Engemann, et al. 2005). Other studies showed that the use of different strains during the preparation of the antigen might result in different sensitivity and specificity, despite the purification of the antigen involved in this methodology. This difference is due to the *O*-glycan residues linked to the molecules (Bernardes-Engemann, et al. 2009).

The development of an enzyme immunoassay using exoantigens produced by the mycelia phase of a *S. schenckii* strain isolated in the zoonotic sporotrichosis endemic area of Rio de Janeiro was also reported (Almeida-Paes et al., 2007a). This antigen was described by Mendoza and collaborators (2002) and showed no cross-reactivity with the antigen and serum samples from patients with coccidioidomycosis, histoplasmosis and paracoccidioidomycosis (Mendoza et al., 2002). The same antigen was used previously in immunodiffusion and immunoelectrophoresis techniques without cross-reactivity with sera from patients with leishmaniasis or chromoblastomycosis (Albornoz et.al., 1984). This test had a sensitivity of 97% and specificity of 89% when performed on 90 sera from patients with different clinical forms of sporotrichosis, 72 sera from patients with other infectious diseases and 76 healthy controls (Almeida-Paes et al., 2007a). The overall efficiency of this test for diagnosis and follow-up of human sporotrichosis is increased when IgG, IgM, and IgA isotypes are also measured providing the most accurate results (Almeida-Paes et al., 2007b).

When the immunoassays probed with different antigenic preparations are compared, the crude exoantigens (Almeida-Paes et al., 2007a) gave values of sensitivity and specificity a little higher than those using the concanavalin A binding fraction of the *S. schenckii* yeast cell wall (Bernardes-Engemann, et al. 2005). A similar observation was found when using this purified antigen and crude exoantigens for the serodiagnosis of feline sporotrichosis. Purified antigens showed 90% sensitivity and 96% specificity, whereas crude exoantigens presented 96% sensitivity and 98% specificity (Fernandes et al., 2011).

2.3.2 Molecular or DNA-based

The *Sporothrix* genus is traditionally identified by phenotypic characteristics, such as macro- and micromorphology and sugar assimilation, but *Sporothrix* spp. colonies grow slowly, and differentiation from other fungi that have similar colony or microscopic morphology is challenging. To confirm the diagnosis, conversion to the yeast phase should be performed, which takes at least 2 to 3 weeks. Methods to identify fungal isolates, such as species-specific DNA, can decrease this time-consuming step while maintaining or improving the specificity, accuracy and sensitivity.

Until now, few molecular methods have been applied to the diagnosis of sporotrichosis to detect *S. schenckii* DNA from clinical specimens, and to identify *Sporothrix* spp. in culture. Diagnosis using the Polymerase Chain Reaction (PCR) is based on the amplification of fungal gene sequences and is a powerful tool for identifying mycoses. One of the pioneering DNA-based methodologies used for the diagnosis of fungal infections was reported by Sandhu and collaborators who developed 21 specific nucleic acid probes targeting the large subunit rRNA gene from several fungi, including *S. schenckii*. The results show a high level of specificity (Sandhu et al., 1995).

In past years, several molecular taxonomic studies using different methodologies, such as restriction fragment length polymorphism (RFLP) from different gene targets, random amplified polymorphic DNA (RAPD), DNA sequencing of internal transcriber spacer (ITS) regions of the ribosomal RNA (rRNA), PCR targeting the DNA topoisomerase II gene, amplified fragment length polymorphism (AFLP), and M13 PCR fingerprinting have demonstrated that *Sporothrix schenckii* isolates have different genetic characteristics, which suggests that they do not belong to the same species (Ishizaki et al., 2000; de Beer et al., 2003; Gutierrez-Galhardo et al., 2008; Kanbe et al., 2005; Mesa-Arango et al., 2002; Neyra et al., 2005; Reis et al., 2009; Watanabe et al., 2004; Zhang et al., 2006). In addition, Marimon and collaborators (2007) supported these findings by suggesting that, according to a combination of phenotypic and genetic features, *S. schenckii* should not be considered a single taxon that causes sporotrichosis in human and animals but should instead be considered a species complex that is comprised of at least four species: *S. brasiliensis, S. globosa, S. luriei,* and *S. schenckii* (Marimon et al., 2006, 2007, 2008). *S. globosa* is distributed worldwide (Madrid et al., 2009; Oliveira et al., 2010), whereas *S. mexicana* is restricted to Mexico and *S. brasiliensis* to Brazil. Also, *S. brasiliensis, S. globosa* and *S. luriei* are related as etiological agents of sporotrichosis (Marimon et al., 2007, 2008). Additionally, other phylogenetic analysis based on the rDNA and the α-tubulin regions from *S. albicans, S. pallida* and *S. nivea* revealed a significant similarity. Therefore, it has been proposed that all the three species were called *S. pallida* when they were first described (de Meyer et al., 2008). An identification key for the *Sporothrix* complex has now been proposed (Marimon et al., 2007) that includes analysis of conidial morphology, auxonogram analysis using raffinose and sucrose, genotyping via PCR amplification, and sequencing of the calmodulin gene. Based on this last analysis, Romeo and collaborators (2011), who were studying the molecular phylogeny and epidemiology of a *S. schenckii* species complex isolated in Italy, demonstrated that 26 environmental strains co-clustered with *S. albicans,* and two clinical isolates grouped with *S. schenckii stricto sensu* (Romeo et al., 2011).

PCR diagnosis based on the amplification of the fungal gene sequences is a powerful tool for identifying invasive mycoses. The first description of PCR for the diagnosis of sporotrichosis was reported by Kano and colleagues (2001). Specific oligonucleotide primers based on the chitin synthase 1 gene were designed, and with this primer pair, PCR was able to detect a 10 pg genomic DNA fragment of *S. schenckii*. A nested PCR assay for the detection of *S. schenckii* was evaluated in clinical samples using the 18S rRNA gene sequence as the target. However, nested PCR could detect *S. schenckii* DNA in tissue samples from infected animals or from clinical specimens from patients with sporotrichosis confirmed by culture or histochemical staining. The test showed high sensitivity and specificity, indicating that the assay could provide rapid diagnosis with sufficient accuracy to be clinically useful for patients with sporotrichosis (Hu et al., 2003). More recently, the same assay was used to detect *S. schenckii* DNA from 38 strains (including all 24 mitochondrial DNA (mtDNA) types) collected from different areas of the world, in the tissues of eight mice infected with the ATCC10268 strain of the fungus, and in skin biopsies of nine patients with sporotrichosis. In addition, the same procedures were used with two strains of *Ceratocystis minor* and isolates of 10 species of other pathogenic fungi. The authors demonstrated that nested PCR could identify *S. schenckii* from all of the mtDNA types and in isolates recovered from different areas of the world, corroborating the data obtained by Hu and collaborators (2003) that the nested PCR assay is highly sensitive and specific and is a rapid method for diagnosis of sporotrichosis under contamination free conditions (Xu et al., 2010).

3. Conclusions

Sporotrichosis is a chronic infection caused by the dimorphic fungus now named the *S. schenckii* species complex. Lymphocutaneous infection is the most common presentation. The diagnosis of sporotrichosis is classically attained by correlation of clinical, epidemiological and laboratorial data. Considerable advances have been made in non-culture-based diagnosis of sporotrichosis with the development of a scarcity of methods for the detection of antibodies, antigens, and nucleic acids. The methods described for the diagnosis of sporotrichosis each have their strengths and weaknesses and require critical analysis by microbiologists and clinicians. However, not all tests described are universally available, which complicates the capacity to diagnose and treat individuals with sporotrichosis. Also, the immunological status of the patient and manifestation of the disease influences the efficacy of the diagnostic test. Continuing efforts to improve or develop diagnostic tests will facilitate our diagnostic aptitude. However, such assays will require validation in populations from diverse regions of the world prior to general applications in routine diagnosis.

Results obtained from a panel of serological diagnostic test play an important role in the diagnosis of sporotrichosis. Nevertheless, nucleotide probes, specific for the *Sporothrix* species complex, and DNA amplification procedures, such as PCR, allow more rapid and precise diagnosis, which can lead to earlier treatment. However, the gold standard in diagnosis continues to be culture and the correlation of molecular data and phenotypic characteristics.

4. References

Albornoz, M.B., Villanueva, E. & Torres, E.D. (1984). Application of immunoprecipitation techniques to the diagnosis of cutaneous and extracutaneous forms of sporotrichosis. *Mycopathologia*, Vol. 85, No. 3, (March, 1984), pp. 177-183, ISSN0301486X .

Almeida-Paes, R., Pimenta, M.A., Pizzini, C.V., Monteiro, P.C.F., Peralta, J.M., Nosanchuk, J.D. & Zancopé-Oliveira, R.M. (2007a). Use of mycelial-phase *Sporothrix schenckii* exoantigens in an Enzyme-linked Immunosorbent Assay for diagnosis of sporotrichosis by antibody detection. *Clinical and Vaccine Immunology*. Vol. 14, No. 3, (March, 2007), pp. 244-249, ISSN 1556-679X.

Almeida-Paes, R., Pimenta, M.A., Monteiro, P.C., Nosanchuk, J.D. & Zancopé-Oliveira, R.M. (2007b). Immunoglobulins G, M, and A against *Sporothrix schenckii* exoantigens in patients with sporotrichosis before and during treatment with itraconazole. *Clinical Vaccine Immunology*. Vol. 14, No.9, (September, 2007), pp.1149-1157, ISSN 1556-679X.

Barros, M.B., Schubach, A.O., Valle, A.C., Galhardo, M.C.G., Conceição-Silva, F., Schubach, T.M.P., Reis, R.S., Wanke, B., Marzochi, K.B.F. & Conceição, M.J. (2004). Cat-transmitted sporotrichosis epidemic in Rio de Janeiro, Brazil: description of a series of cases. *Clinical Infectious Dieases*. Vol. 38, No. 4, (February, 2004), pp. 529-535, ISSN 1058-4838.

Bernardes-Engemann, A.R., Costa, R.C., Miguens, B.R., Penha, C.V., Neves, E., Pereira, B.A., Dias, C.M., Matos, M., Gutierrez-Galhardo, M.C., Schubach, A.O., Oliveira-Neto, M.P., Lazéra, M. & Lopes-Bezerra, L.M. (2005). Development of an enzyme-linked immunosorbent assay for the serodiagnosis of several clinical forms of sporotrichosis. *Medical Mycology*. Vol. 43, No. 6, (September, 2005), pp. 487-493, ISSN 1369-3786.

Bernardes-Engemann, A.R., Loureiro y Penha, C.V., Benvenuto, F., Braga, J.U., Barros, M. L., Orofino-Costa, R. & Lopes-Bezerra, L.M.. (2009). A comparative serological study of the SsCBF antigenic fraction isolated from three *Sporothrix schenckii* strains. *Medical Mycology* . Vol. 47, No. (December, 2008), pp. 874-8, ISSN 1369-3786.

Blumer S.O., Kaufman L., Kaplan W., McLaughlin D.W. & Kraft D. E. (1973). Comparative evaluation of five serological methods for the diagnosis of sporotrichosis. *Applied Microbiology*. Vol. 26, No. 1, (March, 1973), pp. 4-8, ISSN 1472-765X.

Callens, S.F.J., Kitetele, F., Lukun, P., Van Rie, A., Behets, F. & Colebunders, R. (2005). Pulmonary *Sporothrix schenckii* infection in HIV positive child. *Journal of Tropical Pediatrics*, Vol. 52, No. 2, (November, 2005), pp. 144-146, ISSN 0142-6338.

Campos-Macías, P., Arenas, R., Veja-Memije, M. & Kawasaki, M. (2006). *Sporothrix schenckii* type 3D (mtDNA-RFLP): Report of an osteoarticular case. *Journal of Dermatology*. Vol. 33, No. 4, (October, 2005), pp. 295-299, ISSN 0385-2407.

Casserone S., Conti-Diaz I.A., Zanetta E. & Pereira M.E.P. (1983). Serologia de la esporotricosis cutânea. *Sabouraudia*. Vol. 21, No. 2, (March, 1983), pp.317-321, ISSN 0036-2174.

Cooper, C.R., Dixon, D.M. & Salkin, I.F. (1992). Laboratory-acquired sporotrichosis. *Journal Medical Veterinary Mycology*, Vol. 30, (October, 1991), pp. 169-171, ISSN 1365-280X.

Coura J.R. (Ed.). (2005). *Dinâmica das Doenças Infecciosas e Parasitárias*, pp. 1161-1171, Guanabara Koogan, ISBN 85-277-1093-5, Rio de Janeiro – RJ.

de Beer, Z.W., Harrington, T.C., Vismer, H.F., Wingfield, B.D. & Wingfield, M.J. (2003). Phylogeny of the *Ophiostoma stenoceras-Sporothrix schenckii* complex. *Mycologia*. Vol. 95, No. 3, (September, 2002), pp. 434-441, ISSN: 0027-5514.

de Meyer, E.M., de Beer, Z.W., Summerbell, R.C., Moharram, A.M., de Hoog, G.S., Vismer, H.F. & Wingfield, M.J. (2008). Taxonomy and phylogeny of new wood- and soil-inhabiting *Sporothrix* species in the *Ophiostoma stenoceras-Sporothrix schenckii* complex. *Mycologia.* Vol. 100, No. 4, (April, 2008), pp. 647-661, ISSN: 0027-5514.

Dixon, D.M., Salkin, I.F., Duncan, R.A., Hurd, N.J., Haines, J.H., Kemna, M.E. & Coles, F.B. (1991). Isolation and characterization of *Sporothrix schenckii* from clinical and environmental sources associates with the largest U.S. epidemic of sporotrichosis. *Journal of Clinical Microbiology.* Vol. 29, No. 6, (June, 1991), pp. 1106-1113, ISSN 0095-1137.

Fernandes G.F., Lopes-Bezerra L.M., Bernardes-Engemann A.R., Schubach T.M.P., Dias M.A.G., Pereira S.A. & Camargo Z.P. (2011). Serodiagnosis of sporotrichosis infection in cats by enzyme-linked immunosorbent assay using a specific antigen, SsCBF, and crude exoantigens. *Veterinary Microbiology.* Vol. 147, No. 3-4, (July, 2010), pp. 445-449, ISSN 0378-1135.

Freitas, D.F.S., do Valle, A.C.F., Almeida-Paes, R., Bastos, F.I. & Galhardo, M.C.G. (2010). Zoonotic sporotrichosis in Rio de Janeiro, Brazil: a protracted epidemic yet to be curbed. *Clinical Infectious Dieases.* Vol. 50, No. 3, (February, 2010), pp. 453, ISSN 1058-4838.

Galhardo, M.C. , Silva M.T., Lima, M.A., Nunes, E.P., Schettini, L.E., de Freitas, R.F., Paes, R.A., Neves, E.S. &Valle AC.(2010). *Sporothrix schenckii* meningitis in AIDS during immune reconstitution syndrome. *Journal of Neurology, Neurosurgery & Psychiatry.* Vol. 81, No. 6, (April, 2009), pp. 696-699, ISSN 0022-3050.

Gezuele, E., & Rosa, D. (2005). Relevancia del cuerpo asteroide esporotricósico en el diagnóstico rápido de la esporotricosis. *Revista Iberoamericana de Micologia.* Vol. 22, No. 3, (September, 2005), pp. 147-150, ISSN 1130-1406.

Guarro, J., Gene, J. & Stchigel, A.M. (1999). Developments in fungal taxonomy. *Clinical Microbiology Review.* Vol. 12, No. 3, (pp. 454-500, ISSN 0893-8512.

Gutierrez Galhardo, M.C., Zancope-Oliveira, R.M., Valle, A.C.F., Almeida-Paes, R., Tavares, P.M.S., Monzon, A.; Mellado, E. ; Rodriguez-Tudela, J.L. & Cuenca-Estrella, M. (2008). Molecular epidemiology and antifungal susceptibility patterns of *Sporothrix schenckii* isolates from a cat-transmitted epidemic of sporotrichosis in Rio de Janeiro, Brazil. *Medical Mycology.* Vol. 46, No. 2, (November, 2007), pp.141-151, ISSN 1369-3786.

Hajjeh, R., McDonnel, S., Reef, S., Licitra, C., Hankins, M., Toth, B., Padhye, A., Kaufman, L., Passarell, L., Cooper, C.R., Hutwagner, L., Hopkins, R. & McNeil, M. (1997). Outbreak of sporotrichosis among three nursery workers. *Journal of Infectious Diseases.* Vol. 176, No. 2, (March, 1997), pp. 499-504, ISSN 1537-6613.

Hu, S., Chung, W.H., Hung, S.I., Ho, H.C., Wang, Z.W., Chen, C.H., Lu, S.C., Kuo, T.T. & Hong, H.S. (2003). Detection of *Sporothrix schenckii* in clinical samples by a nested PCR assay. *Journal of Clinical Microbiology.* Vol. 41, No. 4, (April, 2003), pp. 1414-1418, ISSN 0095-1137.

Hussein, M.R. (2008). Mucocutaneous Splendore-Hoeppli phenomenon. *Journal of Cutaneous Pathology.* Vol. 35, No. 11, (November, 2008), pp. 979-988, ISSN 0303-6987.

Ishizaki, H., Kawasaki, M., Aoki, M., Vismer, H. & Muir, D. (2000). Mitochondrial DNA analysis of *Sporothrix schenckii* in South Africa and Australia. *Medical Mycology.* Vol. 38, No. 6, (June, 2000), pp. 433–436, ISSN 1369-3786.

Kano, R., Nakamura, Y., Watanabe, S., Tsujimoto, H. & Hasegawa, A. (2001). Identification of *Sporothrix schenckii* based on sequences of the chitin synthase 1 gene. *Mycoses.* Vol.44, No. 2, (February, 2001), pp. 261–265, ISSN 0933-7407.

Kano, R., Matsuoka, A., Kashima, M., Nakamura, Y., Watanabe, S., Mizoguchi, M. & Hasegawa, A. (2003). Detection of *Sporothrix schenckii* chitin synthase 1 (CHS1) gene in biopsy specimens from human patients with sporotrichosis. *Journal of Dermatological Science.* Vol. 33, No. 1, (October, 2003), pp. 73-74, ISSN 0923-1811.

Kanbe, T., Natsume, L., Goto, I., Kawasaki, M., Mochizuki, T., Ishizaki, H. & Kikuchi, A. (2005). Rapid and specific identification of *Sporothrix schenckii* by PCR targeting the DNA topoisomerase II gene. *Journal of Dermatological Science.* Vol. 38, No. 2, (December, 2004), pp. 99–106, ISSN 0923-1811.

Karlin J.V. & Nielsen H.S. (1970). Serologic aspects of sporotrichosis. *Journal of Infectious Diseases.* VOL. 121, No. 3, (March, 1970), pp.316-327, ISSN 1180-2332.

Kauffman, C.A., Bustamante, B., Chapman, S.W. & Pappas, P.G. (2007). Clinical practice guidelines for the management of sporotrichosis: 2007 update by the Infectious Diseases Society of America. *Clinical Infectious Diseases,* Vol. 45, No. 10, (November, 2007), pp. 1255-1265, ISSN 1058-4838.

Kwon-Chung, K.J. & Bennett, J.E., (Ed (s).). (1992). *Medical Mycology.* Lea & Febiger, ISBN 0-8121-1463-9, Philadelphia . London.

Lacaz, C.S., Porto, E., Martins, J.E.C., Heins-Vaccari, E.M., & Melo, N.T. (Ed. (s).). (2002).*Tratado de Micologia Médica.* Sarvier, ISBN 85-7378-123-8, São Paulo – SP.

Larone, D.H. (Ed.). (2002). *Medically Important Fungi: A Guide to identification.* ASM Press, ISBN 1-55581-172-8, Washington, DC.

López-Romero, E., Reyes-Montes, M.R., Pérez-Torres, A., Ruiz-Baca, E., Villagómez-Castro, J.C., Mora-Montes, H.M., Flores-Carreón, A. & Toriello, C. (2011). *Sporothrix schenckii* complex and sporotrichosis, an emerging health problem. *Future Microbiology.* Vol. 6, No. 1, (January, 2011), pp. 85-102, ISSN 1746-0913.

Losman, J.A. & Cavanaugh, K. (2004). Cases from the Osler medical Service at Johns Hopkins University. *The American Journal of Medicine.* Vol. 117, No. 5, (September, 2004), pp. 353-356, ISSN 0002-9343

Loureiro Y Penha C.V. & Lopes-Bezerra L.M. (2000). Concanavalin A-binding cell wall antigens of *Sporothrix schenckii*: a serological study. *Medical Mycology.* Vol. 38, No. 1, (August, 1999), pp. 1-7, ISSN 1369-3786.

McGinnis, M.R. (Ed.). (1980). *Laboratory Handbook of Medical Mycology.*Academic Press, ISBN 0-12-482850-7, New York - NY.

Madrid, H., Cano, J., Gené, J., Bonifaz, A., Toriello, C. & Guarro, J. (2009). *Sporothrix globosa,* a pathogenic fungus with widespread geographical distribution. *Revista Iberoamericana de Micologia.* Vol. 26, No. 3, (February, 2009), pp. 218-222, ISSN 1130-1406.

Marimon, R., Gené, J., Cano, J., Sutton, D.A., Trilles, L., Dos Santos Lazéra, M. & Guarro, J. (2006). Molecular phylogeny of *Sporothrix schenckii. Journal Clinical of Microbiology.* Vol. 44, No. 9, (June, 2006), pp.3251-3256, ISSN 0095-1137.

Marimon, R., Cano, J., Gené, J., Sutton, D.A., Kawasaki, M. & Guarro, J. (2007). *Sporothrix brasiliensis, S. globosa,* and *S. mexicana,* three new *Sporothrix* species of clinical interest. *Journal of Clinical Microbiology.* Vol. 45, No. 10, (July, 2007), pp. 3198-3206, ISSN 0095-1137.

Marimon, R., Gené, J., Cano, J. & Guarro, J. (2008). *Sporothrix luriei*: rare fungus from clinical origin. *Medical Mycology.* Vol. 46, No. 6 (February, 2008), pp.621-625, ISSN 1365-280X.

Mendoza, M., Diaz, A.M., Hung, M.B., Zambrano, E.A., Diaz, E. & Albornoz, M.C. 2002. Production of culture filtrates of *Sporothrix schenckii* in diverse culture media. *Medical Mycology.* Vol. 40, No. 5, (August, 2001), pp. 447-54, ISSN 1365-280X.

Mesa-Arango A.C., Reyes-Montes M.R., Pérez-Mejía A., Navarro-Barranco H., Souza V., Zúñiga G. & Toriello C. (2002). Phenotyping and genotyping of *Sporothrix schenckii* isolates according to geographic origin and clinical form of sporotrichosis. *Journal of Clinical Microbiology.* Vol. 40, No. 8, (August, 2002), pp.3004-3011, ISSN 0095-1137.

Miranda, L.H.M., Quintella, L.P., Santos, I.B., Oliveira, R.V.C., Menezes, R.C., Figueiredo, F.B. & Schubach, T.M.P. (2010). Comparative histopathological study of sporotrichosis and American Tegumentary Leishmaniasis in dogs from Rio de Janeiro. *Journal of Comparative Pathology.* Vol. 143, No. 1, (July, 2010), pp. 1-7, ISSN 0021-9975.

Molinaro E., Caputo L. &Amendoeira R. (Ed. (s)). (2010). *Conceitos e métodos para formação de profissionais em laboratórios de saúde,* pp.399-496, Triunfal Gráfica e Editora, ISBN 978-85-98768-41-0, Assis - SP.

Morris-Jones, R. (2002). Sporotrichosis. *Clinical and Experimental Dermatology.* Vol. 27, No. 6, (April, 2002), pp. 427–431, ISSN: 1365-2230.

Neyra, E., Fonteyne, P. A., Swinne, D., Fauche, F., Bustamante, B. & Nolard, N. (2005). Epidemiology of human sporotrichosis investigated by amplified fragment length polymorphism. *Journal of Clinical Microbiology.* Vol. 43, No. 3, (November, 2004), pp. 1348-1352, ISSN 0095-1137.

Oliveira, M.M.E., Almeida-Paes, R., Muniz, M.M., Barros, M.B.L, Gutierrez-Galhardo, M.C. & Zancopé-Oliveira, R.M. (2010). Sporotrichosis caused by *Sporothrix globosa* in Rio de Janeiro, Brazil: case report. *Mycopathologia.* Vol. 169, No. 5, (January, 2010), pp. 359-363, ISSN 0301-486X.

Orellana, A., Moreno-Coutiño, G., Poletti, E., Veja, M.E. & Arenas, R. (2009). Esporotricosis fija com cuerpo asteroide junto al fragmento vegetal. *Revista Iberoamericana de Micologia.* Vol. 26, No. 4, (December, 2009), pp. 250-251, ISSN 1130-1406.

Queiroz-Telles, F., Nucci, M., Colombo, A.L., Tobón, A. & Restrepo, A. (2011). Mycoses of implantation in Latin America: an overview of epidemiology, clinical manifestations, diagnosis and treatment. *Medical Mycology.* Vol. 49, No. 3, (November, 2010), pp. 225-236, ISSN 1365-280X.

Quintella, L.P., Passos, S.R.L., Valle, A.C.F., Gutierrez-Galhardo, M.C., Barros, M.B.L., Cuzzi, T., Reis, R.S., Carvalho, M.H.G.F., Zappa, M.B., & Schubach, A.O. (2011). Histopathology of cutaneous sporotrichosis in Rio de Janeiro: a series of 119 consecutive cases. *Journal of Cutaneous Pathology.* Vol. 38, No. 1, (September, 2010), pp. 25-32, ISSN 0303-6987.

Ramos-e-Silva, M., Vasconcelos, C., Carneiro, S. & Cestari, T. (2007). Sporotrichosis. *Clinics in Dermatology.* Vol. 25, pp. 181-187, ISSN 0738-081X.

Reis, R. S., Almeida-Paes, R., Muniz, M.M., Tavares, P.M., Monteiro, P.C., Schubach, T.M., Gutierrez-Galhardo, M.C. & Zancopé-Oliveira, R.M. (2009). Molecular characterisation of *Sporothrix schenckii* isolates from humans and cats involved in the sporotrichosis epidemic in Rio de Janeiro, Brazil. *Memórias do Instituto Oswaldo Cruz*. Vol. 104, No. 5, (August, 2009),pp. 769-774, ISSN 0074-0276.

Rippon, J.W. (1988). Sporotrichosis, In: *Medical Mycology: The Pathogenic Fungi and Pathogenic Actinomycetes,* Rippon, J.W., pp. 325-352, WB Saunders, ISBN 0721624448, Philadelphia.

Romeo, O., Scordino, F. & Criseo, G. (2011). New insight into molecular phylogeny and epidemiology of *Sporothrix schenckii* species complex based on calmodulin-encoding gene analysis of Italian isolates. *Mycopathologia.* (March, 2011), Published online: 02 April 2011.

Rohatgi, P.K. (1980). Pulmonary sporotrichosis. *Southern Medical Journal.* Vol. 73, No. 12, (December, 1980), pp. 1611-1617, ISSN 0038-4348.

Sandhu, G.S., Kline, B.C., Stockman, L. & Roberts, G.D. (1995). Molecular probes for diagnosis of fungal infections. *Journal of Clinical Microbiology.* Vol. 33, No. 11, (August, 1995), pp. 2913–2919, ISSN 0095-1137.

Schechtman, R.C. (2010). Sporotrichosis: Part I. *Skinmed.* Vol. 8, No. 4, (July-August, 2010), pp. 216-20, ISSN 1540-9740.

Schenck, B.R. (1898). On refractory subcutaneous abscess caused by a fungus possibly related to the Sporotricha. *Bulletin of the Johns Hopkins Hospital.* Vol.9, pp. 286-290, ISSN 0002-9149.

Schubach, T.M.P., Schubach, A.O., Okamoto, T., Barros, M.B.L., Figueiredo, F.B., Cuzzi, T., Monteiro, P.C.F., Reis, R.S., Perez, M.A., & Wanke, B. (2004). Evaluation of an epidemic of sporotrichosis in cats: 347 cases (1998-2001). *Journal of the American Veterinary Medical Association.* Vol. 224, No. 10, (May, 2004), pp. 1623-1629, ISSN 0003-1488.

Schubach, A., Barros, M.B.L., Schubach, T.M., Francesconi-do-Valle, A.C., Gutierrez-Galhardo, M.C., Sued, M., de Matos Salgueiro, M., Fialho-Monteiro, P.C., Reis, R.S., Marzochi, K.B., Wanke, B. & Conceição-Silva, F. (2005). Primary conjunctival sporotrichosis: two cases from a zoonotic epidemic in Rio de Janeiro, Brazil. *Cornea.* Vol. 24, No. 4, (May, 2005), pp. 491-493, ISSN 0277-7375.

Schubach, T.M.P., Schubach, A.O., Okamoto, T., Barros, M.B.L., Figueiredo, F.B., Cuzzi, T., Pereira, S.A., Santos, I.B., Almeida-Paes, R., Leme, L.R.P. & Wanke, B. (2006). Canine sporotrichosis in Rio de Janeiro, Brazil: clinical presentation, laboratory diagnosis and therapeutic response in 44 cases (1998-2003). *Medical Mycology.* Vol. 44, No. 1, (February, 2006), pp. 87-92, ISSN 1369-3786.

Schubach, A., Barros, M.B.L. & Wanke, B. (2008). Epidemic sporotrichosis. *Current Opinion in Infectious Diseases.* Vol. 21, No. 2, pp. 129-133, ISSN 0951-7375.

Scott, E.N. & Muchmore, H.G. (1989). Immunoblot analysis of antibody responses to *Sporothrix schenckii. Journal of Clinical Microbiology.* Vol. 27, No. 2, (October, 1988), pp. 300-304, ISSN 0095-1137.

Sharma, S., Choudhary, R., Juneja, M., Grover, C. & Nagi-Reddy, B.S. (2005). Cutaneous tuberculosis mimicking sporotrichosis. *Indian Journal Pediatric.* Vol. 72, No. 1, (January, 2005) pp.86, ISSN 0019-5456.

Sigler, L., Harris, J.L, Dixon, D.M., Flis, A.L., Salkin, I.F, Kemna, M. & Duncan, R.A. (1990). Microbiology and potential virulence of *Sporothrix cyanescens,* a fungus rarely isolated from blood and skin. *Journal of Clinical Microbiology.* Vol. 28, No. 5, (January, 1990), pp. 1009-1015, ISSN 0095-1137.

Watanabe, S., Kawasaki, M., Mochizuki, T. & Ishisaki, H. (2004). RFLP analysis of the internal transcriber spacer regions of *Sporothrix schenckii. Japanese Journal Medical Mycology*. Vol. 45, No. 3, (May, 2004), pp. 165-175, ISSN 0916-4804

Xu, T.H., Lin, J.P., Gao, X.H., Wei, H., Liao, W. & Chen, H.D. (2010). Identification of *Sporothix schenckii* of various mtDNA types by nested PCR assay. *Medical Mycology*. Vol. 48, No. 1, (January, 2010), pp. 161–165, ISSN 1369-3786.

Zhang, Z., Liu, X., Yang, G., Gao, X., Jin, L. & An, L. (2006). Genotyping of *Sporothrix schenckii* by analysis of ribosomal DNA regions. *Mycoses*. Vol. 49, No. 4, (February, 2006), pp. 305-310, ISSN 1439-0507

5

Skin Biopsy in Leprosy

Avninder Singh[1], Xiaoman Weng[2] and Indira Nath[1]
[1]*National Institute of Pathology (ICMR), Safdajung Hospital Campus, New Delhi,*
[2]*Beijing Friendship Hospital - Affiliate of Capital University of Medical Sciences, Beijing, Tropical Medicine Research Institute,*
[1]*India*
[2]*China*

1. Introduction

Leprosy is a chronic infectious disease of varying severity caused by *Mycobacterium leprae* (*M. leprae*) a slowly multiplying pathogen. It is primarily a surface disease with lesions mainly involving the skin and peripheral nerves. Rarely visceral organs like liver, lymphnodes, bone marrow, eyes, bones and testes may be involved. Despite the prevalence rate of leprosy having steadily fallen throughout the world, it continues to be a cause of significant public health problem and morbidity in endemic regions. The disease is endemic in many tropical and subtropical countries but is declining in incidence. Globally, 211903 new leprosy cases were detected in 2010 (WHO, 2010). The most affected countries are India and Brazil with some countries in Sub Saharan Africa and Southeast Asia (Noordeen, 1995). The mode of transmission is still unknown but it is believed to be through inhalation of bacilli that are excreted from the nasal passages of the multibacillary patient. Direct person-to-person transmission through skin contact occurs rarely though there have been isolated reports of its transmission from hypodermic needles during skin tattooing or by physical trauma to skin.

2. Clinical and immunopathologic spectrum of leprosy

The sequence of disease pathogenesis in leprosy is complex and depends on the host immunological responses. *M. leprae* is non-toxic and the clinicopathologic manifestations are the result of this host-parasite interaction. (Ridley & Jopling, 1966; Ridley,1974). Leprosy is the classical example of the disease with an immunopathologic spectrum wherein the host immune reaction to the infective agent ranges from none to marked with a consequent range of clinicopathologic manifestations. Tuberculoid leprosy (TT) shows a high cellular response characterized by T-cell and macrophage activation and very few bacilli in the tissues. Lepromatous leprosy (LL) on the opposite pole shows an absent cellular immune response to *M. leprae* antigens with no macrophage activation and abundant bacilli in the tissues. The immunopathologic spectrum is a dynamic continuum in which the patients move in either direction according to the host immune response and treatment. The standard delineation follows the classification of Ridley and Jopling with categories defined along this spectrum by a combination of clinical, microbiological and histopathological indices: TT (tuberculoid), BT (borderline tuberculoid), BB (midborderline), BL (borderline lepromatous) and LL (lepromatous leprosy). The TT and LL group of patients are stable, the former often self-healing and the latter remaining heavily infected unless given chemotherapy. The central point of the spectrum BB is most unstable with patients quickly downgrading to LL if not treated. Apart from these there are some patients who are labeled as 'indeterminate' leprosy and these are the patients with the earliest identifiable skin lesions that cannot be categorized definitely in the immunopathologic spectrum (Table1).

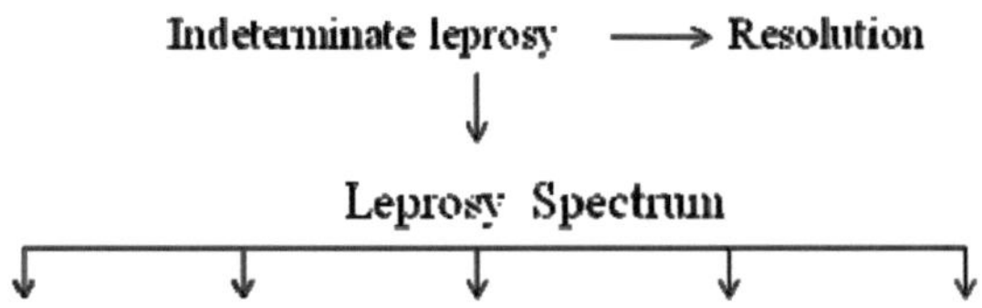

Features	TT	BT	BB	BL	LL
Number of Lesions	single	1- few	several	many	many
AFB	±	+	++/+++	+++/++++	>++++
CMI	+++	+/++	±	–	–
Antibodies	+/±	+	++	+++	+++
Histopathology					
Epitheloid cells	++	++	+	–	–
Macrophages	–	–	+	++/+++	>+++
Lymphocytes	+++	+++	+	+	±

Table 1. Classical features of the leprosy spectrum

3. Leprosy reactions

Leprosy reactions are periodic episodes of acute inflammation caused by immune responses to *M. leprae* or its antigens superimposed on the chronic course of the disease. There are two main types of leprosy reactions depending on the underlying immunological mechanisms.

3.1 Reversal reaction

It is also referred to as type 1 reaction or upgrading reaction and occurs either spontaneously or after a course of chemotherapy and is due to increase in the delayed hypersensitivity reaction. There is influx of lymphocytes that are mainly of CD4+ subtype, especially of the Th1 class (Yamamura et al., 1991; Sreenivasan et al, 1998). During type1 reaction, increases in gene expression of several proinflammatory cytokines have been documented (Scollard et al, 2006). These episodes show cardinal features of inflammation such as erythema, edema, local warmth and tenderness over the skin lesions. The most important effect of a reversal reaction is not the skin but the peripheral nerves which show acute neuritis due to infiltration of lymphocytes and increased intraneural pressure that may result in nerve abscess, necrosis and loss of nerve function.

3.2 Erythema nodosum leprosum (ENL)

It is also known as type 2 reaction and occurs as an acute episode. LL leprosy patients with high bacillary index are more prone to develop ENL as compared to BL leprosy (Pfaltzgraaf et al, 1994). Based primarily on histopathological evidence, it had been proposed that ENL represents an Arthus-like phenomenon mediated by immune complexes (Wemambu et al, 1969). Immunoglobulins and complement deposits have been demonstrated in the skin lesions consistent with this hypothesis. However, neither circulating nor fixed immune complexes have been reproducibly demonstrated in ENL lesions. Other studies have demonstrated evidence of increases in circulating IFN-γ, TNF-α and IL12 and chemokines associated with chemotaxis of neutrophils. Increases in m RNA expression of these cytokines have also been observed in biopsies of skin lesions suggesting that cellular immune activation occurs locally (Sreenivasan et al, 1998; Scollard et al, 2006). Both immune complex deposition and enhanced T-cell reactivity have been demonstrated in peripheral blood and skin lesions. Clinically the skin shows redness, edema, tender plaques and nodules and rarely vesicle formation and ulceration. The eruptions are widespread and associated with constitutional symptoms like fever, arthralgia and involvement of other visceral organs.

3.3 Lucio phenomenon

It occurs in diffuse lepromatous (Lucio) leprosy patients who have either received no treatment or incomplete treatment and have been predominantly observed in Mexican and South American populations. In contrast to ENL, fever, tenderness and leucocytosis are absent. The lesions present as hemorrhagic, sharply marginated irregular crusted plaques that have tendency to ulcerate.

4. Skin biopsy technique

Skin biopsy is a key clinical procedure that is routinely required for the histopathological diagnosis of leprosy and is of paramount importance for correct histopathological classification, bacillary index, and follow-up of treatment response and disease activity. It is also useful for differentiating a relapse from a reversal reaction and to categorize reactions into type 1 or type2.

4.1 Principles of skin biopsy

Before planning a skin biopsy the patients should be informed about the procedure and its side effects. In some countries it is mandatory to obtain a signed consent form. If the patient is illiterate as is common in many endemic countries, care should be taken to explain the procedure verbally and obtain if required a thumbprint on the consent form. Institutional ethical committee's permission is not mandatory for diagnostic biopsies, however whenever the skin biopsy forms part of research project, it is essential to obtain a prior approval from such a committee. Any history of a bleeding disorder or intake of drugs that may interfere with hemostasis should be investigated prior to taking the biopsy.

4.2 Site selection

Deciding the site from where the biopsy will be taken is crucial. Generally the lesions with more advanced inflammatory changes should be chosen. The area from where the biopsy is to be taken should be marked with a skin marker by the physician (Figure 1A).The manifestations of leprosy lesions may vary but generally the site should be active and representative. If a small hypopigmented patch suspected to be indeterminate leprosy is seen, the biopsy should be taken from the center of the lesion where the disease is active. If the lesion is an annular macule then the active spreading edge should be the ideal site of biopsy. If the patient has multiple lesions of different morphology, then more than one biopsy should generally be taken. Even though punch biopsies cause very little scarring care should be taken to avoid wherever possible the cosmetic sites such as face and areas with poor healing characteristics (Alguire & Mathes, 1998).The depth of the biopsy in leprosy should include full depth of the dermis and should extend till the subcutis so as to involve the deeper nerve bundles as well as subcutaneous fat.

4.3 Site preparation

Any common skin antiseptic such as isopropyl alcohol, povidone-iodine solution or chlorohexidine gluconate can be used to prepare the biopsy site (Pariser, 1989). The most commonly used anesthetic agent is 2% lignocaine 1ml of which is injected intradermally in stages while the needle is being inserted in the skin (Figure 1B). Since lignocaine is a vasodilator, small quantity of epinephrine may be added to decrease bleeding and prolong anesthesia. For small lesions the anesthetic can be directly injected into or adjacent to the lesion. For larger lesions a field block is recommended by placing a ring of anesthesia around the intended surgical site (Harrison, 1980).

4.4 Type of skin biopsy

Skin biopsy is a relatively simple procedure that is performed as an outpatient procedure and is essentially of three types

a. Incisional biopsy: is about 12 mm long is in practice, ideal for detection of early lesions. They are reserved for lesions that cannot be removed with a punch owing to their size, depth or location. These need sufficient expertise and invariably require sutures. They are usually reserved for deep inflammatory lesions or lesions involving the panniculus, ex. ENL. After taking the biopsy, the skin tissue is immediately placed in appropriate preservative depending upon type of investigation to be carried out.
b. Punch biopsy: is the most commonly performed skin biopsy and is the biopsy of choice for diagnostic purpose. Biopsy punch is a metal cylinder of variable diameter with a sharp cutting edge and usually attached to a plastic handle (Figure 1C). The diameter ranges from 3-10 mm. Ideally, 4-6mm punches are adequate but 3 mm is the minimum tissue that is considered sufficient for giving a consistently accurate histological diagnosis (Todd, et al., 1996). Biopsy punches blunt easily therefore disposable punches are recommended. Punch biopsies heal by secondary intention though lesions greater than 3mm can sometimes give unacceptable scarring and require 1-2 sutures. The skill required for such biopsies is easily mastered. In comparison to shave biopsies, punch biopsies have a low incidence of bleeding, infection or undesirable scarring (Grekin, 1989). After selecting the punch size, the skin is stabilized with thumb and index finger and slightly stretched perpendicular to the skin tension lines. After placing the punch perpendicular to the skin, a firm downward pressure is applied (Figure 1D). When the punch touches the subcutaneous fat there is a definite 'give' indicating that a full thickness cut has been made. The punch is withdrawn and the cylindrical piece of tissue is gently supported with blunt forceps or a needle tip. The tissue is immediately transferred into a fixative solution and a firm pressure is applied on the wound to prevent bleeding.

c. Shave biopsy: This type of skin sampling is quick, requires little training and sutures for closure are not required. They are usually meant for superficial lesions where the pathology is confined to epidermis and is not of use in leprosy.

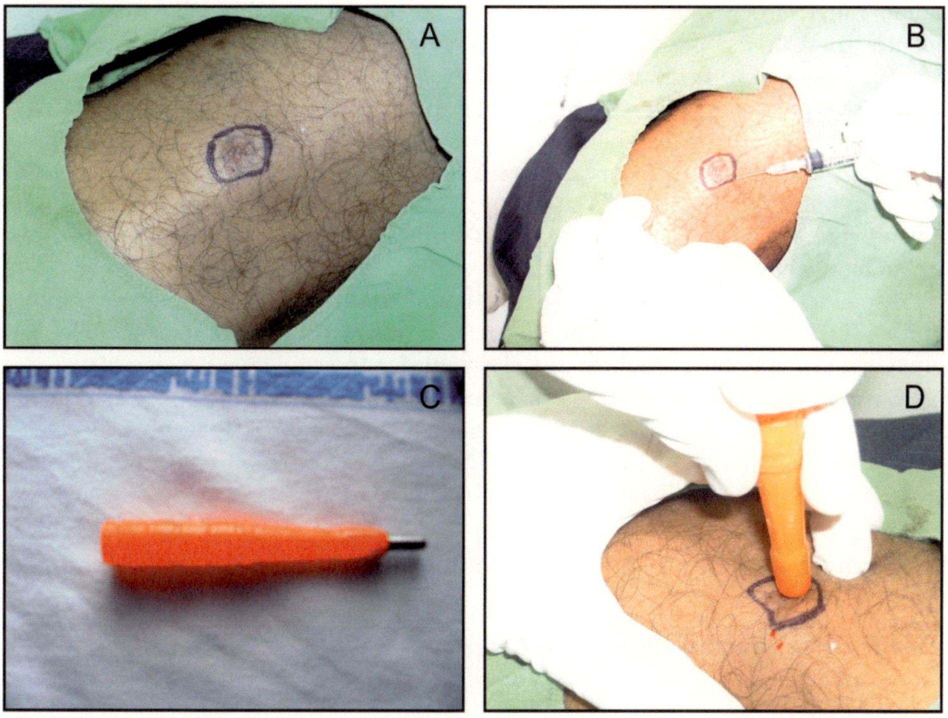

Fig. 1. Selected site for punch biopsy (A), intradermal injection of lignocaine (B), disposable needle punch (C), punch held perpendicular to the skin (D)

4.5 Wound closure

The simplest technique of wound closure is the simple interrupted suture. Primary closure of a punch wound can be accomplished with 1-2 single-layer interrupted sutures. Excisions can be closed in 1-2 layers. The qualities that are most important in suture selection are flexibility, strength, secured knotting and the infection potential (Moy, 1992). There are two broad varieties of sutures absorbable and non-absorbable. Absorbable sutures are made from mammalian-derived collagen (gut) and synthetic absorbable material such as polyglactic acid (vicryl), polyglycolic acid (dexon), poliglecaprone (monocryl) and polydioxanone (PDS). Absorbable sutures have a tensile strength of usually1-2 weeks and are usually placed deep in the wound to reduce skin tension for final closure. Non-absorbable sutures include silk, ethilon (nylon), polypropylene (prolene) and polybutester (dacron). Silk and nylon sutures cause considerable tissue inflammation and have now been largely replaced by synthetic sutures. The latter have a tensile strength ranging from 3 months to 2 years. All biopsy wounds can be dressed with a thin film of a broad spectrum antibiotic ointment and covered with a non adherent dressing topped with gauze dressing and tape (Telfer, 1993). Though skin biopsy is a very safe procedure rarely complications like bleeding, hematoma formation, allergic reaction and infection may still occur.

4.6 Preservation of the skin biopsy

As soon as the biopsy is taken it should be transferred to a preservative to prevent tissue autolysis and drying artifacts. The ideal fixative for standard paraffin embedded histopathological processing is 10% buffered formalin. This fixative is less damaging to the granuloma and works well for preserving the morphology of the AFB. Another fixative frequently used in the past was Lowy's fixative or the FMA (formaldehyde, mercuric chloride, glacial acetic acid) fixative. If properly undertaken FMA fixative gives good cellular details. The biopsy specimen should be completely immersed in the fixative that should be at least 10 times the volume of the skin biopsy. The same fixative can be used for subsequent staining for histochemical characterization and detection of phenolic glycolipid-1 (PGL-1) or lipoarabinomannan (Weng, 2000 ; Verhagen, 1999). For electron microscopy the fixative of choice is 2% glutaraldehyde. If direct fluorescence is to be done within 24 hours then skin biopsy should be thoroughly rinsed with normal saline and preserved at -20^{0} C. If the biopsy is to be used later, then Michel's liquid fixative is the recommended transport medium. This fixative is a proteolytic enzyme inhibitor and is reconstituted by N-ethylmalleimide, ammonium sulfate in a citrate buffer and will give the skin biopsy a shelf life of 4 weeks to 6 months. For molecular techniques like PCR and in-situ hybridization, buffered formalin fixed skin biopsies are considered suitable for PCR as other fixatives may inhibit the reaction (Singh et al, 2004). For RNA studies fresh skin biopsies are preserved immediately in a RNA stabilizing reagent (RNA later) and preserved at -80^{0} C.

5. Protocol for staining of Acid Fast Bacilli (AFB) in paraffin embedded tissue samples

5.1 Modified Fite - Faraco stain (Job & Chacko, 1986)

a. *Ziehl-Neelsens Carbol fuschin solution (200ml) are*
   Basic fuschin: 2 gm
   Melted-phenol: 10 ml
   Absolute alcohol: 20 ml
   Distilled water: 170 ml
b. *5% Sulfuric acid (200ml)*
   Concentrated sulfuric acid (1.0 N):10ml
   Distilled water: 190 ml
c. *Harris Hematoxylin*
   Hematoxylin: 5 gm
   Absolute alcohol: 50 ml
   Potassium alum: 100 gm
   Mercuric oxide: 2.5 gm
   Glacial acetic acid: 25 ml
   Distilled water: 1000 ml

5.2 Staining procedure

- Deparaffinize sections in a mixture of xylene and peanut oil (2 parts of xylene,1 part of peanut oil), two changes of 6 minute each
- Drain, wipe off the excess oil and blot with filter paper
- Wash in running tap water for 4 minutes
- Stain with Ziehl- Neelsen's carbol fuschin solution for 30 minutes at room temperature

- Wash in tap water for 2 minutes
- Differentiate sections in 5% sulfuric acid in 25% alcohol for two changes of 2 minutes each
- Wash in running tap water for 5 minutes
- Drain the excess water, blot dry the sections with a filter paper. Do not dehydrate in alcohol.
- Clear in two changes of xylene and mount

This staining method has two modifications from the standard Fite-Faraco stain for AFB. Firstly, use of alcohol is minimized to prevent excessive decolorization. Secondly, the counterstain is hematoxylin instead of methylene blue. AFB show red colour and nuclei stain dark blue giving the localization of AFB in relation to the cells.

6. Fluorescent microscopy in leprosy

Demonstration of *M. leprae* during histopathological examination of early lesions is an important criterion in the confirmation of leprosy diagnosis. The sensitivity of detection of AFB by histological means remains poor because about 1000 bacilli per cubic centimeter of tissue must be present in order to detect 1 AFB in a section. To enhance the detection rate it is recommended that atleast six sections be examined before declaring them negative. Routine acid fast stains are not so sensitive due to the variability in their ability to decolorize AFB using acid-alcohol. In the search for more sensitivity, a fluorescent method of staining similar to *M. tuberculosis* has been used and is reportedly 1.5 times more sensitive in demonstrating *M. leprae* than Fite-Faraco stain (Nayak, et al., 2003). Immunofluorescence (IF) is also useful in leprosy research where it is a valuable tool in studying localization of antigens like immunoglobulins, HLA-DR, cell surface markers and cytokines on frozen skin biopsies. IF is a better method for studying double labeling of antigens as compared to histochemical staining on formalin fixed paraffin embedded tissue.

7. Numerical indices in a skin biopsy

7.1 Granuloma Fraction (GF)

The fraction of the dermis in a section occupied by a granuloma is observed visually under a low-power objective (x 4) and expressed as fractions. For e.g. 1.0 indicates that the whole of the dermis is occupied by the granuloma, 0.2 that one-fifth is occupied. The range from 1.0-0.1 can be estimated quite accurately if the biopsy specimen extends down up to the subcutis. Being an arithmetic index, GF is sensitive and can adequately reflect the degree of skin infiltration.

7.2 Bacterial Index (BI)

BI is the universally accepted method of assessing the load of acid fast bacilli in a leprosy patient defined by Ridley (Ridley, 1958).The samples tested can be the skin biopsy or slit smears of lesional sites. The latter is obtained as serous fluid by a superficial slit with a sterile blade such that no blood contaminates the fluid. The fluid at the tip of the blade is smeared on to the glass slides which are then stained with Fite-Faraco stain. 3-6 sites from the body are recommended for testing. Slit smear examination is undertaken periodically for assessing improvement with drug therapy and is less invasive than the skin biopsy and is useful in the field sites where facilities for histopathology may not be available.

The bacterial load in skin biopy or slit skin smears is graded using an oil immersion objective as:

0:	No bacilli found in 100 microscopic fields
1+: 1-10	bacilli in 100 microscopic fields
2+: 1-10	bacilli in 10 microscopic fields
3+: 1-10	in one microscopic field
4+: 10-100	in one microscopic field
5+: 100-1000	bacilli in one microscopic field
6+: Over 1000	bacilli and globi in one microscopic field

The BI is calculated as mean BI of the sites tested.

7.3 Histopathological Index (HI)

HI is the logarithmic index of bacilli in a biopsy and makes use of the GF and BI to assess the number of bacilli in the tissue section. The actual number of bacilli in the volume of given tissue can be calculated from the HI

8. Histopathology of leprosy

Taking a skin biopsy from the advancing cutaneous lesion in a patient suffering from leprosy is the single most informative procedure for diagnosis of leprosy spectrum and because of its ability to provide insight into the underlying disease process. The skin biopsy captures the pathology of the lesion at a given point and is a very useful resource that can be used for further investigation of the patient (Figure 2A-F). Standard histopathological examination of the formalin-fixed paraffin embedded skin tissue can provide information regarding cellular morphology, presence of AFB and can be further enhanced by techniques like imunohistochemistry, immunoelectron microscopy and molecular studies. Pure neuritic leprosy is another variant which shows typical tuberculoid or borderline features in nerves. Nerve biopsy is required for diagnosis in such cases but if the subject also shows skin lesions then nerve biopsy is not considered to be essential.

There are several useful applications of histopathological examination of the skin biopsy from a leprosy patient namely:

a. to confirm the diagnosis of leprosy
b. to accurately classify the lesion in the leprosy spectrum
c. for identification of the bacillary load in the tissue
d. in assessment of disease activity and response to treatment
e. for the diagnosis of a leprosy reaction

8.1 Indeterminate leprosy

Indeterminate leprosy is the earliest detectable skin lesion comprising one or few hypopigmented macules with no clear sensory changes. The skin biopsy may show mild accumulation of lymphocytes and macrophages and an occasional AFB either in the non-inflammed nerve, erector pili or in the subepidermal zone in the very early stages. It may show neuritis evidenced by Schwann cell proliferation and infiltration of the nerve fibres with lymphocytes. Nerve infiltration is the most significant feature of leprosy when the rest of the skin shows non specific changes. Moreover, the histological changes are known to precede the clinical manifestations by atleast 3 months (Ridley, 1978). Most indeterminate leprosy cases are known to heal spontaneously (Crawford, et al., 1977) but since it is not possible to predict which indeterminate cases will evolve into full blown leprosy, it is considered ethical to treat all the patients.

8.2 Tuberculoid Leprosy (TT)

Primary polar tuberculoid leprosy has large and compact epitheloid cell granulomas along the neurovascular bundles with lymphocytes. Langhans giant cells are typically scanty or absent and AFB are rare to find. Epitheloid cell granuolmas always erode into the basal layer of the epidermis. The dermal nerves may be either obiliterated and completely effaced or eroded by the dense lymphocyte cuff.

8.3 Borderline Tuberculoid leprosy (BT)

The epitheloid granulomas of BT do not invade into the epidermis and have less lymphocytes in comparison to TT. The granulomas are arranged in a curvilinear pattern along the neurovascular bundle. Nerve erosion by the granuloma is typical and AFB are scanty (ranging from BI 0-2) and are more readily detected in the Schawann cells of the nerves. In addition to nerves, the granuloma can also involve the sweat glands and the erector pili muscle.

8.4 Midborderlne leprosy (BB)

The histopathology in BB shows almost equal admixture of epitheloid cells and macrophages without forming a distinct granuloma. The lymphocytes are scant and scattered and multinucleate giant cells are absent, a feature that helps it to be distinguished from BT. AFB may be frequent (ranging from BI 2-4)

8.5 Borderline Lepromatous leprosy (BL)

The predominant cells in the granulomas are macrophages with occasional epitheloid cells arranged in patches. Lymphocytes are sparse, AFB are abundant (ranging from BI 3-5) but usually not present as globi. Perineural fibroblast proliferation forming an 'onion skin' in cross section is a typical feature. Early evidence of foamy change may be detectable.

8.6 Lepromatous Leprosy (LL)

The typical features consist of a flattened epidermis separated from the dermal infiltrate by a dense zone of normal collagen. The macrophage granuloma of LL is large and expansile consisting of sheets of foam cells with rare presence of lymphocytes. The foam cells harbor abundant AFB (ranging from BI 4-6). The solid bacilli are stacked like cigars and appear as globi. Such appearance is the rule rather than an exception. In contrast to tuberculoid leprosy, the nerves in the skin of LL patients may contain considerable AFB, however, the morphological features of the nerve is fairly well preserved in the earlier phase of the disease before eventually becoming fibrotic.

8.7 Lucio leprosy

The histopathology of this Mexican variant is similar to LL but with a characteristic heavy bacillation of the small blood vessels of the skin leading to thrombosis of vessels and ischemia and ulceration called as the 'lucio' phenomenon.

8.8 Histiod leprosy

This is another variant of LL, which shows the highest load (BI 6) of solid staining AFB arranged in clumps and sheaves. The macrophage reaction is unusual in the sense that the macrophages become spindle shaped and oriented in a storiform pattern reminiscent of a fibrohistiocytoma.

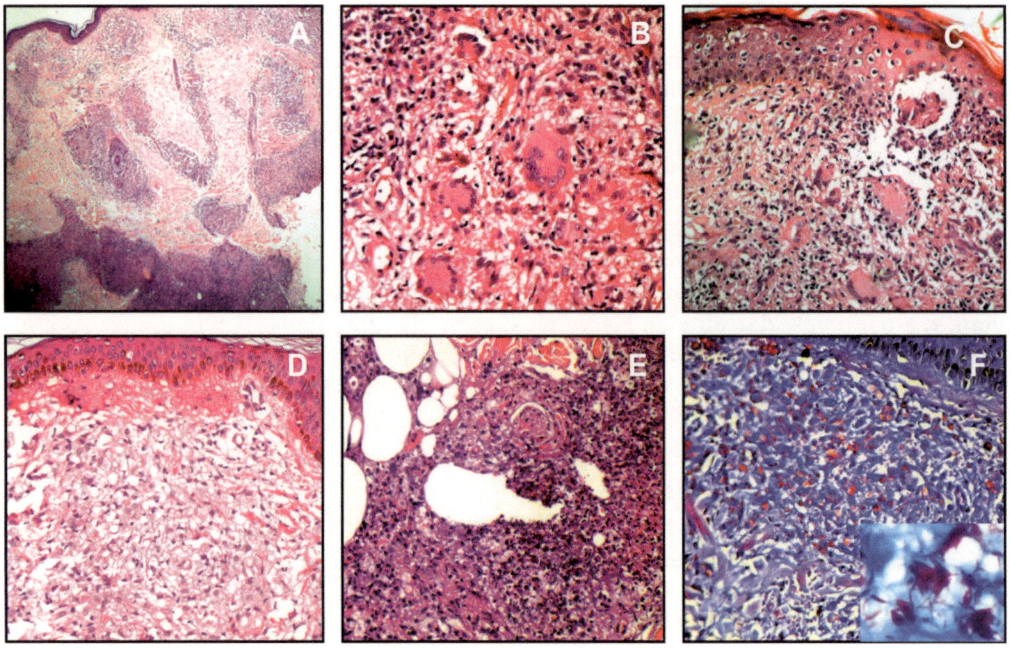

Fig. 2. Photomicrograph showing compact epithelioid granulomas in BT(A), multinucleate Langhans giant cells (B), epidermal erosion in leprosy reversal reaction (C), foamy macrophage granuloma of LL (D), ENL showing infiltration in subcutis along with neutrophils (E), Fite stain showing numerous globi (F) and AFB (inset) (magnification 40X except for inset which is 100X oil immersion)

9. Histopathological differential diagnosis

Tuberculoid leprosy needs to be differentiated from other granulomatous dermatitides. Cutaneous tuberculosis is the most important differential diagnosis which has to be excluded. The epidermis in tuberculoid leprosy is usually flat and not hyperplastic as in tuberculosis. The arrangement of the granulomas in leprosy is along the neurovascular bundles giving an oblong pattern to the granuloma unlike tuberculosis where there is intense and sometimes lichenoid pattern of the chronic granulomatous infiltrate. The dermal nerve twigs are spared by the infiltrate in tuberculosis. The presence of granuloma or AFB in the nerve is a conclusive proof of leprosy. Cutaneous sarcoidosis may sometimes be confused with tuberculoid leprosy as fibrinoid necrosis may be found in both these entities. The granuloma of sarcoidosis show paucity of lymphocytes and are more confluent and show fibrosis around the granuloma. Other granulomatous lesions like leishmaniasis or granulomatous post kala azar dermal leishmaniasis also need to be excluded by demonstration of Leishman-Donovan bodies and frequent presence of plasma cells. Borderline lepromatous and pure lepromatous leprosy may be confused with histocyte-rich lesions like xanthomas, however demonstration of AFB in these lesions usually solves the diagnostic dilemma.

10. Histopathology of leprosy reactions

Histopathological examination of a skin biopsy of reversal reaction will show dermal and intragranuloma edema. The granulomas become more epitheloid, show infiltration of lymphocytes within and around them and the Langhans giant cells become increased in number and bigger in size and may also show bizarre shapes. The granulomas also erode into the epidermis representing the upgrading reaction. In addition caseous necrosis may be evident in the nerves. At the molecular level, the events in type 1 reaction are responses to an array of cytokines secreted by the lymphocytes and macrophages. The skin and nerves are infiltrated by interferon-γ and tumor necrosis factor-α secreting CD4+ lymphocytes and are responsible for the inflammation and tissue damage.
On histopathology, a type 2 reaction is characterized by varying degree of polymorphonuclear infiltration superimposed on already existing lepromatous granuloma. The influx of neutrophils can be intense so as to form neutrophilic microabscess. Edema is frequently present in the dermis. Deposition of immune complexes in the small cutaneous capillaries, arterioles and venules result in necrotizing vasculitis. The downgrading reaction is reflected by deeper infiltration of foamy histiocytes into the subcutaneous fat. The AFB are fragmented and granular. Superficial ulceration, bulla formation and necrosis may sometimes supervene.

11. Skin biopsy in relapse

Relapse in paucibacillary (PB) leprosy may be defined as appearance of a new skin lesion or increase in the size of a pre-existing skin lesion provided there is a strong clinical and/or histopathological evidence of leprosy in such a lesion (Boeriggter, 1991). The difficulty in relapse in PB is to differentiate relapse from a type 1 reaction or drug resisitance. A true relapse can be detected histopathologically only after recording complete histological resolution of the earlier lesion in a previous biopsy. A relapse indicates that the AFB have survived despite antileprosy therapy and have multiplied and released antigens to produce fresh granulomas at the site of original lesion and show solid staining viable AFB. Alternatively, a fresh infection or reinfection may have occurred on reexposure. The cause of relapse may be irregular, inadequate therapy, presence of high initial BI, presence of 'persistors' bacilli that had remained dormant. Relapse in multibacillary (MB) leprosy are characterized in the early stage of relapse by emergence of foci of spindle shaped macrophages with granular, eosinophilic cytoplasm along with small foci of persisting foamy histiocytes and solid staining AFB in these patients who have not completely become smear negative. In late stage of relapse perineural thickening, fibrosis along with Schwann cell and endothelial cells packed with solid AFB are detectable.
A relapse can be differentiated from a reversal reaction by the fact that reversal reaction usually occurs within 6 months of release from treatment while relapse occurs after a year of release. The reversal reaction additionally shows erythema, edema, neuritis and fewer new lesions unlike relapse. Reactions respond well to steroids and show complete subsidence of lesions in 2-4 weeks whereas the relapse will show only partial or no response. Owing to chronic course and long duration of treatment, drug resistance is an emerging problem in leprosy. Drug resistance can be primary or secondary due to mutant bacilli surviving in a

setting of monotherapy as in dapsone resistance or irregular therapy as seen in rifampicin resistance. While there is appearance of new lesions and patient downgrades in drug resistance, in relapse there is reappearance over the old lesions but the patient rarely downgrades.

12. Use of molecular tools in leprosy

Definitive identification of *M. leprae* is somewhat problematic since the organism is not cultivable. This problem is further confounded by increased prevalence of other mycobacterial infections of skin. Molecular tests like real time PCR are being used for the rapid detection and quantification of bacterial DNA content from the clinical biopsy samples in which AFB were not detectable by conventional histopathological staining (Martinez et al., 2006). Molecular methods can help in rapid direct identification of drug resistance. Mutations in the *M. leprae* genome that are associated with resistance to several drugs have been identified and DNA analysis to detect these mutations has largely replaced the mouse footpad technique. Mutations in targeted genes can be identified by molecular approaches such as probe assays and sequencing and the magnitude of drug resistant mutants can be assessed from the biopsy samples (Honore & Cole, 2001)). Decrease in PCR signals have been shown to correlate with effect of therapy and cases showing persistence of signals for longer periods have been shown to correlate with higher relapses. (Wood & Cole, 1989; Gupta et al, 2001; Singh et al,1999). These molecular tools therefore can be useful adjuncts to clinical and histopathologic diagnosis of leprosy.

Molecular tools are also being increasingly used for research. Pathogenesis of leprosy is being explored by studying the expression of cell markers, cytokines and growth factors. *M. leprae* being noncultivable by conventional means constrained information on its metabolism and strain variations. Subsequent to the sequencing of its genome from an Indian strain, it has become possible to understand its genetic makeup. In addition, it has become possible to characterize strains of *M. leprae* using short tandem repeats of nucleotides in the genome sequence of the bacillus. Global studies are underway to study the distribution of strains as well as pathogen transmission by DNA based signatures of the bacilli. Since *M. leprae* is noncultivable, such strains are obtained from skin biopsies. DNA is extracted and amplified by PCR and probed with appropriate probes. Using archival material it has been possible to investigate the evolution of *M. leprae* as well as its origin in man in Africa and its subsequent spread to other parts of the world along with its human host (Monot et al, 2009; Singh & Cole, 2011). Recent evidence indicates that the organism from disseminated lepromatous leprosy endemic to Mexico and Latin America has different molecular signatures to *M. leprae* and has thus been given the new nomenclature of *M. lepromatosis* (Han et al, 2009).

13. Conclusion

Skin biopsy is integral to the understanding of leprosy, its causative organism and for monitoring its relapse and drug resistance. Diagnosis of leprosy has been based on classical cardinal signs, characteristic histopathological findings and demonstration of acid-fast bacilli both from the skin smears and skin biopsies of these lesions. The current primary goal is early diagnosis of this disease in order to interrupt the transmission by early treatment. Histopatholgical examination of the lesional skin is still the gold standard in confirmation of its diagnosis and its classification based on the immunopatholgic status. As new serological and molecular tests become available for the early diagnosis of leprosy, its reactions and resistance to drugs, skin biopsies will continue to compliment these emerging tools for providing more insights into the pathology of this fascinating disease.

14. References

Alguire CA, Mathes BM. (1998) Skin biopsy techniques for the internist. *J Gen Intern Med* 1: 46-54

Boeriggter G, Ponnighaus JM, Fine PEM, et al. (1991) Four-year follow-up results of a WHO-recommended multiple-drug regimen in pucibacillary leprosy patients in Malawi. *Int J Lep* 59:255-261

Crawford CL, Hardwicke PMD, Evans DHL, et al. (1977) Granulomatous hypersensitivity induced by sensory peripheral nerve. *Nature* 265:457-459

Gupta UD, Katoch K, Sharma RK, et al. (2001) Analysis of quantitative relationship between viability determination in leprosy by MFP, ATP bioluminescence and gene amplification assays. *Int J Lep Other Mycobact Dis* 69:328-334

Grekin RC. (1989) Simple dermatological surgical procedures. *Res Staff Phys* 35:61-67

Han XY, Sizer KC, Thompson EJ, et al. (2009) Comparative sequence analysis of *M. leprae* and the new leprosy-causing *Mycobacterium lepromatosis. J Bact.*191:6067-6074

Harrison PV. (1980) A guide to skin biopsies and excisions. *Clin Exp Dermatol* 5: 235-243

Honore N, Cole ST. (2001) A method for rapid detection of rifampicin-resistant isolates of *Mycobacterium leprae. Lep Rev* 172:441-448

Job CK, Chacko CJG (1986). A modification of Fite's stain for demonstration of *M. leprae* in tissue sections. *Ind J Lepr* 58:17-18

Martinez AN, Britto FPCC, Nery JAC, et al. (2006) Evaluation of real time and conventional PCR targeting complex 85 genes for detection of *Mycobacterium leprae* DNA in skin biopsy samples from patients diagnosed with leprosy. *J Clin Microbiol* 44: 3154-3159

Monot M, Honroe N, Garnier T, et al. (2009) Comparative genomic and phylogeographic analysis of *M. leprae. Nat Genet* 41:1282-1289

Moy RL, Waldman B, Hein DW. (1992) A review of sutures and suturing technique. *J Dermatol Surg Oncol* 18:785-795

Nayak SV, Sivarudrappa AS, Mukkamil AS. (2003) Role of fluorescent microscopy in detecting *M. leprae* in tissue sections. *Ann Diag Patho* 7:78-81

Noordeen SK. (1995). Eliminating leprosy as a public health problem.; why the optimism is justified. *Int J Lep;* 63:559-566

Pariser RJ.(1989). Skin biopsy: lesion selection and optimal technique. *Mod Med* 57: 82-90

Pfaltzgraff RE, Ramu G. (1991) Clin Leprosy. In: Hastings RC(ed). *Leprosy.* Churchill Livingston, Edinburgh.

Ridley DS. (1958) Therapeutic trials in leprosy using serial biopsies. *Lep Rev* 29:45-82

Ridley DS, Jopling WH (1966). Classification of leprosy according to immunity: A five group system. *Int J Lep* 34:255-273

Ridley DS. (1974) Histological classification and the immunological spectrum of leprosy. *Bull World Health Organization* 51: 451-465

Ridley DS. (1978). Classification of leprosy. In: *Window in leprosy.* Gandhi Memorial Leproy foundation, Wardha.

Scollard DM, Adams LB, Gillis TP, et al (2006). Continuing Challenges of leprosy. *Clin Microbiol Rev* 19:338-381

Sreenivasan P, Misra RS, Wilfred D, et al. (1998) Lepromatous patients show T helper1-like cytokine profile with differential expression of interleukin-10 during type 1 and 2 reactions. *Immunology* 95: 529-536

Singh HB, Katoch K, Gupta UD, et al.(1999) Effect of PCR positivity in MB patients treated with conventional and newer drugs ofloxacin and minocycline. *Acta Leprol* 11:179-182

Singh HB, Katoch VM, Natrajan M, et al. (2004) Improved protocols for PCR detection of *Mycobacterium leprae* in buffered formalin fixed skin biopsies. *Int J Lep Other Mycobact. Dis* 72:175-178

Singh P, Cole ST.(2011) *M. leprae,* genes, pseudogenes and genetic diversity. *Future Microbiol* 6:57-71

Telfer NR, Moy RL. (1993) Wound care after office procedures. *J Dermatol Surg Oncol* 19:722-731

Todd P, Garioch JJ, Humphreys S, et al.(1996) Evaluation of the 2-mm punch biopsy in dermatological diagnosis. *Clin Exp Dermatol* 21:11-17

Verhagen C, Faber W, Klatser P, et al. (1999) Immunohistological analysis of in situ expression of Mycobacterial antigen in skin lesions of leprosy patients across the histopathological spectrum. Association of Mycobacreial lipoarabinomannan(LAM) and *M. leprae* phenolic glycolipid-1(PGL-1) with leprosy reactions. *Am J Pathol* 154:1793-1804

Weng XM, Chen SY, Ran SF, et al. (2000) Immunohistopathology in the diagnosis of early leprosy. *Int J Lep* 68 :426-433

Wemambu SN, Turk JL, Waters MF, et al. (1969) Erythema nodosum leprosum: a clinical manifeastation of the arthus phenomenon. *Lancet* 2:933-935

World Health Organization. (2010). Global leprosy situation. *Wkly Epidemiol Record* 85:337-348

Wood SA, Cole ST. (1989) A rapid method for detection of potentially viable *Mycobacterium leprae* in human biopsies: A novel application of PCR. *FEMS Microbiol Lett* 65:305-310

Yamamura M, Uyemura K, Deans RJ, et al. (1991) Defining protective responses to pathogens: cytokine profiles in leprosy lesions. *Science* 254:277-279.

Yamamura M, Wang XH, Ohmen JD, et al. (1992) Cytokine patterns of immunologically mediated tissue damage. *J Immunol* 42:149:1470-1481

6

Severe Drug-Induced Skin Reactions: Clinical Pattern, Diagnostics and Therapy

Mirjana Ziemer[1] and Maja Mockenhaupt[2]
[1]*Department of Dermatology, Venereology, and Allergology, University Hospital of Leipzig,*
[2]*Department of Dermatology, Dokumentationszentrum schwerer Hautreaktionen – (dZh), Freiburg University - Medical Center, Germany*

1. Introduction

Cutaneous drug eruptions are common, with a prevalence of approximately 2 % to 3 % in hospitalized patients.[Bigby, 2001, Bigby, et al., 1986] It has been estimated that 1 of every 1000 hospitalized patients has a serious cutaneous drug reaction.[Roujeau and Stern, 1994] In clinical practice, the diagnosis of a cutaneous drug eruption is based on a clinical history suggesting that the rash is temporally related to the consumption of a new drug, the gross morphology of the rash, and, often, the histopathologic examination of a skin biopsy. The diversity of cutaneous drug eruptions is broad.[Kaplan, 1984, Roujeau, 2005, Wintroub and Stern, 1985] The vast majority of drug reactions is represented by morbilliform (scarlatiniform or rubeoliform) exanthemas (40%).[Gerson, et al., 2008] Followed by urticaria and angioedema, they account for up to 95% of cutaneous reactions.[Crowson, et al., 2003, Kauppinen and Stubb, 1984, Stubb, et al., 1994] Although generalized and often developing fast with some systemic symptoms such as pruritus, burning or shiver, these drug reactions are not severe and usually stop rapidly without much intervention after cessation of the culprit drug.

Histopathologically, drug reactions may simulate each of the patterns of inflammatory diseases of the skin and subcutaneous fat. However, by far the most common pattern evoked by them is "interface dermatitis".[Ackerman, et al., 2005] That pattern usually is joined by an infiltrate that encircles only the venules of the superficial plexus, but, episodically, the infiltrate is present around venules of both vascular plexuses. Of the two types of interface dermatitis induced by drugs, namely, vacuolar and lichenoid, the vacuolar is the most common.

Severe drug-induced skin reactions include Stevens-Johnson syndrome (SJS) and toxic epidermal necrolysis (TEN), moreover, generalized bullous fixed drug eruption (GBFDE), acute generalized exanthematous pustulosis (AGEP), and drug reaction with eosinophilia and systemic symptoms (DRESS). Furthermore, toxic erythemas after chemotherapy and drug-induced linear-IgA-dermatosis should be listed among them. Within the following chapter they will be elucidated from a clinical but in particular histopathologic point of view.

2. Stevens-Johnson syndrome and toxic epidermal necrolysis

2.1 Clinical presentation

SJS and TEN are viewed as a single disease entity of different severity.[Bastuji-Garin, et al., 1993] Both are characterized by a macular confluent erythema evolving into sometimes extensive blistering or epidermolysis that resembles a second degree burn (figures 1A and 2A). This is accompanied by mucosal erosions, especially affecting the mouth, the lips, the

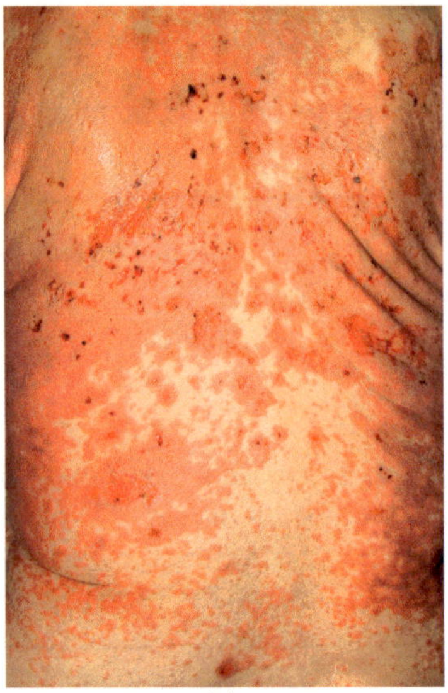

(a)

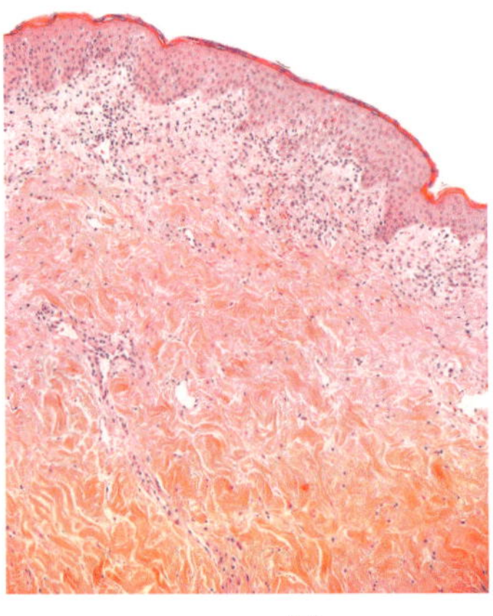

(b)

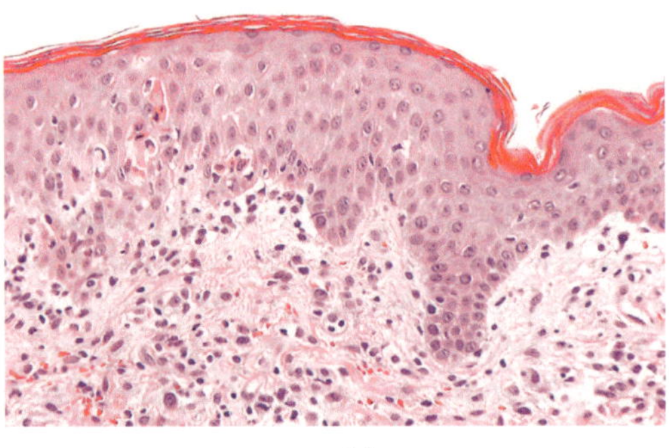

(c)

Fig. 1. A: SJS/TEN, early stage, with confluent erythematous macules, atypical targets and localized epidermolysis. The patient later developed more extensive epidermolysis.
B and C: Normal cornified layer. Dermal, superficial, sparse, perivascular and interstitial infiltrate of lymphocytes. Focal vacuolar alteration along the dermoepidermal junction in company with some lymphocytes. Focally scattered necrotic keratinocytes throughout the lower part of the epidermis. Extravasated erythrocytes. (B: hematoxylin-eosin, original magnification x100, C: hematoxylin-eosin, original magnification x400).

conjunctiva, and the genitals. The reactions are often accompanied by fever and malaise. SJS is characterized by a preference for the trunk or generalized dissemination of rather atypical target lesions and maculae. These are confluent and form blisters which may merge. Detachment of the skin affects less than 10 % of body surface area. The largest percentage of skin detachment, more than 30 %, occurs in TEN with maculae, whereas in the very rare form of TEN with widespread erythema the amount of blisters and erosions often affects little more than 10% of body surface area. A transitional form called SJS/TEN-overlap has been defined with blisters and erosions affecting 10 % to 30 % of body surface area.[Bastuji-Garin, et al., 1993].

Whereas SJS, SJS/TEN-overlap and TEN are considered as a single disease of different severity, erythema (exsudativum) multiforme majus (EM with mucosal involvement; E(E)MM) is different not only in terms of the clinical pattern, but also in terms of etiology. Especially shared histologic characteristics lead to the original thinking of a common disease spectrum. Typical or atypical raised targets are characteristic for EMM. They appear mainly on the limbs, but sometimes also on face and trunk, especially in children. Severe mucosal involvement is found in both, EMM and SJS/TEN, and does not allow a differentiation. Skin detachment in EMM is usually very limited, since only small blisters appear on the target lesions. While the minor and major form of EM are mainly triggered by infectious agents, such as acute or recurrent eruptions of herpes simplex, mycoplasma pneumonia, as well as other infections of the upper respiratory tract, flu, and flu-like infections, SJS/TEN are predominantly caused by drugs. [Auquier-Dunant, et al., 2002] Drugs with a high risk to induce SJS/TEN are allopurinol, antibacterial sulfonamides, non-steroidal anti-inflammatory drugs of the oxicam-type, various antiepileptic drugs, such as carbamazepine, lamotrigine, phenobarbital, phenytoin,, and the non-nucleoside reverse-transcriptase inhibitor nevirapine. [Mockenhaupt, et al., 2008]) SJS/TEN may end fatally in only a few days and mortality is more than 40% in TEN.[Mockenhaupt, 2008, Mockenhaupt and Norgauer, 2002] Despite the fact that a diagnosis of EMM and SJS/TEN in most cases can be made clinically and histopathologically with confidence, no judgment can be made, on morphologic grounds alone, about the cause of it. Moreover, there are currently no in vivo or in vitro tests that can identify the causative agent in SJS/TEN with certainty. Thus, causality assessment is mainly based on a thorough history of drug exposure and infection of the individual patient.

2.2 Histology

SJS and TEN share a particular histological pattern.[Ackerman, et al., 2005, Rzany, et al., 1996] In early erythematous macules, papules, or plaques a sparse to moderate perivascular and interstitial infiltrate of lymphocytes is present in the superficial dermis. Occasional eosinophilic granulocytes may be found. Vacuolar alteration is found along the dermoepidermal junction (DEJ) often in company with some lymphocytes. Necrotic keratinocytes are scattered throughout the lower part of the epidermis (figures 1B and 1C). Infundibular epidermis and acrosyringia of eccrine ducts may be involved. Slight ballooning of keratinocytes and spongiosis may be present. The cornified layer shows a normal basket-weave configuration. In fully developed stages of the disease, when epidermal detachment/epidermolysis appears, in addition to the above mentioned changes subepidermal vesiculation secondary to extensive vacuolar alteration and confluent necrosis of keratinocytes develops. Confluent necrosis can involve the upper part of infundibular epidermis and acrosyringia of eccrine ducts. Variable numbers of extravasated erythrocytes are present. As the process develops rapidly, usually neither melanophages nor siderophages are found in the upper part of the dermis. The cornified layer remains unchanged (figures 2B, 2C, and 2D). In late hyperpigmented macules and patches a sparse superficial perivascular infiltrate of lymphocytes may still be present. Slight vacuolar alteration remains at the DEJ. Melanophages are scattered in variable numbers in the papillary dermis, optionally together with some siderophages. Re-epithelialization of the epidermis beneath a subepidermal blister can be mentioned. Cornified layer shows slight parakeratosis or sometimes scale-crust. In areas of epidermal necrosis and epidermolysis the dermis may be covered by a fibrinoid crust containing neutrophilic granulocytes. Some neutrophilic granulocytes may also be present in the adjacent dermis.

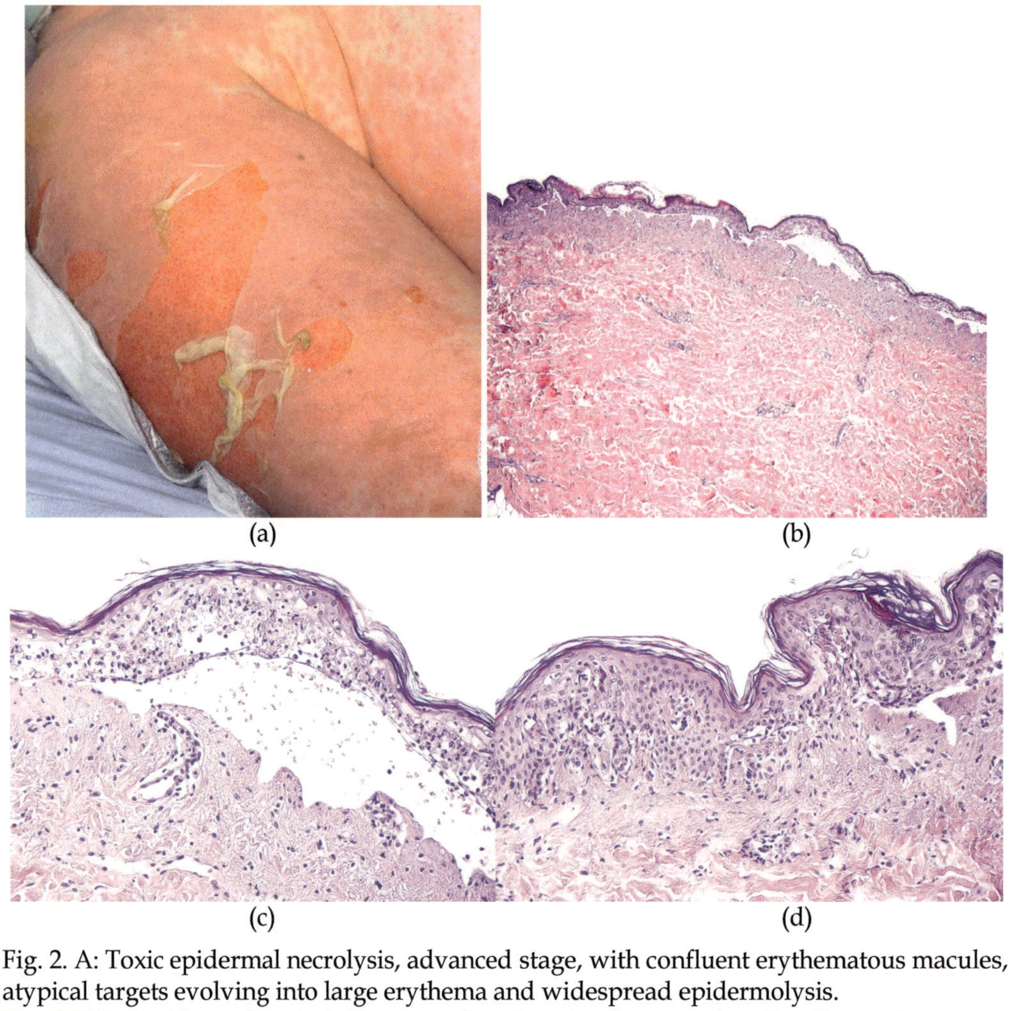

(a) (b) (c) (d)

Fig. 2. A: Toxic epidermal necrolysis, advanced stage, with confluent erythematous macules, atypical targets evolving into large erythema and widespread epidermolysis.
B and C: Subepidermal vesiculation secondary to extensive vacuolar alteration and confluent necrosis of keratinocytes. A dermal, superficial, very sparse, perivascular and interstitial infiltrate of lymphocytes. Unchanged cornified layer. (B: hematoxylin-eosin, original magnification x40, C: hematoxylin-eosin, original magnification x400)
D: Changes from the erythematous edge of a blister. Features correspond to early changes mentioned in figure 1B and C (hematoxylin-eosin, original magnification x400).

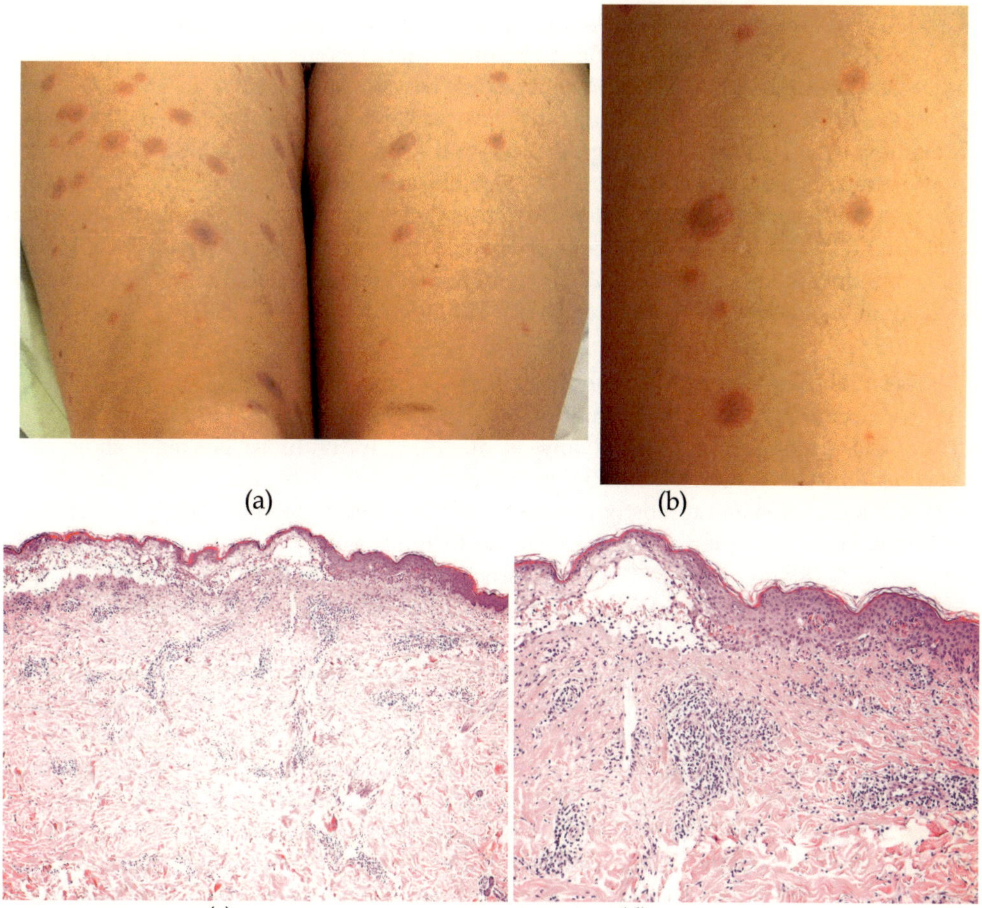

(a) (b) (c) (d)

Fig. 3. A and B: Erythema multiforme with target lesions on the extremities.
C and D: Subepidermal vesiculation secondary to extensive vacuolar alteration and confluent necrosis of keratinocytes. Dermal, superficial, moderate, perivascular and interstitial infiltrate of lymphocytes. Unchanged cornified layer. Changes are indistinguishable from those of Stevens-Johnson syndrome or toxic epidermal necrolysis. (C: hematoxylin-eosin, original magnification x40, D: hematoxylin-eosin, original magnification x200).

Immunohistochemically, there is a predominance of CD4+ cells in the dermis and CD8+ cells in the epidermis similar to graft-versus-host disease (GVHD). Cytotoxic T cells can initiate apoptosis, exacerbated by the release of perforins, cytokines such as tumor necrosis factor-alpha (TNF-α) and FAS-ligand.[Abe, et al., 2003, Chang, et al., 2004, Nassif, et al., 2004a, Nassif, et al., 2002] Recent findings demonstrate that secretory granulysin is a key molecule responsible for the disseminated keratinocyte death in SJS/TEN and highlight a mechanism for cytotoxic T lymphocyte- and natural killer cell-mediated cytotoxicity that does not require direct cellular contact.[Chung, et al., 2008] Granulysin concentrations in the blister fluids were two to four orders of magnitude higher than perforin, granzyme B or soluble FAS-ligand concentrations, therewith being the most highly expressed cytotoxic molecule.[Chung, et al., 2008] It is also thought that proteins such as FAS-antigen (CD95) and p55-TNF-α-receptors promote keratinocyte apoptosis.[Abe, et al., 2003, Chang, et al., 2004, Viard, et al., 1998] In blister fluid obtained from patients with sulfonamide-induced TEN, it has been shown that the lymphocytes were only cytotoxic in the presence of cotrimoxazole or sulfamethoxazole, but not toward hydroxylamine metabolites of sulfamethoxazole. This is the first sign that lesional T lymphocytes exhibit a direct cytotoxic response towards autologous cells without prior re-stimulation.[Nassif, et al., 2004b] In addition, ligands such as TRAIL (tumor necrosis factor related apoptosis inducing ligand) and TWEAK (TNF-like weak inducer of apoptosis) are secreted by CD1a+ and CD14+ cells capable of inducing keratinocyte death in an MHC class I-independent manner, also seem to be present in the blister fluids of patients with TEN.[de Araujo, et al., 2011]

2.3 Differential diagnoses histopathologically

Erythema (exsudativum) multiforme majus (E(E)MM) and SJS/TEN share a similar histology.[Ackerman, et al., 2005, Rzany, et al., 1996] Individual cases may show minor differences, but these concern mostly quantitative aspects. The dermal infiltrate in EM, SJS/TEN is a superficial and mostly perivascular. However, it decreases with the severity of the disease, being intermediate or even dense in the majority of cases of EM and rather sparse in TEN.[Rzany, et al., 1996] Erythrocyte extravasation is found more often in EM.[Rzany, et al., 1996] Nevertheless, histopathologic differentiation is impossible (figures 3A, 3B, 3C, and 3D).

The most important differential diagnoses for SJS/TEN are 'generalized bullous fixed drug eruption' (GBFDE) and 'staphylococcal scalded skin syndrome' (SSSS). The clinical presentation of GBFDE differs from SJS/TEN, as described below, and the Nikolsky sign is negative on healthy skin in GBFDE. Also in GBFDE and SSSS there may be limited involvement of mucous membranes. Histopathologically, differentiation may be hindered based on the fact that features of GBFDE show great overlap with those of EM, or SJS/TEN. To what extent histopathologic characteristics of localized fixed drug eruption can be transferred for GBFDE and therewith being helpful in differentiation from SJS/TEN has not yet been clarified. The dermal inflammatory infiltrate in localized fixed drug eruption is usually a superficial and deep, perivascular, lymphocytic infiltrate with some eosinophilic and neutrophilic granulocytes, the latter being dispersed also interstitially. However, it seems that those features are not necessarily present in GBFDE (data based on experience of the authors). Unlike the macular confluent exanthema seen in SJS/TEN, in SSSS there is widespread erythema sometimes evolving into erythroderma (figure 4A). The Nikolsky sign is often positive, but skin detachment is very superficial. SSSS is far less common than SJS/TEN and has a variable age distribution with peak incidences in early childhood and in adulthood.[Mockenhaupt, et al., 2005] The disease was previously known as pemphigus acutus neonatorum Ritter von Rittershain. Histology in SSSS shows acantholytic blistering within the stratum granulosum. There is either no or only a sparse superficial lymphocytic infiltrate (figures 4B and 4C). In order to determine the level of epidermal separation as quickly as possible and differentiate between TEN and SSSS, the Tzanck smear may be used, which employs exfoliative cytology of the blister fluid, which is spread on a slide and stained with Giemsa. In SSSS, wide epithelial cells with a small nucleus/cytoplasm ratio are seen; in TEN, cuboidal cells with a large cell nucleus/cytoplasm ratio are found. Rapid histopathologic diagnosis of a cryostat section is certainly more reliable for rapid differentiation between SSSS and TEN. In SSSS, the removed roof of the blister demonstrates subcorneal separation, while in TEN the separation is deeper, in the stratum spinosum.

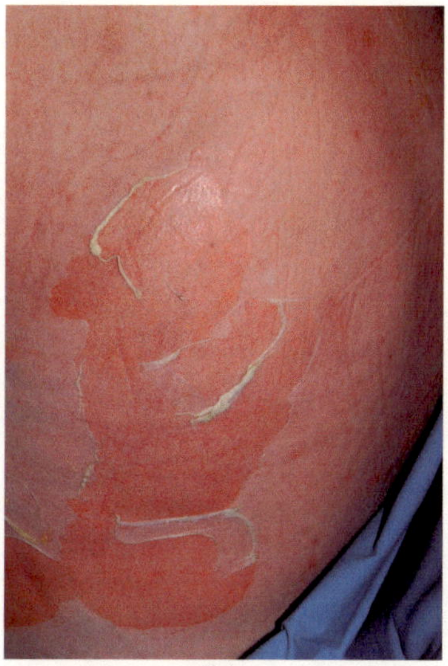

(a)

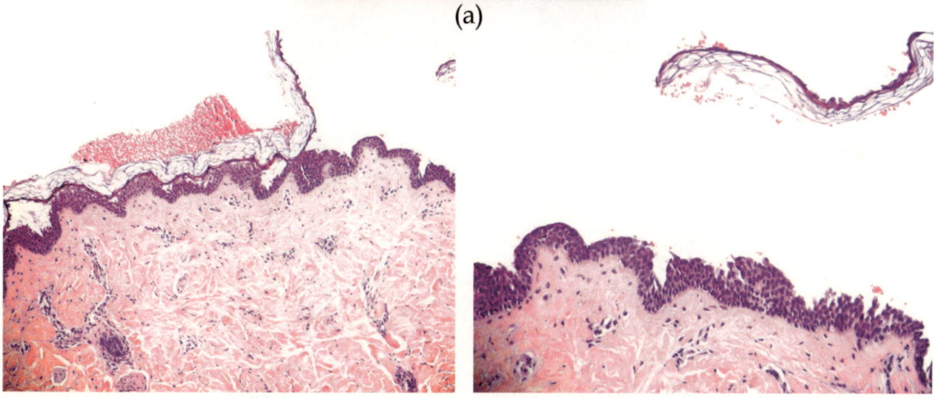

(b) (c)

Fig. 4. A: Staphylococcal scalded skin syndrome with generalized erythema and widespread superficial epidermolysis.
B and C: Acantholytic blistering within the stratum granulosum. Very sparse superficial lymphocytic infiltrate (B: hematoxylin-eosin, original magnification x100, C: hematoxylin-eosin, original magnification x200).

Further, drug-induced exanthemas which sometimes demonstrate a multiform, target-like appearance without mucosal erosions, and which are histopathologically distinct must be considered as differential diagnoses. In particular, cyclooxygenase-2 inhibitors are able to induce widespread erythematous target-like skin reactions with certain additional symptoms, especially dyspnea and facial edema, and often also more widespread dermal edema (figure 5A).[Ziemer, et al., 2007] The exanthema is not accompanied by mucous membrane involvement and usually shows no or only very localized blisters (< 5% of the body surface). Histopathologically, biopsy specimens show a normal epidermis. Necrotic keratinocytes are not found. In the superficial dermis, there is a sparse perivascular and interstitial lymphocytic infiltrate, sometimes accompanied by a few eosinophilic granulocytes (figure 5B). A few lymphocytes may be found in the epidermis; which may in some cases focally be detached from the underlying skin as a result of severe edema in the papillary dermis.[Ziemer, et al., 2007]

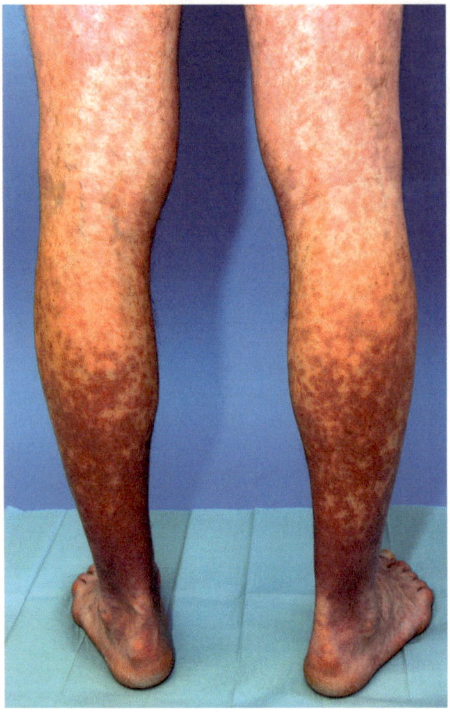

(a)

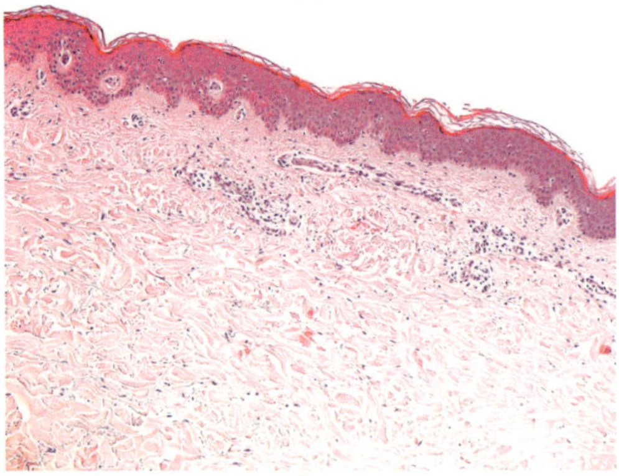

(b)

Fig. 5. A: Target-like or multiforme-like drug eruption. Extensive, confluent, erythematous-violaceous, target-like macules cover the entire body. (Reprinted with permission from JAMA & Archives) Cutaneous adverse reactions to valdecoxib distinct from Stevens-Johnson syndrome and toxic epidermal necrolysis. Arch Dermatol. 2007;143(6):711-6. Copyright© (2007), American Medical Association. All rights reserved.
B: Normal epidermis. Note a sparse perivascular and interstitial lymphocytic infiltrate in the superficial dermis and a few lymphocytes in the epidermis (hematoxylin-eosin, original magnification x40). (Reprinted with permission from JAMA & Archives) Cutaneous adverse reactions to valdecoxib distinct from Stevens-Johnson syndrome and toxic epidermal necrolysis. Arch Dermatol. 2007;143(6):711-6. Copyright© (2007), American Medical Association. All rights reserved.

Another, essentially distinct, severe and potentially fatal condition is 'drug reaction with eosinophilia and systemic symptoms' (DRESS). Although clinically well characterized, histology has not been studied systematically for this disease entity and reported findings are not consistent. If necrotic keratinocytes and basal cell vacuolar degeneration predominate together with a superficial lymphocytic infiltrate, histologic differentiation from SJS/TEN may be problematic. However, if present, necrotic keratinocytes in DRESS are scattered solitary within the epidermis, never provoking blister formation or epidermolysis (see subchapter 5).

In some instances differentiation from autoimmune bullous skin disorders may be necessary. Although histopathologically usually distinctive, in such cases immunofluorescence should be performed. This may be helpful in differentiating bullous drug eruptions from autoimmune-blistering diseases, such as bullous pemphigoid or pemphigus. In particular this can be of importance in diagnosing drug-induced linear-IgA-dermatosis, showing IgA-depositions along the basal membrane zone (see subchapter 7).

In a few further particular situations the diagnosis of SJS/TEN may be complicated to a maximum. This is the case in differentiation of SJS/TEN from advanced acute graft-versus-host disease of the skin and in differentiation of SJS/TEN from some manifestations of acute lupus erythematosus. In lupus erythematosus, vacuolar alteration of the DEJ and damage to keratinocytes are helpful in establishing diagnosis. Depending on the stage of evolution, necrotic keratinocytes can be seen either scattered throughout the lower part or in the entire epidermis in lupus erythematosus and SJS/TEN, leading to histopathologic misinterpretation. Because of the paucity of the rather superficial perivascular lymphocytic infiltrates and less epidermal atrophy, hyperkeratosis, basal membrane zone thickening and pigmentary incontinence, especially subacute-cutaneous lupus erythematosus and acute cutaneous lupus erythematosus may show considerable histopathologic overlap with SJS/TEN. However, the sum of changes and the notice of subtle histopathologic findings often allow differentiation [unpublished data from the German Registry of Severe Skin Reactions (Dokumentationszentrum schwerer Hautreaktionen, dZh), [Rzany, et al., 1996]). The same difficulty concerns clear histopathologic distinction of SJS/TEN from acute GVHD, where a morbiliform rash may rapidly progress to severe erythema and blisters (figure 6A). Histologically, in severe acute GVHD scattered necrotic keratinocytes predominate in the deeper epidermis. There may or may not be an accompanying lymphocytic infiltrate. Apart from a few investigations - none of them performed with an essentially necessary clinical correlation - considerable histopathologic studies do not exist.[Paquet, et al., 2001] The importance of a lymphocytic infiltrate is disputed and may not be compulsary for the diagnosis of GVHD.[Snover, 1990] Nevertheless, in GVHD a few eosinophilic granulocytes may be found within the infiltrate, a feature rarely observed in SJS/TEN. Moreover, adnexal involvement in SJS/TEN seems to be restricted to infundibular epidermis and epithelia of acrosyringia, whereas in GVHD lower parts of the hair follicle and epithelia of sebaceous glands may be involved (figures 6B and 6C).[Elliott, et al., 1987]

3. Generalized bullous fixed drug eruption

3.1 Clinical presentation

Generalized bullous fixed drug eruption (GBFDE) may be differentiated clinically from SJS/TEN.[Kauppinen, 1972] Classically, in GBFDE there are disseminated brownish violaceous patches on which flaccid blisters arise. However, some cases present with bright erythematous patches, lacking the brownish discoloration (figures 7A and 7B).

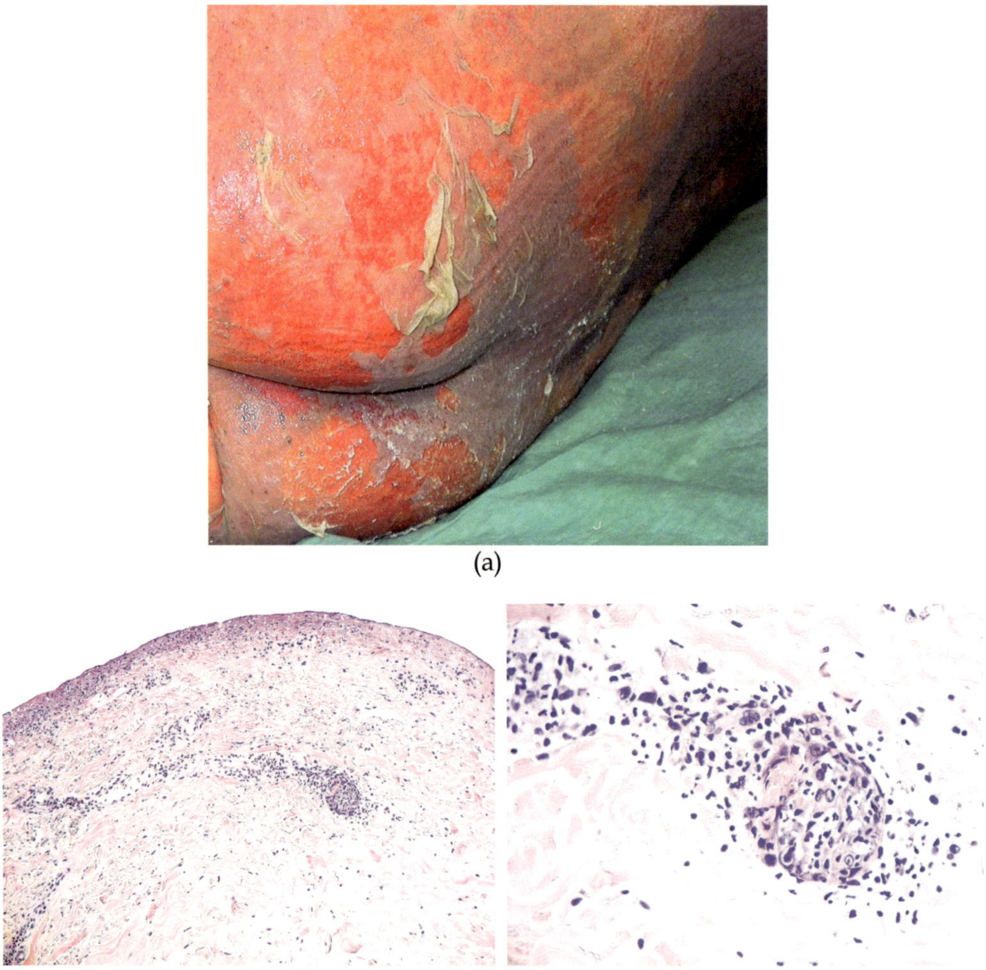

(a) (b) (c)

Fig. 6. A: Severe acute cutaneous graft-versus-host disease with confluent erythematous macules evolving into large erythema and widespread epidermolysis.
B: Completely lost epidermis due to subepidermal blister formation. Superficial, dermal, perivascular and periadnexal infiltrate of lymphocytes and occasionally eosinophilic granulocytes. (hematoxylin-eosin, original magnification x40)
C: Scattered necrotic keratinocytes and vacuolar alteration throughout the lower part of eccrine duct in company with lymphocytes. (hematoxylin-eosin, original magnification x400).

Blistering usually affects only a small percentage of body surface area and between the large blisters there are sizable areas of intact skin. Erosive mucosal involvement was reported as being rare and rather mild. However, recent data show that in 77% of patients with GBFDE mucous membranes were affected with a predominance of genitalia in both men (58%) and women (48%).[Mockenhaupt, et al., 2010] Patients usually do not feel sick, however, a fever may occur. Most patients report a history of a similar, often local reaction (fixed drug eruption).[Mockenhaupt, et al., 2010, Mockenhaupt and Norgauer, 2002] Nearly always GBFDE develops after re-exposure of the drug, possibly worsening with repeated use. This clearly distinguishes GBFDE from SJS/TEN, which generally appear during the first cycle of medication use, that is, without prior sensitization. Nevertheless, repeated GBFDE events can lead to increasingly widespread detachment of the skin and thus to serious disease. The overall mortality in such cases within six weeks after the onset of the reaction was reported to be 21%; all but one patient with lethal outcome were more than 70 years old.[Mockenhaupt, et al., 2010] Cotrimoxazole has been identified as the most common cause of GBFDE.[Mahboob and Haroon, 1998] In the recent case series most frequently associated drugs were co-trimoxazole (50%), followed by analgesics such as paracetamol (20%) and metamizole (18%).[Mockenhaupt, et al., 2010] The average duration between beginning of drug use and onset of the disease ranged from one day to about five days.[Mockenhaupt, et al., 2010]

3.2 Histology

As mentioned above it is still unclear to what extent histopathologic characteristics of localized fixed drug eruption are identical with those of GBFDE. Early lesions of localized fixed drug eruption show a sparse superficial and usually deep perivascular and interstitial mixed-cell infiltrate of lymphocytes with neutrophilic and eosinophilic granulocytes scattered interstitially. The papillary dermis may reveal some edema. Lymphocytes in company with neutrophilic and/or eosinophilic granulocytes sprinkled along the DEJ in conjunction with vacuolar alteration. The epidermis shows slight spongiosis and ballooning. Individual necrotic keratinocytes are found in the basal and spinous layers. The cornified layer is normal. In fully developed lesions vacuolar alteration at the DEJ is more extensive and may eventuate in subepidermal clefts and subepidermal vesicles. Spongiosis is more marked with intraepidermal vesicles. Necrotic keratinocytes are more numerous and the entire epidermis sometimes becomes necrotic (figures 7C and 7D). In late stages a sparse superficial perivascular infiltrate of lymphocytes with numerous melanophages remains in the papillary and sometimes upper reticular dermis. Melanophages at the base of a thickened papillary dermis in the context of a mixed infiltrate of inflammatory cells that includes neutrophils and eosinophils and of an epidermis that houses necrotic keratinocytes are a clue to fixed drug eruption recurrent at a particular site. [Ackerman, et al., 2005]

3.3 Differential diagnoses histopathologically

SJS/TEN displays changes at the DEJ and in the epidermis identical to those of fixed drug eruption, but the perivascular infiltrate usually is superficial only and is made up almost exclusively of lymphocytes. Eosinophils usually are few, if they are present at all, and neutrophils are absent unless confluent necrosis of the epidermis is prominent and attracts them chemotactically. Fixed drug eruption, in contrast to SJS/TEN, usually affects the venules of the deep as well as the superficial plexus, and the infiltrate of inflammatory cells is mixed, consisting of lymphocytes, eosinophils, and neutrophils perivascular, in the interstitium, along the DEJ, and in the epidermis.[Ackerman, et al., 2005]

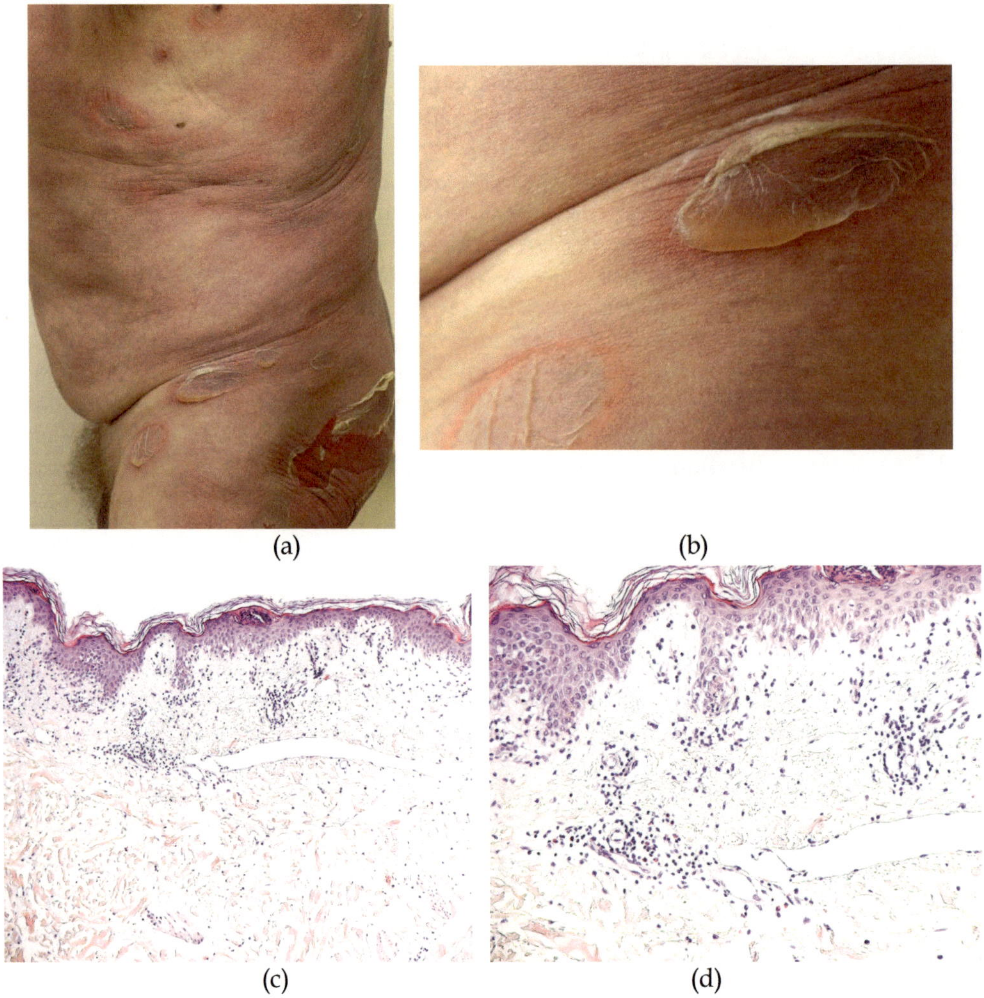

Fig. 7. A and B: Disseminated violaceous patches with flacid blisters on trunk and extremities.
C and D: Superficial, perivascular and interstitial, mixed-cell infiltrate of lymphocytes with neutrophilic and eosinophilic granulocytes scattered interstitially also in deeper parts of the dermis. Lymphocytes in company with some neutrophilic granulocytes sprinkled along the DEJ in conjunction with vacuolar alteration. Epidermis shows slight spongiosis. Individual necrotic keratinocytes are found in the basal and spinous layers. (C: hematoxylin-eosin, original magnification x100, D: hematoxylin-eosin, original magnification x200).

4. Acute generalized exanthematous pustulosis

4.1 Clinical presentation

In AGEP there is very acute widespread erythema with hundreds of small, flaccid, confluent, non-follicular pustules, especially along the skin folds and on the flexor surfaces (figure 8A). The reaction rarely involves mucous membranes, and when it does, symptoms are mild. Patients have acute fever and neutrophilia on blood tests.[Roujeau, et al., 1991, Sidoroff, et al., 2001] AGEP shows spontaneous resolution in less then 15 days with characteristic desquamation. The main causes for AGEP are aminopenicillins, quinolones, macrolides, diltiazem, and antimalarial drugs such as (hydroxy-)chloroquine. Pristinamycine, which is approved for use in selected countries, is associated with a high relative risk of AGEP.[Mockenhaupt, et al., 2008, Sidoroff, et al., 2007] The latency period between initiation of the drug and onset of the cutaneous reaction is only a few days.

4.2 Histology

Histology typically shows non-follicular, spongiform, subcorneal and/or intraepidermal pustules, sometimes with marked edema of the papillary dermis. The epidermis is otherwise normal with an orthokeratotic stratum corneum, housing in foci neutrophilic granulocytes. The adjacent dermis shows superficial, perivascular and interstitial lymphocytic infiltrates with neutrophilic (figure 8B) and in most instances eosinophilic granulocytes.[Burrows and Russell Jones, 1993, Halevy, et al., 2010, Kardaun, et al., 2010a, Sidoroff, et al., 2001] Apart from neutrophils a few eosinophilic granulocytes may be found within the epidermis. [Sidoroff, 2001] Vasculitis and/or a small number of necrotic keratinocytes[Kardaun, et al., 2010a, Sidoroff, et al., 2001] have been reported in a few cases, however, such features are not typical for the disease. Moreover, presence of vasculitis could not be confirmed in a recent histopathologic study.[Kardaun, et al., 2010a] In summary, comparing AGEP and generalized pustular psoriasis, the presence of eosinophils, necrotic keratinocytes, a mixed perivascular and interstitial mid-dermal infiltrate and absence of tortuous or dilated blood vessels are in favor of AGEP.[Kardaun, et al., 2010a] Immunohistology shows neutrophilic leukocytes in subcorneal pustules that are surrounded by activated CD4+ and CD8+ T cells. The keratinocytes, as well as T-cells that have migrated to the epidermis, express interleukin-8 (IL-8), which attracts neutrophils. Presumably drug-specific T-cells migrate first, induce blistering, and then recruit neutrophilic leukocytes.[Britschgi, et al., 2001, Pichler, et al., 2002]

4.3 Differential diagnoses histopathologically

The main clinical differential diagnosis of an acute developing generalized pustular rash is acute generalized (exanthematous) pustular psoriasis. The morphology of the pustules is indistinguishable in both diseases. For the differentiation of AGEP from pustular psoriasis, criteria for histopathologic distinction have been proposed, i.e. papillary edema, vasculitis, exocytosis of eosinophils and single-cell necrosis of keratinocytes in AGEP and acanthosis and papillomatosis in pustular psoriasis.[Sidoroff, et al., 2001] However, acanthosis and papillomatosis are never suspected findings in acute generalized pustular psoriasis. Moreover, vasculitis and single-cell necrosis of keratinocytes, have only eventually been observed in AGEP. The fact that in patients with AGEP the allele HLA-DR-B1*07 has been detected, which is also present in psoriasis patients, might explain the interaction between T-cells and neutrophilic leukocytes in both diseases.[Britschgi, et al., 2001, Pichler, et al., 2002] Discrimination is impossible on the basis of histological criteria, but rather depending on the clinical course, since AGEP ameliorates rapidly following discontinuation of the trigger in contrast to pustular psoriasis that frequently exhibits a prolonged course and is characterized by a difficult therapeutic management.[Sidoroff, et al., 2001, Ziemer and Böer, 2006].

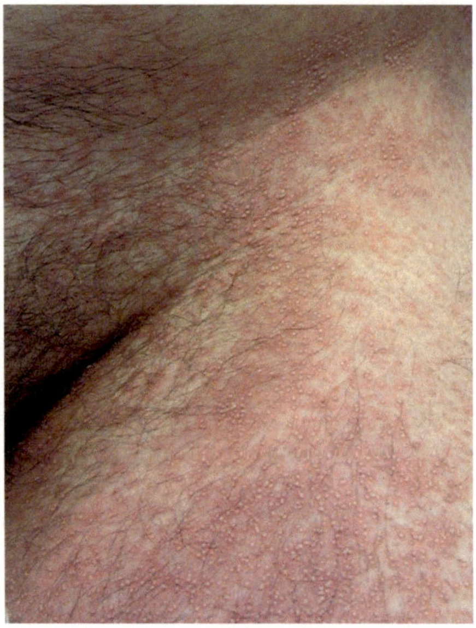

(a)

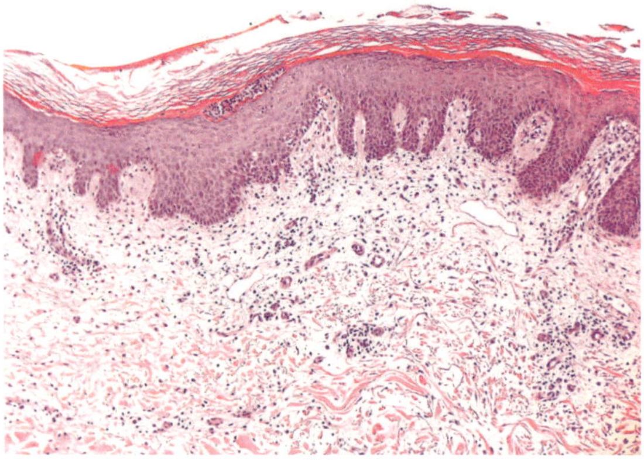

(b)

Fig. 8. A: Acute generalized exanthematous pustulosis. Widespread erythema with hundreds of small, flaccid, confluent, non-follicular pustules, especially along the groins and on the flexor surfaces of the legs.
B: Subcorneal pustules. The epidermis is slightly acanthotic with an orthokeratotic stratum corneum. The adjacent dermis shows superficial, perivascular and interstitial lymphocytic infiltrates with some neutrophilic granulocytes. Features are practically indistinguishable from acute eruptive lesions in pustular psoriasis (hematoxylin-eosin, original magnification x200).

Histopathologically, subcorneal and intraepidermal pustules are moreover the pathognomic feature in IgA-pemphigus.[Harman, et al., 1999] IgA-pemphigus is a rare intraepidermal autoimmune disease characterized by tissue-bound and circulating IgA autoantibodies that target the desmosomal proteins of the epidermis, mainly desmocollin 1 and desmogleins. The main clinical characteristics are erythematous skin lesions with vesiculopustules, erosions, crusts and desquamation favoring the trunk, groins, axillas, and proximal extremities (figures 9A and 9B). The average age of onset is approximately 50 years. Histological hallmarks of IgA-pemphigus are subcorneal or intraepidermal pustules, and neutrophilic infiltration. Scant epidermal acantholysis may be found, however, acantholysis is not as characteristic as it is in classic pemphigus (figures 9C and 9D). Finally, histologic discrimination of AGEP from IgA-pemphigus is only possible by immunofluorescence. Direct immunofluorescence reveals IgA deposits in the intercellular space throughout the epidermis, more intense in superficial layers and less intense in lower layers. Nevertheless, in some cases IgA autoantibodies do not react with desmogleins or desmocollins.[Niimi, et al., 2000]

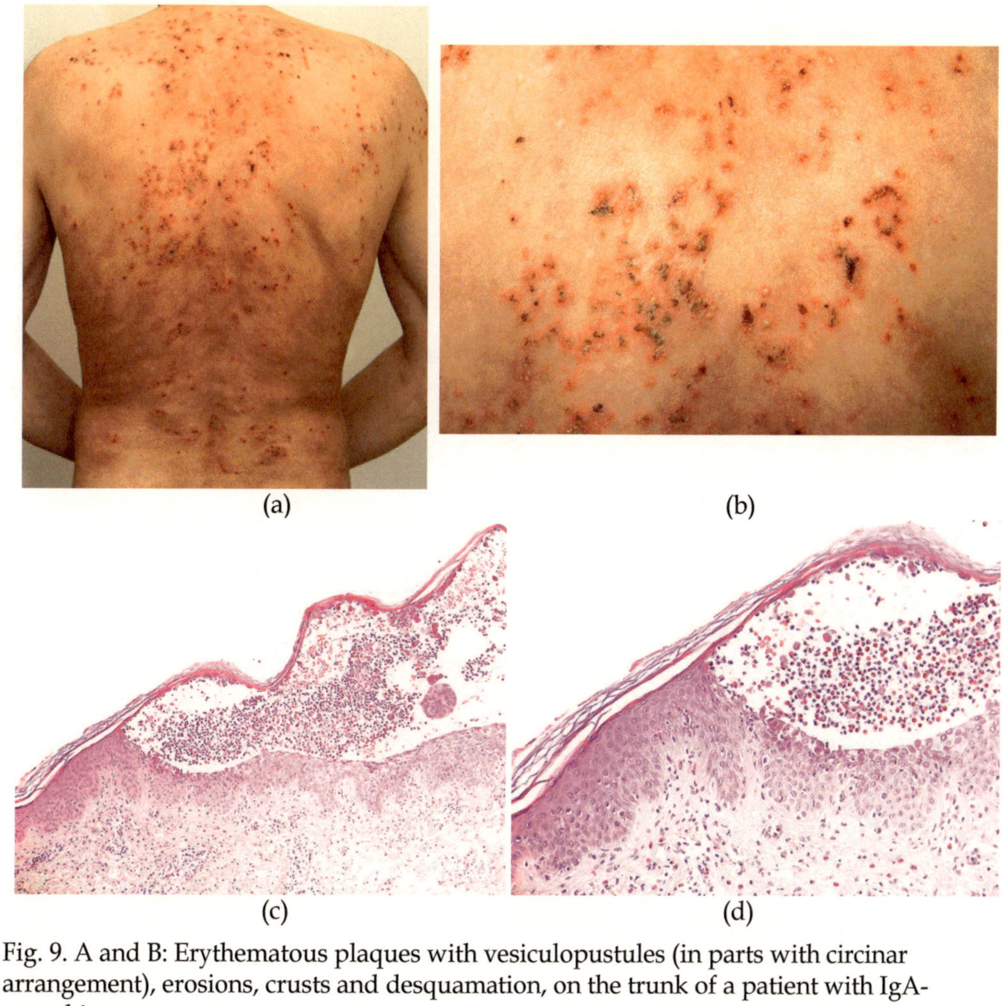

Fig. 9. A and B: Erythematous plaques with vesiculopustules (in parts with circinar arrangement), erosions, crusts and desquamation, on the trunk of a patient with IgA-pemphigus.
C and D: Subcorneal pustules and neutrophilic infiltration (subcorneal pustular dermatosis type of IgA-pemphigus). Superficial epidermal acantholysis. Dermal superficial mixed cell infiltrate with lymphocytes, eosinophilic and neutrophilic granulocytes, with lymphocytes and eosinophilic granulocytes being also in blister content (C: hematoxylin-eosin, original magnification x100, D: hematoxylin-eosin, original magnification x200).

Within the spectrum of intraepidermal neutrophilic dermatoses is subcorneal pustular dermatosis of Sneddon and Wilkinson.[Sneddon and Wilkinson, 1956] Sneddon and Wilkinson reported a chronic disease with flaccid and aseptic pustules developing predominantly on the trunk and in the groins, axillae and submammary areas. However, subcorneal pustulosis Sneddon-Wilkinson no longer seems to be considered an authentic clinical entity, since under this term unrelated diseases such as pustular psoriasis and IgA-pemphigus are subsumed.[Ziemer and Böer, 2006]
Finally, dermatophyte infections may present with intracorneal and intraepidermal pustules together with a superficial perivascular lymphocytic infiltrate containing neutrophilic granulocytes. Histochemical staining with periodic acid-Schiff (PAS) may be helpful in revealing fungi (figures 10A and 10B).

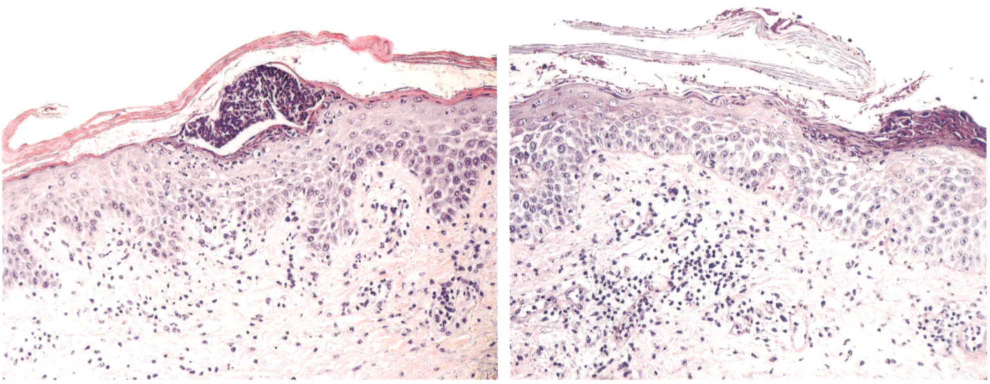

(a) (b)

Fig. 10. A: Tinea corporis. Intra- and subcorneal as well as intraepidermal pustules together with spongiosis and a superficial perivascular lymphocytic infiltrate containing neutrophilic granulocytes. Numerous hyphae within the stratum corneum (hematoxylin-eosin, original magnification x200).
B: Numerous intracorneal hyphae (periodic acid-Schiff, original magnification x200).

5. Hypersensitivity syndrome / drug reaction with eosinophilia and systemic symptoms

5.1 Clinical presentation

In 1996, Bocquet et al. coined the term 'drug rash with eosinophilia and systemic symptoms' (DRESS) for a cutaneous adverse drug reactions associated with fever, exanthema and facial edema, lymphadenopathy, hematologic abnormalities and organ involvement.[Bocquet, et al., 1996] This clinical entity was reported under various names including 'anticonvulsant hypersensitivity syndrome' (HSS), 'drug-induced delayed multiorgan hypersensitivity syndrome' (DIDMOHS) and DIHS (drug-induced hypersensitivity syndrome). The clinical presentation of DRESS includes beside exanthema (figure 11A), hematologic abnormalities, enlargement of lymph nodes and organ involvement.[Bocquet, et al., 1996] The initial exanthema in DRESS may have a morbilliform, sometimes target-like appearance, but then often evolves into erythroderma. Patients have facial edema, which often is more pronounced in the periorbital region. Sometimes the reaction is accompanied by cheilitis and redness of the pharynx and small erosions on the oral mucosa. Most commonly aromatic anti-convulsant drugs such as phenytoin, carbamazepine, and phenobarbital as well as allopurinol have been reported as triggering DRESS.[Kardaun, et al., 2010b] There are also numerous reports of DRESS after administration of minocycline, thalidomide, and sulfonamides.[Bocquet, et al., 1996] Furthermore, a variety of other drugs, such as lamotrigine as well as valproic acid and non-steroidal anti-inflammatory drugs (NSAIDs) have been associated with this clinical entity.[Wolf, et al., 2005a, Wolf, et al., 2005b] It has also been suggested that virus reactivation may play an important role in the development of DRESS, and possibly also in a recurrent course or persistence of disease.[Kano, et al., 2006] Japanese research groups have consistently shown that human herpes virus 6 (HHV-6) reactivation can be detected in the vast majority of their patients who meet the criteria for DRESS.[Shiohara, et al., 2007, Shiohara, et al., 2006] These authors included HHV-6 reactivation as a diagnostic criterion and coined the term 'drug-induced hypersensitivity syndrome' (DHIS). They speculate that patients fulfilling the criteria of DIHS may represent those with a more severe form of DRESS.[Shiohara, et al., 2007, Shiohara, et al., 2006] However, it has still not been conclusively explained whether the reactivation of HHV-6 and other members of the human herpes virus family are part of the disease itself or whether they are better interpreted as a complication.

To date, various diagnostic criteria have been identified: maculopapular rash developing more than 3 weeks after starting a drug, prolonged clinical symptoms 2 weeks after discontinuation of the causative drug, fever (> 38°C), hematological abnormalities such as eosinophilia (> 1.5×10^9/l), leukocytosis (>$11x10^9$L) and/or the presence of atypical lymphocytes in peripheral blood (> 5%), systemic involvement with lymph node enlargement and involvement of at least one internal organ such as hepatitis (more than twofold increase in transaminase values), interstitial nephritis, interstitial pneumonia, and carditis.[Kardaun, et al., 2007, Shiohara, et al., 2007] Along with the previously mentioned changes seen in blood work, patients may also experience thrombocytopenia and a drop in hemoglobin levels. Pathological liver, kidney, and other laboratory values should be present for several days. Lymph node enlargement should be present at a minimum of two different sites. In organ manifestations, interstitial inflammation (kidney, lung) predominates. Furthermore, joint pain and myositis, including myocarditis may occur.

5.2 Histology

The skin changes seen in DRESS are highly variable, and so is histology, which has not been studied systematically for this disease entity. A variety of histopathologic features has been described in patients with DRESS. Histology in many cases shows solitary to many scattered necrotic keratinocytes with basal cell vacuolar degeneration and papillary edema. The accompanying lymphocytic infiltrate (drug-specific T-cells also play a role in DRESS) may be dense lichenoid with melanophages and some eosinophilc granulocytes, resembling the pattern of a lichenoid drug eruption, or very sparse making the findings compatible with early features of EM (figure 11B). Dermal edema may be present, but is not necessarily so. Sometimes a band-like infiltrate consisting of atypical lymphocytes with epidermotropism is noted that resembles mycosis fungoides.[Bocquet, et al., 1996] Furthermore, leukocytoclastic vasculitis and pseudolymphomatous histology were described in patients with DRESS.[Bocquet, et al., 1996, Chiou, et al., 2008]

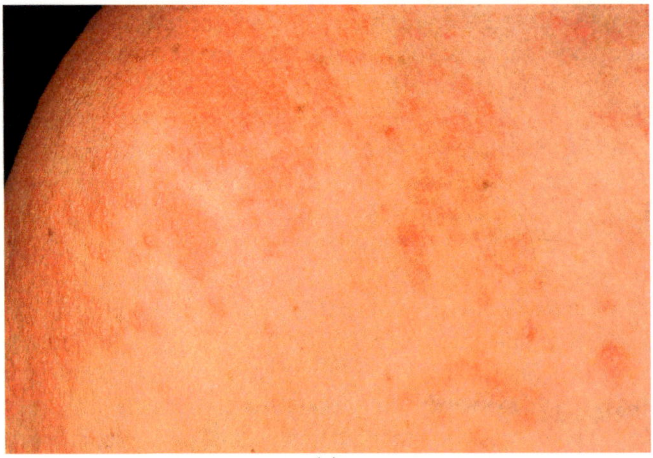

(a)

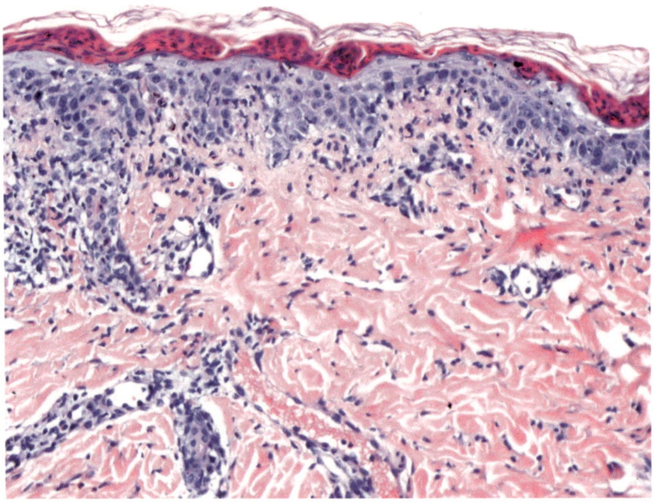

(b)

Fig. 11. A: Generalized erythematous confluent maculo-papules. Detail from the shoulder. B: One of the possible histopathologic presentations of DRESS. A confluent zone of parakeratosis below a basket-weave cornified layer. Dermal, superficial, sparse, perivascular and interstitial infiltrate of lymphocytes. Focal vacuolar alteration along the dermoepidermal junction in company with some lymphocytes. Scattered necrotic keratinocytes throughout the entire epidermis. Necrotic keratinocytes also along an acrosyringium. (hematoxylin-eosin, original magnification x200).

5.3 Differential diagnoses histopathologically

As the histopathologic findings in DRESS are very heterogeneous, final diagnosis is mainly based on clinical criteria and specific lab values as indicated by the diagnostic score published by Kardaun and colleagues. [Kardaun, et al., 2007].

6. Toxic erythemas after chemotherapy

6.1 Clinical presentation

Usually toxic erythema after chemotherapy develops on the palms, soles, as well as fingers and toes beginning with dysesthesia followed by edema and erythema. Such condition is known as palmoplantar erythrodysesthesia (PPE). Fissuring and ulceration develop in severe cases, observed in about one third of treated patients, associated with extreme pain, impeded walking and grasping.[Fabian, et al., 1990, Lokich and Moore, 1984, Muggia, et al., 1997, Vogelzang and Ratain, 1985, Zuehlke, 1974] Apart from palms and soles, or rather hands and feet in general, lesions may develop on any other skin area. Severe involvement has been reported on buttocks[Lopez, et al., 1999] and os sacrum.[Muggia, et al., 1997, Uziely, et al., 1995] Further locations are mentioned occasionally. Such changes have been reported under different names, to wit, "chemotherapy-induced toxic erythema" or intertriginous epidermal dysmaturation".[English, et al., 2003, Skelton, et al., 2002] However, proceeding from the influence of mechanical stress in the pathogenesis of palmoplantar erythrodysesthesia and the increased accumulation of the drug in sweat glands, involvement of more extensive parts of the body is most likely. Flexural areas are predisposed due to lasting influence of friction and dense distribution of sweat glands (figures 12A and 12B). Such clinical manifestations are in the spectrum of chemotherapy-induced epidermal changes, showing identical clinical as well as histopathologic features.

6.2 Histology

Despite the numerous publications, histopathologic features have not systematically been described. Typical features include a vacuolar degeneration of the basal layer of the epidermis together with necrotic keratinocytes and mild spongiosis. Dermal changes may include slight papillary edema, dilated blood vessels and a sparse superficial perivascular lymphocytic infiltrate.[Nagore, et al., 2000] Other authors described the condition as marked by hyperkeratosis.[Comandone, et al., 1993, Gordon, et al., 1995] However, hyperkeratosis is not related to the drug reaction but simply explained by the volar location of the lesions. In cases of PPE developing on non-volar skin, this feature is not present. Histopathologic changes of PPE are indistinguishable from other chemotherapy-induced toxic erythemas such as generalized erythema [Hymes, et al., 1985b, Yokel, et al., 1987] or lesions reported as "intertriginous epidermal dysmaturation".[English, et al., 2003] Those conditions show similar epidermal changes with vacuolization and necrotic keratinocytes that are disposed solitary or in clusters near the junction and sometimes also within the middle and upper spinous layers. Often chemotherapeutics cause epidermal maturation disturbances with individual enlarged keratinocytes with abnormally large nuclei and prominent nucleoli (figure 12 C).

6.3 Differential diagnoses histopathologically

Similar changes, however without keratinocyte maturation disturbances, are also present in SJS/TEN or fixed drug eruption. Fixed drug eruptions comparatively show a superficial perivascular, and interstitial infiltrate that includes eosinophilic and neutrophilic granulocytes in most instances. SJS/TEN is best differentiated by clinical impression; however, diagnosis might be difficult in early stages. Principally, it is true that similar histologic features appear in acute graft-versus-host disease.[Beard, et al., 1993] However, graft-versus-host disease is distinguishable, in particular together with the patient's history of stem cell or bone marrow transplantation.

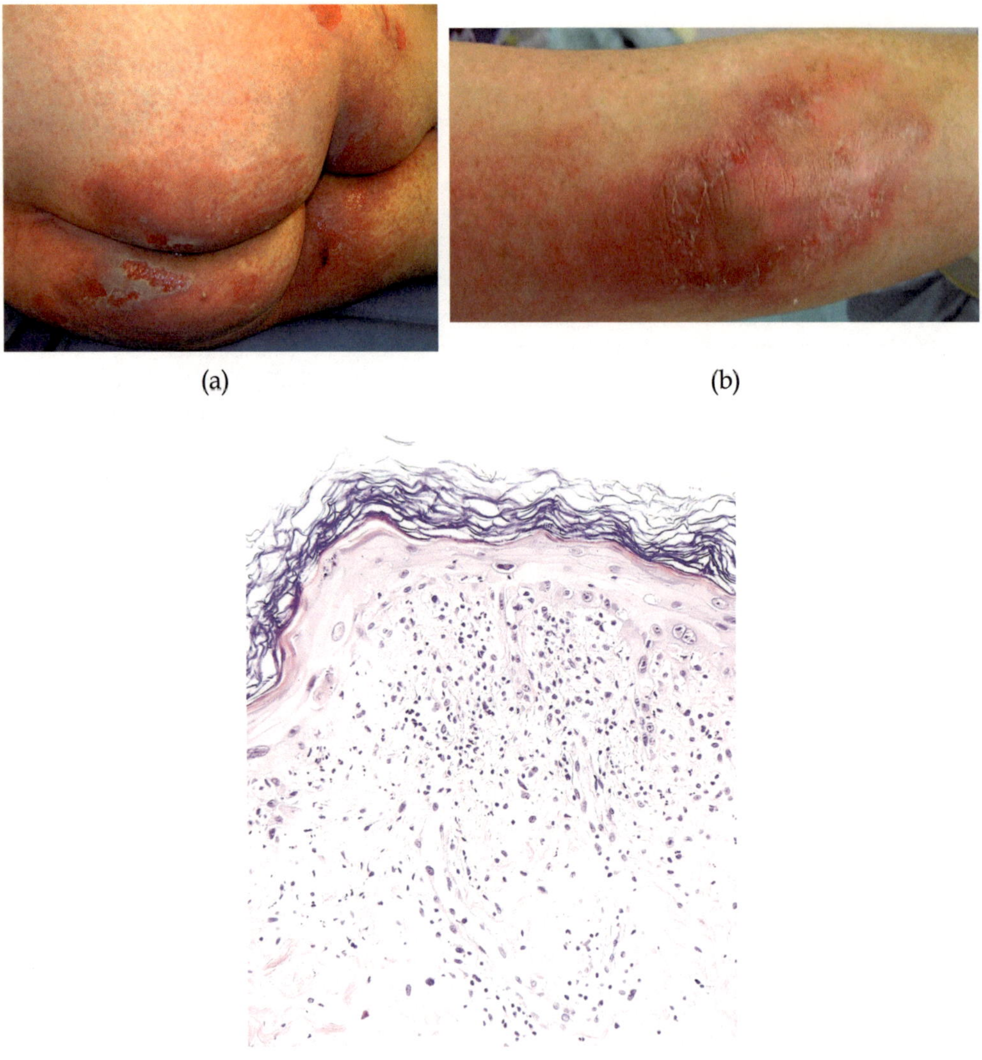

Fig. 12. A and B: Toxic erythema after chemotherapy with pegylated doxorubicine. Confluent erythematous macules to large erythemas with epidermolysis. Severe involvement of mechanically stressed areas such as the buttocks, sacrum and elbows. C: Vacuolization and necrotic keratinocytes disposed solitary near the junction. Epidermal maturation disturbances with individual enlarged keratinocytes with prominent nucleoli (hematoxylin-eosin, original magnification x40).

7. Drug-induced linear-IgA dermatosis

7.1 Clinical presentation

Linear IgA dermatosis (LAD) is a rare autoimmune subepidermal blistering disorder. Although in most instances idiopathic, LAD may be drug-related. Multiple drugs have been reported to cause LAD, but vancomycin is reported most frequently.[Brinkmeier, et al., 2003] Classically, LAD shows tense blisters with a linear or annular arrangement on erythematous or normal appearing skin (figures 13A and 13B). Sites of predilection are the trunk, lower extremities, face, perineum and groins. Mucous membrane involvement, reported in idiopathic LAD with about 50%, is observed less often. However, the clinical presentations of both idiopathic and drug-related LAD are variable and may mimic other blistering disorders, such as bullous pemphigoid, dermatitis herpetiformis, and SJS/TEN. In drug-induced LAD, the onset of blisters usually occurs within 7–15 days after beginning of drug use with a mean onset of 8 days and resolution within 2–7 weeks upon drug withdrawal.[Nousari, et al., 1999] Circulating IgA-antibodies are found in less than 40% of cases.[Nousari, et al., 1999] Antigenic targets are heterogeneous.[Wojnarowska, et al., 1999] Patient's sera react against the basement membrane similar to the pattern observed with antibodies to the hemidesmosome components, the alpha6beta4 integrin and the bullous pemphigoid antigens BP230 and BP180, 255-kD and 285-kD proteins as well as collagen VII.[Wojnarowska, et al., 1999]

7.2 Histology

Histologically, LAD shows subepidermal blisters most often with an infiltrate primarily consisting of neutrophils (figures 13C and 13D). As much as clinically, LAD is variable histopathologically, resembling bullous pemphigoid, dermatitis herpetiformis, or epidermolysis bullosa aquisita. Even LAD under the clinical picture of SJS/TEN has been reported.[Schneck, et al., 1999] Direct immunofluorescence of perilesional skin shows linear deposition of IgA along the basement membrane zone, usually in a homogenous pattern (figure 13E). Examples of granular linear deposition at the BMZ have also been identified.[Kuechle, et al., 1994] In addition, C3 deposition at the BMZ is also found on occasion.[Kuechle, et al., 1994]

7.3 Differential diagnoses histopathologically

The diagnosis of LAD cannot be made exclusively based on histopathology. Clinical data as well a results form direct and indirect immunofluorescence have to be considered. Differentiation has to be made in particular from bullous pemphigoid, dermatitis herpetiformis, and epidermolysis bullosa aquisita.

8. Principles and techniques of skin biopsies in drug eruptions [Ackerman, et al., 2005, Weyers and Diaz, 2002]

In patients with severe skin reactions, a skin biopsy should be taken whenever possible. The clinician is obliged to present rudimentary information to the dermatohistopathologist. In several instances histopathologic diagnosis is impossible without any clinical information. Such information is: age and gender of the patient, duration of the disease/biopsied lesion, distribution, configuration and arrangement of lesions, morphology of the individual lesion, localization and type of biopsy, suggested clinical diagnosis and differential diagnosis. The skin biopsy itself follows an essential sequence beginning with the selection of one or more lesions for biopsy, sampling of the tissue with optimal technique, correct fixation of the tissue and finally the accurate histopathologic diagnosis.

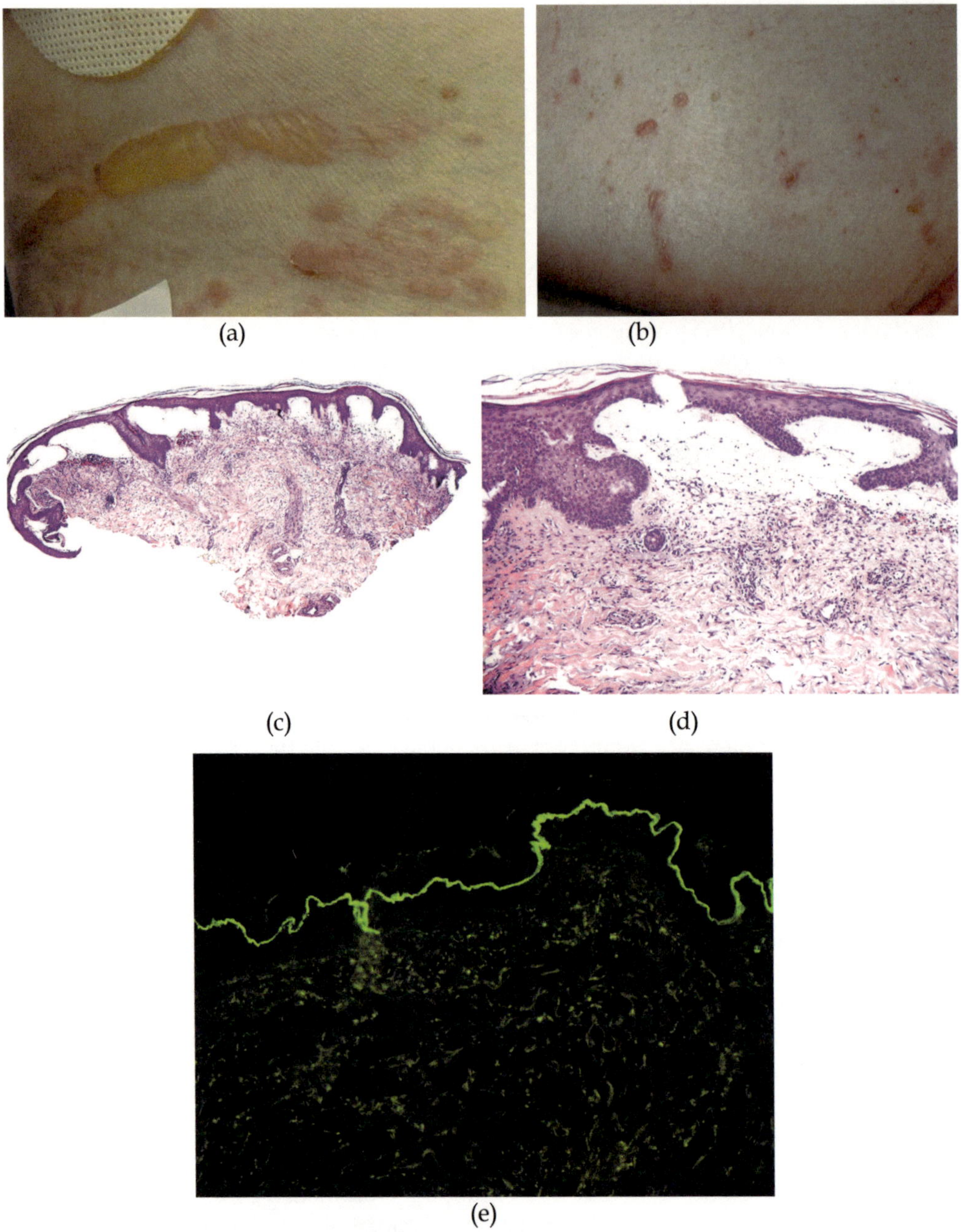

Fig. 13. A and B: Tense blisters with a linear or annular arrangement on erythematous but mostly normal appearing skin.
C and D: Subepidermal blisters with an infiltrate of neutrophilic and eosinophilic granulocytes (B: hematoxylin-eosin, original magnification x40, C: hematoxylin-eosin, original magnification x200).
E: Direct immunofluorescence of perilesional skin with linear homogenous deposition of IgA along the basement membrane zone (original magnification x200).

The very-first criterion for the selection of the biopsy-site is the appearance of the efflorescence. As a general rule, biopsies should not be performed from excoriated or scarred lesions, and postinflammatory pigmentary changes. Those, in most instances, do not provide enough information for evaluation of the nature of the underlying inflammatory process. Preferentially, a fresh primary lesion should be selected, without secondary changes. Such are: macules and papules (papules are preferred to macules), papulovesicles, vesicles or pustules. If similar lesions are present on the legs and elsewhere, the biopsy should not be taken from the legs below the knee. In the latter localization changes could be superimposed by stasis dermatitis, complicating the correct histopathologic diagnosis. The biopsy should be performed in the most inflamed area. In some situations it could be helpful to take several or sequential biopsies, in particular if primary lesions are present in different stages of evolution. In cases of vesicular or bullous lesions or even widespread epidermolysis the biopsy should be performed at the periphery of the blister/bulla including larger parts of the surrounding erythema. A biopsy from the blister itself or from the surrounding of older blisters has to be avoided. If the biopsy is taken from the blister itself, the roof of the blister usually gets lost and consequently is not available for histopathologic evaluation. However, even if present, the blister roof is mostly already totally necrotic. Moreover, direct immunofluorescence (where necessary for differential diagnosis) from the blister itself gives false negative results. Furthermore, older blisters are often contaminated with bacteria, show signs of re-epithelialization and again do not allow for direct immunofluorescence. In most instances a punch biopsy is adequate. The biopsy punch is penetrated up to the subcutaneous adipose tissue. The dermis easily separates from the subcutis and the tissue cylinder can be removed gently (to avoid squeezing artefacts) with anatomic forceps. The resulting defect is in most instances closed with a simple suture. A sufficient size (advised are at least 6mm) of the biopsy punch has to be chosen. It has to be kept in mind that subsequent formalin fixation and paraffin embedding reduce the tissue-volume up to one third. Alternatively an excision biopsy with a scalpel can be performed. In particular, biopsies from bullous skin diseases have, apart from tiny tense vesicles, to be performed with a scalpel since a punch biopsy leads to the loss of the epidermis. Shave biopsies *are inadequate*. A shave in general is not a proper technique for biopsy of inflammatory dermatoses. Moreover, histopathologic analysis of a biopsy taken from a blister only does not allow the various types of reaction to be distinguished. After removal of the specimen it should be added to a fixative solution. The common fixative for skin tissue is 4 % or 10 % buffered formalin (formaldehyde). The amount of formalin should excess the volume of the specimen by about 20times. Before further technical preparation, the specimen should be kept in formalin at least for several hours to obtain optimal fixation. No refrigeration is needed. Formalin is inappropriate as transport medium for direct immunofluorescence. Diverse electrolyte solutions have been suggested for immunofluorescence and vary in laboratories of different countries (e.g. Michel´s medium; isotonic sodium chloride solution; or a ready-to-use 'electrolyte solution 77 with glucose 5', Serumwerk Bernburg AG; Germany). In the vast majority of cases histopathologic diagnosis is based on a few hematoxylin & eosin sections. Slides should be systematically screened in all its layers. Further histochemical stainings (such as periodic-acid-Schiff (PAS), Masson Fontana, Giemsa) are usually not necessary, but can be helpful for differential diagnosis. Immunhistochemical stainings are not routinely performed. Immunhistochemical stainings, using polyclonal or monoclonal antibodies binding specifically to tissue antigens, may be of scientific interest concerning CD-antigens or antibodies against cytokines or cytokine receptors. If differential diagnosis includes autoimmune bullous skin disorders, immunofluorescence should be performed and an additional biopsy specimen (or part of a biopsy) should be taken for direct immunofluorescence. Direct immunofluorescence uses single antibodies which are chemically linked to a fluorophore which can be detected via microscope. Routinely, IgG, IgM, IgA, complement factors (C3) and fibrin are used to detect intra- and subepidermal, basal membrane zone, or perivascular depositions. These may be helpful in differentiating bullous drug eruption from primarily autoimmune-blistering diseases, such as bullous pemphigoid or pemphigus. In particular, this can be of importance in diagnosing drug-induced linear-IgA-dermatosis. For sampling of tissue for direct immunofluorescence the following has to be considered: a biopsy for direct immunofluorescence is more suitable from direct perilesional skin. The biopsy of a blister itself has to be avoided.

Sine qua non, however, prior to any sophisticated technique, is a close contact to the clinician and whenever possible a clinical-histopathologic correlation. In case direct consultation of the patient is not possible, means of teledermatology can be used. Dermatology is ideally suited for telemedicine techniques, as has been shown in a number of recent studies investigating feasibility and reliability of teledermatology.[Massone, et al., 2008] It has generally demonstrated high levels of concordance in diagnoses compared with face-to-face consultations. Moreover, the implementation of virtual slide systems for teledermatopathology has allowed avoiding the limitations imposed by conventional microphotography.[Massone, et al., 2008]

9. Conclusion

Severe cutaneous adverse reactions - mainly related to drugs - include several distinct clinical entities. Within the past decades enormous endeavor has been made to clinically classify SJS, TEN and transitional forms and separate them clinically from EMM. In addition, new disease entities have been described, among them AGEP and DRESS, formerly referred to as hypersensitivity syndrome. GBFDE has been recognized as a severe form of the well known localized fixed drug eruption. In clinical terms, for all those entities substantiated classification criteria have been developed and established in clinical practice. However, despite all these efforts, some diagnostic gaps still exist from a histopathologic point of view. This is based on the fact that several entities of severe cutaneous adverse reactions have histopathologic features in common, impeding the exact separation among each other. In addition, superficially or insufficiently performed biopsies complicate the diagnosis. Generally accepted standards of biopsy and sample processing including (additional) stainings or techniques are still missing. Histopathologic assessment and report of findings is still arbitrary with many inter-observer variations. Since all named entities are quite rare, the quality of histopathologic assessment depends mainly on the experience of the histopathologist. Besides this, difficulties may occur in differentiation of severe cutaneous adverse reactions from unrelated inflammatory skin diseases.

10. References

Abe, R, Shimizu, T, Shibaki, A, Nakamura, H, Watanabe, H and Shimizu, H. (2003). Toxic epidermal necrolysis and Stevens-Johnson syndrome are induced by soluble Fas ligand. *Am J Pathol.* 162(5): 1515-1520.

Ackerman, AB, Böer, A, Bennin, B and Gottlieb, JG. Histologic Diagnosis of Inflammatory Skin Diseases. An Algorithmic Method Based on Pattern Analysis. 3 edn., ed.: ArdorScribendi. 2005.

Ackerman, AB, Kerl, H, Sánchez, J, et al. A Clinical Atlas of 101 Common Skin Diseases with histopathologic correlation. 2 edn., ed. New York City: Ardor Scribendi. 2000.

Ackerman, AB and Ragaz, A. The lives of lesions: chronology in dermatopathology ed. New York: Lea & Febiger. 1984

Auquier-Dunant, A, Mockenhaupt, M, Naldi, L, Correia, O, Schroder, W and Roujeau, JC. (2002). Correlations between clinical patterns and causes of erythema multiforme majus, Stevens-Johnson syndrome, and toxic epidermal necrolysis: results of an international prospective study. *Arch Dermatol.* 138(8): 1019-1024.

Bastuji-Garin, S, Rzany, B, Stern, RS, Shear, NH, Naldi, L and Roujeau, JC. (1993). Clinical classification of cases of toxic epidermal necrolysis, Stevens-Johnson syndrome, and erythema multiforme. *Arch Dermatol.* 129(1): 92-96.

Beard, JS, Smith, KJ and Skelton, HG. (1993). Combination chemotherapy with 5-fluorouracil, folinic acid, and alpha-interferon producing histologic features of graft-versus-host disease. *J Am Acad Dermatol.* 29(2 Pt 2): 325-330.

Bigby, M. (2001). Rates of cutaneous reactions to drugs. *Arch Dermatol.* 137(6): 765-770.

Bigby, M, Jick, S, Jick, H and Arndt, K. (1986). Drug-induced cutaneous reactions. A report from the Boston Collaborative Drug Surveillance Program on 15,438 consecutive inpatients, 1975 to 1982. *JAMA.* 256(24): 3358-3363.

Bocquet, H, Bagot, M and Roujeau, JC. (1996). Drug-induced pseudolymphoma and drug hypersensitivity syndrome (Drug Rash with Eosinophilia and Systemic Symptoms: DRESS). *Semin Cutan Med Surg.* 15(4): 250-257.

Brinkmeier, T, Angelkort, B, Frosch, PJ and Herbst, RA. (2003). [Vancomycin-induced linear IgA dermatosis]. *J Dtsch Dermatol Ges.* 1(3): 212-214.

Britschgi, M, Steiner, UC, Schmid, S, et al. (2001). T-cell involvement in drug-induced acute generalized exanthematous pustulosis. *J Clin Invest.* 107(11): 1433-1441.

Burrows, NP and Russell Jones, RR. (1993). Pustular drug eruptions: a histopathological spectrum. *Histopathology.* 22(6): 569-573.

Chang, HY, Cooper, ZA, Swetter, SM and Marinkovich, MP. (2004). Kinetics and specificity of fas ligand induction in toxic epidermal necrolysis. *Arch Dermatol.* 140(2): 242-244.

Chiou, CC, Yang, LC, Hung, SI, et al. (2008). Clinicopathological features and prognosis of drug rash with eosinophilia and systemic symptoms: a study of 30 cases in Taiwan. *J Eur Acad Dermatol Venereol.* 22(9): 1044-1049.

Chung, WH, Hung, SI, Yang, JY, et al. (2008). Granulysin is a key mediator for disseminated keratinocyte death in Stevens-Johnson syndrome and toxic epidermal necrolysis. *Nat Med.* 14(12): 1343-1350.

Comandone, A, Bretti, S, La Grotta, G, et al. (1993). Palmar-plantar erythrodysestasia syndrome associated with 5-fluorouracil treatment. *Anticancer Res.* 13(5C): 1781-1783.

Crowson, AN, Brown, TJ and Magro, CM. (2003). Progress in the understanding of the pathology and pathogenesis of cutaneous drug eruptions : implications for management. *Am J Clin Dermatol.* 4(6): 407-428.

de Araujo, E, Dessirier, V, Lapree, G, et al. (2011). Death ligand TRAIL, secreted by CD1a+ and CD14+ cells in blister fluids, is involved in killing keratinocytes in toxic epidermal necrolysis. *Exp Dermatol.* 20(2): 107-112.

Elliott, CJ, Sloane, JP, Sanderson, KV, Vincent, M, Shepherd, V and Powles, R. (1987). The histological diagnosis of cutaneous graft versus host disease: relationship of skin changes to marrow purging and other clinical variables. *Histopathology.* 11(2): 145-155.

English, JC, 3rd, Toney, R and Patterson, JW. (2003). Intertriginous epidermal dysmaturation from pegylated liposomal doxorubicin. *J Cutan Pathol.* 30(9): 591-595.

Fabian, CJ, Molina, R, Slavik, M, Dahlberg, S, Giri, S and Stephens, R. (1990). Pyridoxine therapy for palmar-plantar erythrodysesthesia associated with continuous 5-fluorouracil infusion. *Invest New Drugs.* 8(1): 57-63.

Gerson, D, Sriganeshan, V and Alexis, JB. (2008). Cutaneous drug eruptions: a 5-year experience. *J Am Acad Dermatol.* 59(6): 995-999.

Gordon, KB, Tajuddin, A, Guitart, J, Kuzel, TM, Eramo, LR and VonRoenn, J. (1995). Hand-foot syndrome associated with liposome-encapsulated doxorubicin therapy. *Cancer.* 75(8): 2169-2173.

Halevy, S, Kardaun, SH, Davidovici, B and Wechsler, J. (2010) The spectrum of histopathological features in acute generalized exanthematous pustulosis: a study of 102 cases. *Br J Dermatol.* 163(6): 1245-1252.

Harman, KE, Holmes, G, Bhogal, BS, McFadden, J and Black, MM. (1999). Intercellular IgA dermatosis (IgA pemphigus)--two cases illustrating the clinical heterogeneity of this disorder. *Clin Exp Dermatol.* 24(6): 464-466.

Horn, TD. (1994). Acute cutaneous eruptions after marrow ablation: roses by other names? *J Cutan Pathol.* 21(5): 385-392.

Horn, TD, Zahurak, ML, Atkins, D, Solomon, AR and Vogelsang, GB. (1997). Lichen planus-like histopathologic characteristics in the cutaneous graft-vs-host reaction. Prognostic significance independent of time course after allogeneic bone marrow transplantation. *Arch Dermatol.* 133(8): 961-965.

Hymes, SR, Farmer, ER, Lewis, PG, Tutschka, PJ and Santos, GW. (1985a). Cutaneous graft-versus-host reaction: prognostic features seen by light microscopy. *J Am Acad Dermatol.* 12(3): 468-474.

Hymes, SR, Simonton, SC, Farmer, ER, Beschorner, WB, Tutschka, PJ and Santos, GW. (1985b). Cutaneous busulfan effect in patients receiving bone-marrow transplantation. *J Cutan Pathol.* 12(2): 125-129.

Kano, Y, Hiraharas, K, Sakuma, K and Shiohara, T. (2006). Several herpesviruses can reactivate in a severe drug-induced multiorgan reaction in the same sequential order as in graft-versus-host disease. *Br J Dermatol.* 155(2): 301-306.

Kaplan, AP. (1984). Drug-induced skin disease. *J Allergy Clin Immunol.* 74(4 Pt 2): 573-579.

Kardaun, SH, Kuiper, H, Fidler, V and Jonkman, MF. (2010a). The histopathological spectrum of acute generalized exanthematous pustulosis (AGEP) and its differentiation from generalized pustular psoriasis. *J Cutan Pathol.* 37(12): 1220-1229.

Kardaun, SH, Sekula, P, Mockenhaupt, M and Roujeau, JC. (2010b); Drugs inducing DRESS (Drug Reaction with Eosinophilia and Systemic Symptoms): the RegiSCAR experience. Proceedings of the 26th International Conference for Pharmacoepidemiology; Brighton, UK, 19. - 22. August 2010: *Pharmacoepidem Dr S;* 19, S1-S347: S39.

Kardaun, SH, Sidoroff, A, Valeyrie-Allanore, L, et al. (2007). Variability in the clinical pattern of cutaneous side-effects of drugs with systemic symptoms: does a DRESS syndrome really exist? *Br J Dermatol.* 156(3): 609-611.

Kauppinen, K. (1972). Cutaneous reactions to drugs with special reference to severe bullous mucocutaneous eruptions and sulphonamides. *Acta Derm Venereol Suppl (Stockh).* 68: 1-89.

Kauppinen, K and Stubb, S. (1984). Drug eruptions: causative agents and clinical types. A series of in-patients during a 10-year period. *Acta Derm Venereol.* 64(4): 320-324.

Kuechle, MK, Stegemeir, E, Maynard, B, Gibson, LE, Leiferman, KM and Peters, MS. (1994). Drug-induced linear IgA bullous dermatosis: report of six cases and review of the literature. *J Am Acad Dermatol.* 30(2 Pt 1): 187-192.

Lokich, JJ and Moore, C. (1984). Chemotherapy-associated palmar-plantar erythrodysesthesia syndrome. *Ann Intern Med.* 101(6): 798-799.

Lopez, AM, Wallace, L, Dorr, RT, Koff, M, Hersh, EM and Alberts, DS. (1999). Topical DMSO treatment for pegylated liposomal doxorubicin-induced palmar-plantar erythrodysesthesia. *Cancer Chemother Pharmacol.* 44(4): 303-306.

Mahboob, A and Haroon, TS. (1998). Drugs causing fixed eruptions: a study of 450 cases. *Int J Dermatol.* 37(11): 833-838.

Massone, C, Wurm, EM, Hofmann-Wellenhof, R and Soyer, HP. (2008). Teledermatology: an update. *Semin Cutan Med Surg.* 27(1): 101-105.

Mockenhaupt, M. (2008). *Severe cutaneous adverse reactions.* In: Burgdorf, WHC, Plewig, G, Wolff, HH and Landthaler, M, ed.^eds. Braun-Falco's Dermatology. Heidelberg, Germany: Springer Medizin Verlag, 473-483.

Mockenhaupt, M, Herb, T, Liß, Y, Bork, K and Haustein, UF. (2010). Generalized bullous fixed drug eruption: analysis of 62 cases. 4th International Drug Hypersensivity Meeting, Rome, 22. - 25. April 2010. *European Annals of Allergy and Clinical Immunology.* 42(2): 43.

Mockenhaupt, M, Idzko, M, Grosber, M, Schöpf, E and Norgauer, J. (2005). Epidemiology of staphylococcal scalded skin syndrome in Germany. *J Invest Dermatol.* 124(4): 700-703.

Mockenhaupt, M and Norgauer. (2002). Cutaneous adverse drug reactions: Stevens-Johnson syndrome and toxic epidermal necrolysis. *Allergy Clin Immunol Int: J World Allergy Org.* 14: 143-150.

Mockenhaupt, M, Viboud, C, Dunant, A, et al. (2008). Stevens-Johnson syndrome and toxic epidermal necrolysis: assessment of medication risks with emphasis on recently marketed drugs. The EuroSCAR-study. *J Invest Dermatol*. 128(1): 35-44.

Muggia, FM, Hainsworth, JD, Jeffers, S, et al. (1997). Phase II study of liposomal doxorubicin in refractory ovarian cancer: antitumor activity and toxicity modification by liposomal encapsulation. *J Clin Oncol*. 15(3): 987-993.

Nagore, E, Insa, A and Sanmartin, O. (2000). Antineoplastic therapy-induced palmar plantar erythrodysesthesia ('hand-foot') syndrome. Incidence, recognition and management. *Am J Clin Dermatol*. 1(4): 225-234.

Nassif, A, Bensussan, A, Boumsell, L, et al. (2004a). Toxic epidermal necrolysis: effector cells are drug-specific cytotoxic T cells. *J Allergy Clin Immunol*. 114(5): 1209-1215.

Nassif, A, Bensussan, A, Dorothee, G, et al. (2002). Drug specific cytotoxic T-cells in the skin lesions of a patient with toxic epidermal necrolysis. *J Invest Dermatol*. 118(4): 728-733.

Nassif, A, Moslehi, H, Le Gouvello, S, et al. (2004b). Evaluation of the potential role of cytokines in toxic epidermal necrolysis. *J Invest Dermatol*. 123(5): 850-855.

Niimi, Y, Kawana, S and Kusunoki, T. (2000). IgA pemphigus: a case report and its characteristic clinical features compared with subcorneal pustular dermatosis. *J Am Acad Dermatol*. 43(3): 546-549.

Nousari, HC, Kimyai-Asadi, A, Caeiro, JP and Anhalt, GJ. (1999). Clinical, demographic, and immunohistologic features of vancomycin-induced linear IgA bullous disease of the skin. Report of 2 cases and review of the literature. *Medicine (Baltimore)*. 78(1): 1-8.

Paquet, P, Arrese, JE, Beguin, Y and Pierard, GE. (2001). Clinicopathological differential diagnosis of drug-induced toxic epidermal necrolysis (Lyell's syndrome) and acute graft-versus-host reaction. *Curr Top Pathol*. 94: 49-63.

Pichler, WJ, Yawalkar, N, Britschgi, M, et al. (2002). Cellular and molecular pathophysiology of cutaneous drug reactions. *Am J Clin Dermatol*. 3(4): 229-238.

Roujeau, JC. (2005). Clinical heterogeneity of drug hypersensitivity. *Toxicology*. 209(2): 123-129.

Roujeau, JC, Bioulac-Sage, P, Bourseau, C, et al. (1991). Acute generalized exanthematous pustulosis. Analysis of 63 cases. *Arch Dermatol*. 127(9): 1333-1338.

Roujeau, JC and Stern, RS. (1994). Severe adverse cutaneous reactions to drugs. *N Engl J Med*. 331(19): 1272-1285.

Rzany, B, Hering, O, Mockenhaupt, M, et al. (1996). Histopathological and epidemiological characteristics of patients with erythema exudativum multiforme major, Stevens-Johnson syndrome and toxic epidermal necrolysis. *Br J Dermatol*. 135(1): 6-11.

Schneck, B, Termeer, C, Mockenhaupt, M, Augustin, M and Schopf, E. (1999). [Linear IgA dermatosis in an adult with clinical signs of Stevens-Johnson syndrome]. *Hautarzt*. 50(4): 288-291.

Shiohara, T, Iijima, M, Ikezawa, Z and Hashimoto, K. (2007). The diagnosis of a DRESS syndrome has been sufficiently established on the basis of typical clinical features and viral reactivations. *Br J Dermatol.* 156(5): 1083-1084.

Shiohara, T, Inaoka, M and Kano, Y. (2006). Drug-induced hypersensitivity syndrome (DIHS): a reaction induced by a complex interplay among herpesviruses and antiviral and antidrug immune responses. *Allergol Int.* 55(1): 1-8.

Sidoroff, A, Dunant, A, Viboud, C, et al. (2007). Risk factors for acute generalized exanthematous pustulosis (AGEP)-results of a multinational case-control study (EuroSCAR). *Br J Dermatol.* 157(5): 989-996.

Sidoroff, A, Halevy, S, Bavinck, JN, Vaillant, L and Roujeau, JC. (2001). Acute generalized exanthematous pustulosis (AGEP)--a clinical reaction pattern. *J Cutan Pathol.* 28(3): 113-119.

Skelton, H, Linstrum, J and Smith, K. (2002). Host-vs.-altered-host eruptions in patients on liposomal doxorubicin. *J Cutan Pathol.* 29(3): 148-153.

Sneddon, IB and Wilkinson, DS. (1956). Subcorneal pustular dermatosis. *Br J Dermatol.* 68(12): 385-394.

Snover, D. The pathology of acute graft-vs-host disease. Burakoff, S, ed. New York: M. Decker. 1990. 337-353.

Stubb, S, Heikkila, H and Kauppinen, K. (1994). Cutaneous reactions to drugs: a series of in-patients during a five-year period. *Acta Derm Venereol.* 74(4): 289-291.

Sviland, L, Pearson, AD, Eastham, EJ, Hamilton, PJ, Proctor, SJ and Malcolm, AJ. (1988). Histological features of skin and rectal biopsy specimens after autologous and allogeneic bone marrow transplantation. *J Clin Pathol.* 41(2): 148-154.

Uziely, B, Jeffers, S, Isacson, R, et al. (1995). Liposomal doxorubicin: antitumor activity and unique toxicities during two complementary phase I studies. *J Clin Oncol.* 13(7): 1777-1785.

Viard, I, Wehrli, P, Bullani, R, et al. (1998). Inhibition of toxic epidermal necrolysis by blockade of CD95 with human intravenous immunoglobulin. *Science.* 282(5388): 490-493.

Vogelzang, NJ and Ratain, MJ. (1985). Cancer chemotherapy and skin changes. *Ann Intern Med.* 103(2): 303-304.

Weyers, W and Diaz, C. (2002). [Basic principles of skin biopsy]. *Pathologe.* 23(1): 4-8.

Wintroub, BU and Stern, R. (1985). Cutaneous drug reactions: pathogenesis and clinical classification. *J Am Acad Dermatol.* 13(2 Pt 1): 167-179.

Wojnarowska, F, Allen, J, Collier, PM and Leigh, IM. (1999). A comparison of the expression of known basement membrane components with the linear IgA disease antigens using the novel substrate cylindroma. *Br J Dermatol.* 141(1): 62-70.

Wolf, R, Matz, H, Marcos, B and Orion, E. (2005a). Drug rash with eosinophilia and systemic symptoms vs toxic epidermal necrolysis: the dilemma of classification. *Clin Dermatol.* 23(3): 311-314.

Wolf, R, Orion, E, Marcos, B and Matz, H. (2005b). Life-threatening acute adverse cutaneous drug reactions. *Clin Dermatol.* 23(2): 171-181.

Yokel, BK, Friedman, KJ, Farmer, ER and Hood, AF. (1987). Cutaneous pathology following etoposide therapy. *J Cutan Pathol.* 14(6): 326-330.

Ziemer, M and Böer, A. (2006). Pustular psoriasis - A historical perspective. *Dermatopathol: Pract & Conc.* 2006;12(3):8. Available at: http://derm101.com/content/32494

Ziemer, M, Wiesend, CL, Vetter, R, et al. (2007). Cutaneous adverse reactions to valdecoxib distinct from Stevens-Johnson syndrome and toxic epidermal necrolysis. *Arch Dermatol.* 143(6): 711-716.

Zuehlke, RL. (1974). Erythematous eruption of the palms and soles associated with mitotane therapy. *Dermatologica.* 148(2): 90-92.

7

Severe Cutaneous Adverse Reactions

Suran Fernando
Sydney University
Australia

1. Introduction

Severe cutaneous adverse reactions (SCARs) are generally induced by drugs and encompass the conditions of Stevens-Johnson syndrome (SJS) and toxic epidermal necrolysis (TEN), drug induced eosinophilia and systemic syndrome (DRESS) also known as drug induced hypersensitivity syndrome (DIHS), and acute generalized exanthematous pustulosis (AGEP). These conditions, although rare, cause significant morbidity and are potentially fatal. It is therefore important for the treating physician to promptly recognize SCARs through the identification of their characteristic clinical features so that the offending drug is promptly withdrawn and supportive and adjunctive therapies are administered. SCARs are accompanied by particular abnormalities on routine laboratory investigations and skin biopsy that enables confirmation of the diagnosis and provision of useful prognostic information. Data bases have been established, predominantly in Europe, since the 1980s to characterize the epidemiology of SCARs including the identification of drugs with the highest relative risk and the latency between the commencement of drug intake and the onset of clinical manifestations. The pathogenesis of the various SCARs involves delayed T cell-mediated inflammation in a genetically predisposed individual and in the case of DIHS, may involve viral factors. The emerging field of the genetic susceptibility to SCARs has raised the important issue of pharmacogenetic screening as a method of predicting an individual's risk of developing SCAR to a certain drug.

2. Stevens-Johnson syndrome/toxic epidermal necrolysis

2.1 History and nosology

Stevens-Johnson syndrome (SJS) and toxic epidermal necrolysis (TEN) were once considered as variants of erythema multiforme (EM), a condition first described by Ferdinand von Hebra in 1860 as a mild and relapsing eruption of target lesions affecting the acral regions. Mucosal involvement occurs in up to 70 % of cases of EM. In 1922, Albert Stevens and Frank Johnson described two cases of fever, stomatitis, purulent conjunctivitis, and a generalized eruption of purple papules in boys aged 7 and 8 years, respectively (Stevens and Johnson 1922). Both cases were distinguished from EM by the prolonged high fever, and the generalized distribution and heavy terminal crusting of the skin lesions. Bernard Thomas proposed two categories of EM in 1950: erythema multiforme minor, as described by von Hebra, and erythema multiforme major, a severe form that encompassed SJS (Thomas 1950). Alan Lyell termed the condition toxic epidermal necrolysis (TEN) after reporting four cases of an acute life threatening mucocutaneous disorder characterized by diffuse erythema followed by extensive epidermal detachment manifesting as blistering and sloughing of the skin (Lyell 1956). Although SJS and TEN were initially considered distinct entities, it was later proposed that they form a continuum along the same disease process and differ mainly in the extent of involvement. It was also proposed that EM major and SJS are distinct conditions, with EM major characterised by acral target-like lesion typical of EM minor but with mucosal involvement. SJS was applied to cases of mucous membrane involvement and a more extensive eruption of atypical targetoid lesions, blisters or sloughing of the skin (Bastuji-Garin, Rzany et al. 1993). The distinction between EM and SJS are consistent with observations regarding differences in etiology, demography and histopathology and not just confined to variations in the severity of disease. Most cases of EM are related to infection especially those with recurrent disease, which is related to herpes simplex virus (HSV) infection (Ng, Sun et al. 2003) in contrast to SJS which usually is an idiosyncratic reaction to drugs (Mockenhaupt, Viboud et al. 2008). EM typically affects young adults in their 20s and 30s although approximately 20% of cases involve children (Lam, Yang et al. 2004) whereas SJS/TEN occurs at any age (Mockenhaupt, Viboud et al. 2008). Histopathology in EM in contrast to SJS/TEN consists of a denser infiltrate of lymphocytes and less apoptosis of keratinocytes (Cote, Wechsler et al. 1995).

In 1993, a classification scheme was proposed that is widely but not universally adopted that arbitrarily defines SJS and TEN according to the extent of epidermal detachment (Bastuji-Garin, Rzany et al. 1993). In SJS, epidermal loss affects less than 10% of the total body surface area (TBSA) whereas TEN involves greater than 30% of the TBSA. Epidermal detachment between 10 and 30% of the TBSA is classified as SJS/TEN overlap.

2.2 Epidemiology

The epidemiology of SJS/TEN and other severe cutaneous adverse reactions (SCARs) has been more accurately determined in recent years due to registries that have been established mainly across Europe comprising cases that are reviewed by expert committees and based on predefined and validated criteria. A population-based registry was commenced in Germany in 1990 to collect all hospitalised cases of SJS, TEN and EM major. An international case-control study was conducted between 1989 and 1995 in France, Germany, Italy and Portugal (SCAR study) focusing on cases of SJS/TEN requiring hospitalisation. A European case-control surveillance study of SCARs (EuroSCAR study) was conducted between 1997 and 2001 in Austria, France, Germany, Israel, Italy, and the Netherlands investigating both SJS/TEN and AGEP that resulted in admission to hospital. In 2003, the European registry on SCARs (RegiSCAR) was commenced collecting biological samples across the same countries that participated in the EuroSCAR study. This network, which is focused on SJS/TEN and AGEP, has spawned numerous studies on epidemiology, pharmacogenetics and histopathology and includes community cases that required hospitalisation as well as cases that developed during hospital admissions. These registries not only provide valuable information on the epidemiology of SCAR but they have enabled close scrutiny of the availability and prescription of high-risk drugs. For example, the SCAR study resulted in the withdrawal of chlormezanone from the market and restricted indications for cotrimoxazole and phenobarbitol (Roujeau 2005).

The incidence of SJS/TEN is 1-2 cases/million inhabitants/year (Rzany, Mockenhaupt et al. 1996). The EuroSCAR study published in 2008 comprised 379 cases that included 134 cases of SJS, 136 cases of SJS/TEN overlap, and 109 cases TEN spanning a geographical area encompassing over a 100 million inhabitants. The median age of cases was found to be 50 years (range 1-95 years), and a female preponderance (62% of cases) was noted (Mockenhaupt, Viboud et al. 2008).

2.3 Etiology

2.3.1 Drugs

Drugs are nearly always the cause of SJS/TEN. Over 220 medications have been implicated but only relatively a few are responsible for the majority of cases. The EuroSCAR study comprised 379 cases of SJS/TEN and 1505 age-matched controls, who were patients admitted to hospital for other acute illnesses (Mockenhaupt, Viboud et al. 2008). Univariate relative risk (uRR) and multivariate relative risk (mRR) were calculated for each drug suspected of causing SJS/TEN. The drugs found to confer the highest risk were cotrimoxazole (uRR 102), other anti-bacterial sulphonamides (uRR 53), carbamazepine (mRR 72), nevirapine (uRR >22), allopurinol (mRR 18), phenytoin (mRR 17), oxicam-NSAIDs (mRR 16), lamotrigine (uRR >14), and sertraline (mRR 11). Drugs that were found to have a significant but lower risk included acetic acid-NSAIDs, macrolides, quinolones, cephalosporins, tetracyclines and aminopenicillins. SJS/TEN typically occurs with drugs that are taken on a long-term basis. The median latency between the onset of medication use and the occurrence of SJS/TEN in the EuroSCAR study was found to be less than 4 weeks (range 1-8 weeks): carbamazepine 15 days, phenobarbitol 17 days, allopurinol 20 days, phenytoin 24 days. Pantoprazole and tramadol were associated with high uRRs, 18 and 20, respectively, but the frequent co-medication with highly suspected drugs and the timing of the onset of SJS/TEN were not suggestive of a true risk. Commonly used medications not associated with a risk of SJS/TEN included beta-blockers, ACE-inhibitors, calcium channel blockers, thiazide diuretics, furosemide, propionic acid-NSAIDs, sulphonylureas, and insulin. Interestingly, valproic acid was not shown to have a significant risk, which is contrast to previous observations (Roujeau, Kelly et al. 1995; Rzany, Correia et al. 1999). The most likely explanation is that valproic acid was frequently coadministered with high-risk drugs.
A pooled analysis of the SCAR and EuroSCAR data was performed for children under 15 years of age and showed that anti-bacterial sulphonamides, phenobarbitol, lamotrigine and carbamazepine were strongly associated with SJS/TEN in this paediatric population (Levi, Bastuji-Garin et al. 2009).

2.3.2 Other causes

Infection with *Mycoplasma pneumoniae* is a known cause of SJS especially in the paediatric population and a few cases of TEN have been reported to complicate infection with this agent (Lam, Yang et al. 2004). However, the EuroSCAR study, failed to show that infection was a risk factor either on its own although there is a suggestion that is may modestly increase the risk of SJS/TEN from medication. SJS/TEN has been reported in association with vaccinations (Ball, Ball et al. 2001) and exposure to industrial chemicals and fumigants (House, Jakubovic et al. 1992).

2.4 Clinical presentation

SJS/TEN is characterized, as per the original descriptions, by fever, blistering skin eruption and severe mucositis. The skin lesions initially appear as atypical target -like or targetoid lesions, which are erythematous macules that contain a central purpuric blister (Fig. 1). Lesions are symmetrically distributed often starting on the face and thorax before spreading to other areas. The scalp is typically spared. Blisters result from epidermal detachment and they are easily breached resulting in dark red oozing erosions. Lesions exhibit Nikolsky's sign, which is epidermal separation induced by gentle lateral pressure applied to the skin surface. The skin then sloughs rapidly over several days as a result of separation of large sheets of the epidermis from the dermis. Fulminant cases of TEN have been reported where total loss of the epidermis occurs within 24 hours. New lesions may continue to erupt for up to 4 weeks. However, the growth of a new epithelium occurs after several days and individual lesions are completely re-epithelialized after a mean of 3 weeks. Cicatrization of the mucous membranes may take longer to complete.

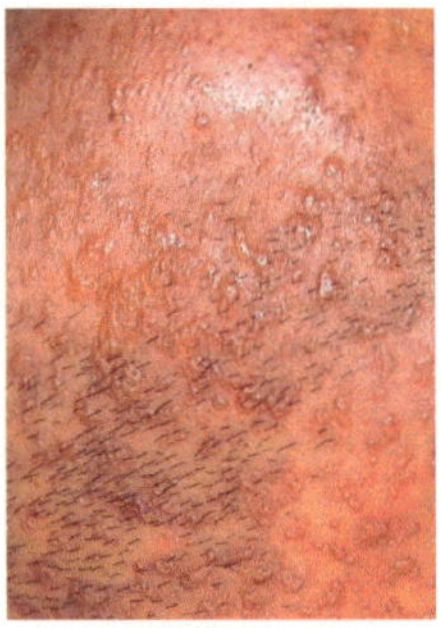

Fig. 1. Atypical target-like or targetoid lesions in a patient with SJS characterized by an erythematous macule with a central blister.

At least two mucosal surfaces are involved in 90% of cases of SJS/TEN (Letko, Papaliodis et al. 2005). Oropharyngeal involvement causes severe pain and odynophagia as a result of erosion and crusting (Fig. 2). Ocular regions may show a purulent conjunctivitis, pseudomembrane formation and corneal ulceration as a result of sloughing of conjunctival and corneal epithelia (Fig. 3). Urethritis may result in dysuria and even urinary retention. Sloughing of the tracheal and bronchial epithelium occurs in up to 30% of cases and may result in hypoxia, bronchial hypersecretion, pulmonary edema and bronchiolitis obliterans and the need for mechanical ventilation (Lebargy, Wolkenstein et al. 1997). The gastrointestinal tract can also be involved resulting in per rectal bleeding (Sugimoto, Mizutani et al. 1998).

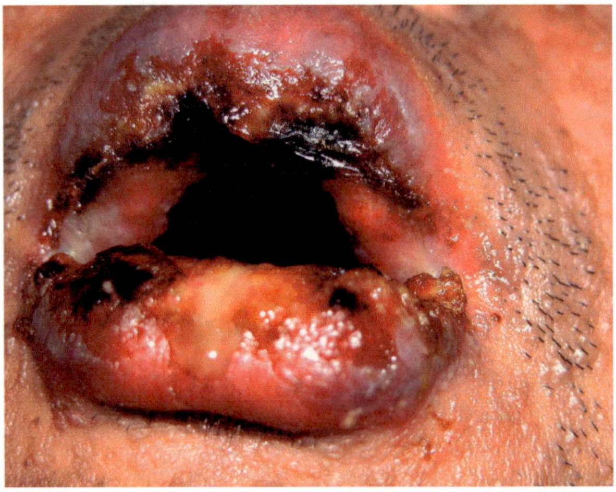

Fig. 2. Oral mucositis in a patient with SJS depicted as sloughing, necrosis and crusting of the inner labial surfaces.

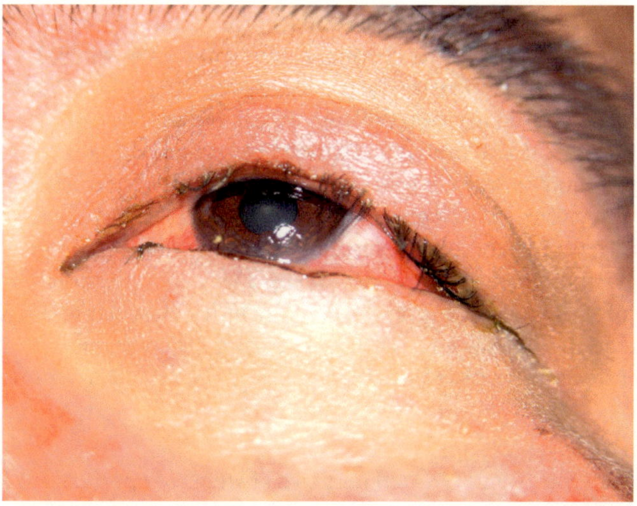

Fig. 3. Purulent conjunctivitis in a patient with SJS accompanied by pseudomembrane formation, which results from sloughing of conjunctival and corneal surfaces.

The mortality of SJS is generally below 10% whereas 30-50% of TEN patients die in the acute phase of the illness mostly as a result of skin failure. Infection and sepsis with multiorgan failure is the most common of death. The causative organisms are usually *Staphylococcus aureus* and *Pseudomonas aeruginosa* (Atiyeh, Dham et al. 2003). Fluid and electrolyte imbalances occur as a result of increased transepidermal water loss and impaired intake of nutrition due to odynophagia from stomatitis. Less common fatal complications include adult respiratory distress syndrome, pulmonary embolism and gastrointestinal haemorrhage (Wolkenstein and Revuz 2000; Abood, Nickoloff et al. 2008). Mortality is accurately predicted by the SCORTEN scale (Table 1) and should be computed within 24 hours and 3 days following admission (Bastuji-Garin, Fouchard et al. 2000; Guegan, Bastuji-Garin et al. 2006).

Parameter	Score
Age >40 years	1
Presence of malignancy	1
Heart rate >120/min	1
TBSA involved >10%	1
Serum urea > 10 mmol/L (28 mg/dL)	1
Serum glucose >14 mmol/L (252 mg/dL)	1
Serum bicarbonate <20 mmol/L (20 mEq/L)	1

SCORTEN	Mortality (%)
0-1	3.2
2	12.1
3	35.3
4	58.3
≥5	90

Table 1. SCORTEN

Chronic complications occur frequently following the acute phase of SJS/TEN. The most serious sequelae relate to the eye. The chronic ocular consequences are that of a cicatrization of the conjunctiva and symblepharon formation, severe dry eye, trichiasis, eyelid margin keratinization, and limbal stem cell deficiency, all of which combine to cause corneal ulceration and scarring and loss of vision. Patients may also experience chronic photophobia and eye pain. Skin sequelae include scarring, pigmentation abnormalities, and shedding of hair and nails. Vulvovaginal involvement can result in stenosis. Vulvar adenosis can occur in young women several years after resolution of the acute episode and can present with tender, erosive, haemorrhagic lesions. Phimosis can occur in men. Bronchopulmonary complications confer a poor prognosis and include chronic bronchitis, bronchiolitis obliterans, bronchiolitis obliterans with organizing pneumonia, and bronchiectasis. Oesophageal stricture and webbing has also been described and can result in dysphagia.

2.5 Pathogenesis

SJS/TEN results from the T- and NK-cell mediated extensive apoptosis of keratinocytes. The pharmaco-immune (p-i) concept, the mechanism by which the drug binds directly with the T cell receptor (TCR) causes activation of proapoptotic pathways. Granulysin is the major mediator of apoptosis in SJS/TEN. Apoptosis is also mediated through Fas-FasL interaction, and the release of granzyme and perforin.

2.5.1 The pharmaco-immune (p-i) concept

It is generally accepted that in SJS/TEN, the parent drug binds directly and non-covalently to the MHC and the TCR of primed effector and memory T cells (Pichler, Adam et al. 2010). Naïve T cells are not sufficiently stimulated by a p-i drug and additional signals are required (Pichler 2005). T cells may be primed by infection or autoimmune disease resulting in high cytokine levels such as IL-2 and IFN-γ resulting in increased expression of MHC and costimulatory molecules. This may provide an explanation for the increased incidence of drug hypersensitivity in inflammatory and infectious diseases. The drug may also bind to toll-like receptors resulting in the expression of costimulatory molecules by dendritic cells. For drugs such as cotrimoxazole, lamotrigine, and carbamazepine, the p-i concept may not be the sole mechanism involved; metabolites may also play a role through haptenization (Sanderson, Naisbitt et al. 2007).

2.5.2 Granulysin

A recent study by Chung et al using global gene expression profiling showed that granulysin RNA was the most significant cytotoxic molecule expressed in blister cells from patients with SJS/TEN. Granulysin protein concentrations were 2-4 times higher than perforin, granzyme B, and FasL and depleting granulysin reduced cytotoxicity (Chung, Hung et al. 2008). Granulysin is a cationic cytolytic protein produced by CTL, NK and NKT cells (Fig. 4A) (Gamen, Hanson et al. 1998). The 15-kDa-precursor form, found in blister fluid, induced skin necrosis when injected into mice and exhibited significant cytotoxicity in vitro. This contrasted with the minimal cytotoxicity induced by perforin, granzyme B, and FasL (Chung, Hung et al. 2008). Granulysin is also a proinflammatory molecule that causes an increase in the expression of chemokines (RANTES/CCL5, MCP-1, MCP-3, MIP-1α/CCL3) and cytokines (IL-1, IL-6, IFN-α) resulting in the recruitment of T cells, monocytes and other inflammatory cells (Deng, Chen et al. 2005).

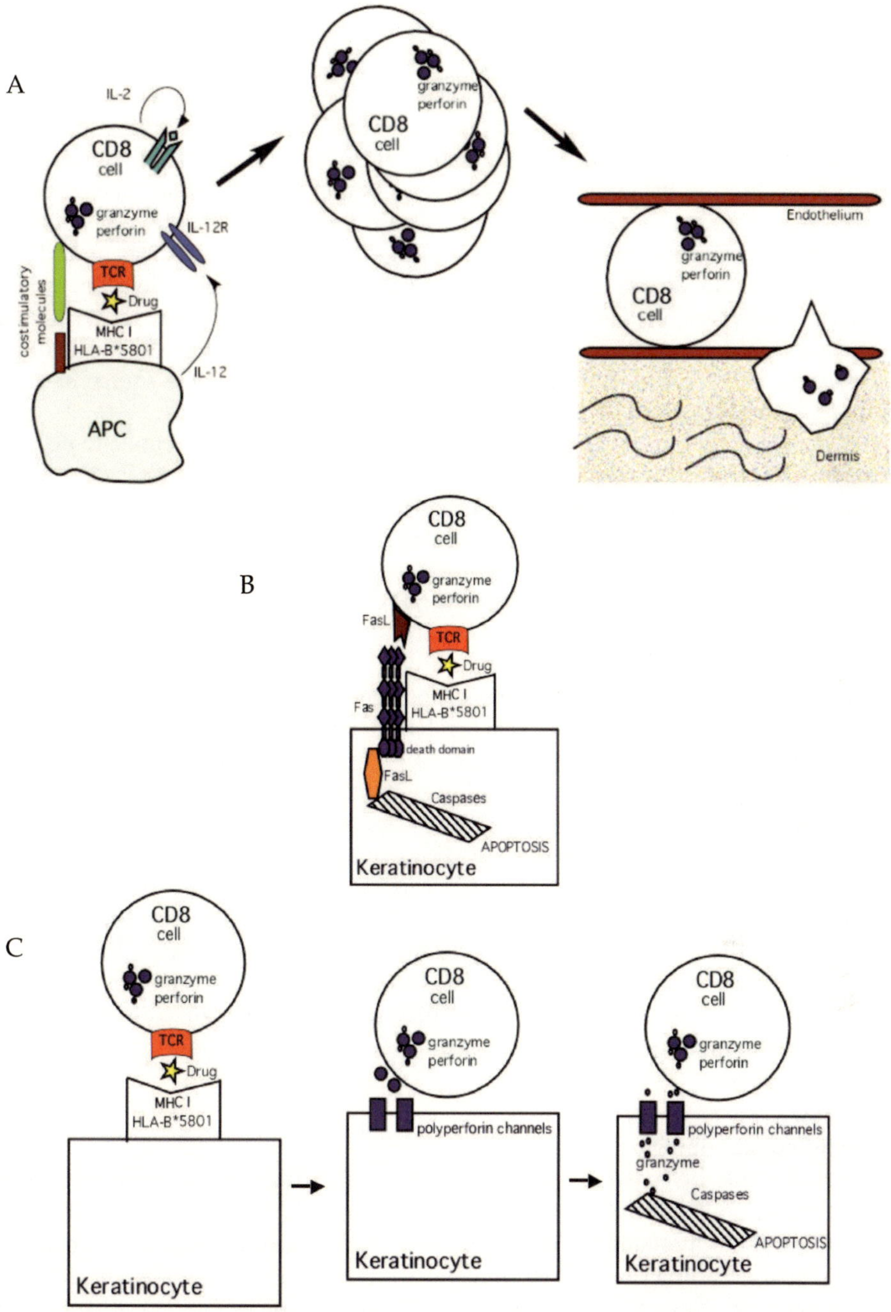

Fig. 4. SJS/TEN is primarily mediated by cytotoxic T cells. The drug binds to the CD8 T cell receptor and MHC via the pi concept resulting in their proliferation, activation and infiltration of these effector cytotoxic T cells (CTLs) into the skin (A). These CTLs may also bind drug that also binds to MHC class I molecules expressed on keratinocytes. Apoptosis of keratinocytes in SJS/TEN is caused primarily by the release of granulysin (A), but the ligation of Fas by FasL (B), and the degranulation of perforin and granzyme (C) may also play a role.

Fas-FasL, perforin/ granzyme and TNF pathways

Viard et al, showed that the binding of FasL to Fas expressed on the surface of keratinocytes resulted in their apoptosis (Fig. 4B) (Viard, Wehrli et al. 1998). The cytoplasmic death domain of Fas undergoes conformational changes and trimerization upon recognition of FasL. This results in the recruitment of the Fas-associated death domain (FADD), which binds to procaspase 8 resulting in triggering of the caspase cascade and apoptosis. The source of the FasL is unclear. Viard et al showed that the FasL was is present on the surface of keratinocytes and in the serum of patients with TEN but not on the surface of keratinocytes or in the serum of patients with maculopapular exanthems and normal controls (Viard, Wehrli et al. 1998). A further study demonstrated that FasL was not constitutively expressed on the surface of keratinocytes but are transported to the cell membrane after damage to the keratinocyte (Viard-Leveugle, Bullani et al. 2003). Abe et al, however, found that the source of FasL was PBMCs and not keratinocytes (Abe, Shimizu et al. 2003).

Nassif et al showed that mononuclear cells from blister fluid induce cytotoxicity via perforin and granzyme B (Nassif, Bensussan et al. 2002). This cytotoxicity was blocked by inhibiting perforin/granzyme but not by inhibiting Fas. Perforin and granzyme are proteins stored in the granules of CTLs. Upon recognition of a target cell, the CTL releases perforin, which create 16-nm channels in the target cell membrane. Granzyme B, a protease passes through these channels to activate the caspase cascade (Fig. 4C). The loss of T regulatory cell function in the acute stage of SJS/TEN may further contribute to the epidermal damage caused by effector T cells (Takahashi, Kano et al. 2009).

Posadas et al, showed that both Fas-FasL and perforin/granzyme pathways may be involved in SJS/TEN. They found a direct correlation between disease severity and levels of perforin and granzyme B in patients with maculopapular exanthems, SJS and TEN. FasL was detected in the PBMCs and blister fluid of patients in SJS and TEN but not in those in maculopapular exanthema, suggesting that Fas-FasL is involved in more severe reactions (Posadas, Padial et al. 2002). Nassif et al, also showed a potential role for cytokines in the pathogenesis of SJS/TEN. He found elevated levels of IFN-γ, soluble TNF, IL-10, soluble FasL in the blister fluid of TEN patients. Although they disputed the central role of FasL, they hypothesised that drug specific CTLs secrete IFN-γ, which activates keratinocytes to produce TNF, a cytokine that upregulates MHC class I molecules. This increases exposure of keratinocytes to CTL resulting in perforin/granzyme-mediated apoptosis. IL-10 serves to downregulate the inflammatory reaction (Nassif, Bensussan et al. 2004).

2.6 Risk factors for SJS/TEN

2.6.1 Genetic susceptibility

It was observed in the 1990s that the most commonly offending drugs vary among different ethnic populations. In Western countries, the most commonly implicated agents of SJS/TEN were NSAIDs and sulphonamides (Roujeau, Kelly et al. 1995). In contrast, carbamazepine was found to be the leading cause of SJS/TEN in Southeast Asian countries, including India, Malaysia, Singapore, Taiwan and Hong Kong (Hung, Chung et al. 2005a). Interestingly, carbamazepine in Western countries causes more cases of DIHS than SJS/TEN. Allopurinol is also a frequent case of SJS/TEN and DIHS but does not appear to have a racial bias (Hung, Chung et al. 2007).

The most striking genetic association was detected in a cohort of Han Chinese in Taiwan, where the *HLA-B*1502* allele was found in 100% of the 44 patients with carbamazepine-induced SJS/TEN and only 3% of the carbamazepine-tolerant individuals; OR 2504 [126–

49522] (Chung, Hung et al. 2004). These findings were replicated in an extended cohort of subjects of Chinese descent originating from separated geographic areas of China, Taiwan, and the United States (Hung, Chung et al. 2006). This association with carbamazepine-induced SJS/TEN, however, was not found in individuals with European (Lonjou, Thomas et al. 2006) and Japanese ancestries (Kaniwa, Saito et al. 2008), respectively, and therefore the allele appears relevant in the context of ethnicity. In a recent study comprising 12 patients of Northern European ancestry with carbamazepine-induced SJS/TEN, 5 (42%) carried the *HLA-A*3101* allele, as compared with 10 (4%) of the 257 control subjects; OR 25.93 [4.93-116.18] (McCormack, Alfirevic et al. 2011). The results of this study are yet to be replicated in other cohorts of subjects with Northern European ancestry. In a Japanese study, The *HLA-A*3101* allele was found in 5/6 (83.3%) carbamazepine-induced SJS/TEN compared to 47/376 (12.5%) carbamazepine-tolerant patients; OR 33.9 [3.9-295.6]. Larger patient sample sizes are required to confirm this association in the Japanese where the allele frequency is 9% (Ozeki, Mushiroda et al. 2011). Interestingly the *HLA-A*3101* allele was shown to be associated with maculopapular exanthem (OR 17.5 [4.6-66.5]) but not SJS/TEN in a Han Chinese population (Wen, Lai et al. 2008).

A study comprising a Han Chinese cohort in Taiwan demonstrated the presence of the *HLA-B*5801* allele in all 51 patients with allopurinol-induced SCAR (21 with TEN, 30 with DIHS) compared with only 15% (20/135) in allopurinol-tolerant subjects; OR 580.3 [34.4-9780.9] (Hung, Chung et al. 2005b).

The role of these HLA alleles in the pathogenesis of SCAR is unclear. Certain HLA alleles may bind to particular drugs more robustly than other alleles. Furthermore, the binding of the drug in SJS/TEN is MHC class I restricted, which is consistent with the prominent role of CD8 cells in the pathogenesis of the disease. If an allele has a functional effect that may play a role in the pathogenesis of disease, this association will be consistently observed across different populations. The differences observed between the Chinese and European studies may be partly explained by the fact that pharmacogenetic studies are likely to yield positive results when conducted in a population with a high frequency of such an allele. The risk of disease from a genetic polymorphism is influenced by its prevalence. The *HLA-B*1502* allele frequency is 4.8 to 12.8% in Southeast Asians compared to 0-0.1% observed in Northern Europeans (Fig. 5). Therefore, *HLA-B*1502* is of low prevalence in Caucasians and hence, if it is a true susceptibility allele, a very large sample size is required in this population to detect a significant odds ratio of sufficient power. In contrast, the allele frequency of *HLA-A*3101* is 2-5% in Northern Europeans and the sample size required to demonstrate an association in a sufficiently powered study is less than that for the *HLA-B*1502* allele. The *HLA-B*5801* allele, in contrast to *HLA-B*1502* is more evenly distributed among different racial groups (Fig. 6) and hence, associations, albeit weaker, have been demonstrated in other ethnic groups such as the Southern Japanese (Kaniwa, Saito et al. 2008) and in whites (OR 80 [34-157]) (Lonjou, Borot et al. 2008). Another explanation is that *HLA-B*1502,* is a marker of a true disease contributing allele through strong linkage disequilibrium, which varies between populations. In other words, the same high-risk allele may have a different pattern of association with marker alleles and therefore *HLA-B*1502* is in strong linkage disequilibrium in the Han Chinese population, but not in a European population. It is also plausible that SJS/TEN is a polygenic disorder, with many susceptibility and protective alleles in genes involved in the pathogenesis of the disease. Polymorphisms in the proapoptotic gene *Fas-L*, the toll-like receptor 3 gene, and in the IL-4 receptor/IL-13 signalling pathway have all been recently described in a Japanese study (Ueta, Sotozono et al. 2008). Such alleles may also vary in different populations.

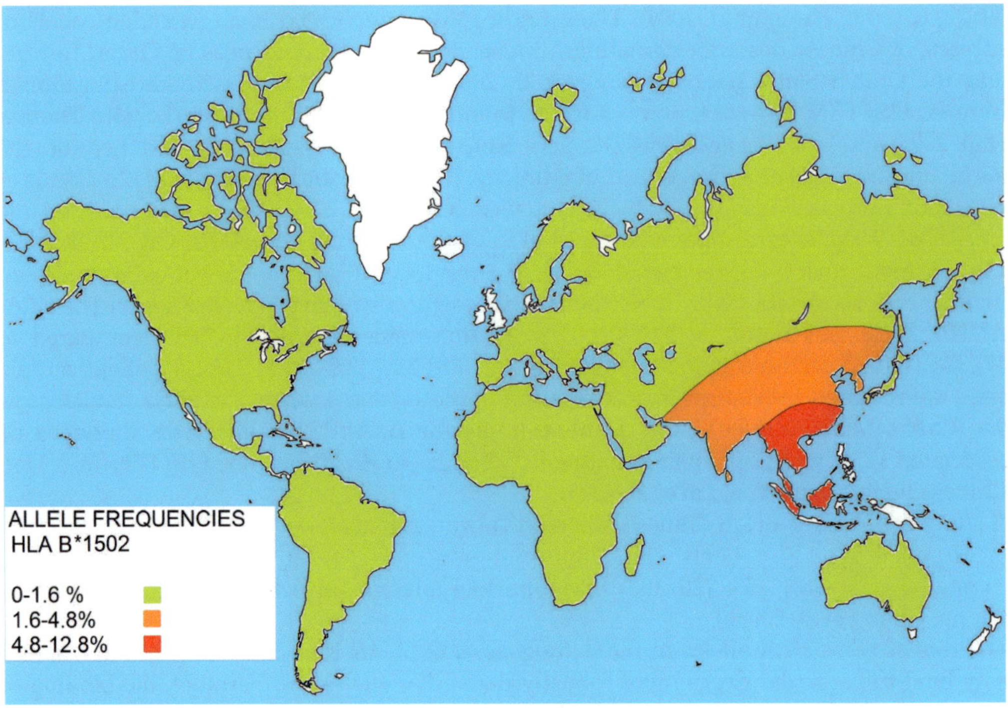

Fig. 5. The high variation in the prevalence of *HLA-B*1502* across geographical regions.

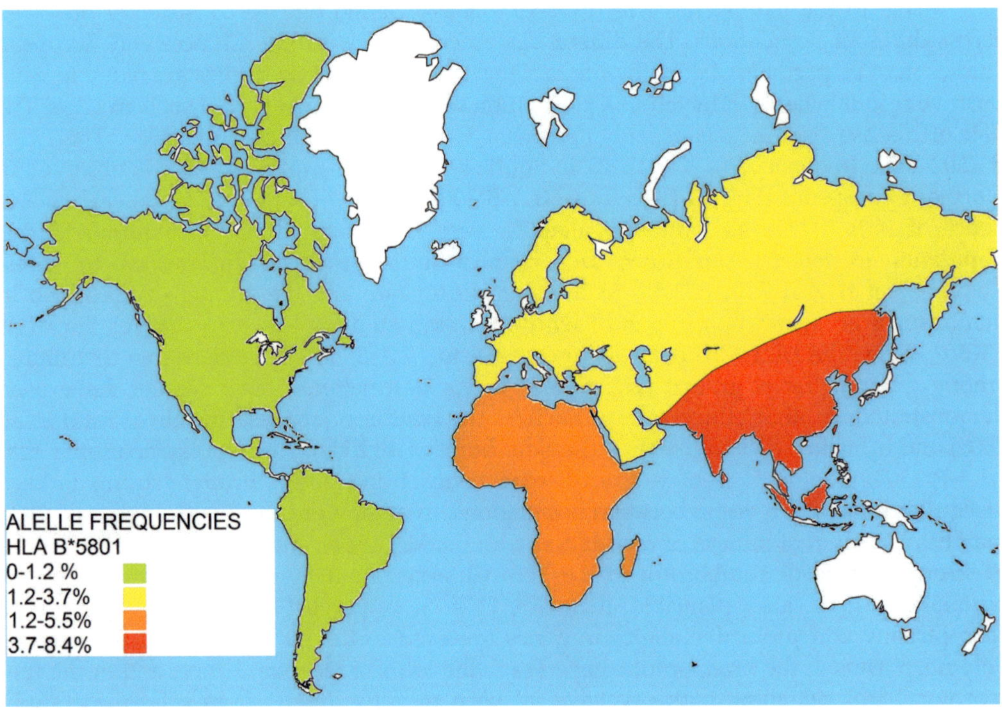

Fig. 6. The low variation in the prevalence of *HLA-B*5801* across geographical regions.

The FDA and Health Canada have issued warnings for carbamazepine stating that persons with ancestry in genetically at-risk populations should be screened for the presence of *HLA-B*1502* prior to initiating treatment. Genetic screening for *HLA-B*1502* in a high risk population such as the Han Chinese has a 100% sensitivity and 97% specificity and its presence confers a 7.7% positive predictive value for carbamazepine-induced SJS/TEN whereas its absence has a 100% negative predictive value (Hung, Chung et al. 2005a). A recent study demonstrated the benefit of genetic screening; in a Taiwanese population, screening for the *HLA-B*1502* allele resulted in no cases of SJS/TEN in 4501 patients who were negative for the allele (Chen, Lin et al. 2011). The authors concluded that this would have prevented 10 cases of SJS/TEN. Despite the FDA recommendations, screening is not routinely performed partly because of the lack of availability of cost effective and rapid methods of detection (Fernando and Broadfoot 2010). However, many laboratories have now developed high resolution genetic testing using a sequence-specific primer assay method for the detection of this allele from whole blood samples and buccal swabs. The assay can be performed within 3-4 hours. Such a strategy has been very successful in virtually abolishing the incidence of *HLA-B*5701*-associated abacavir hypersensitivity in HIV-infected patients (Rauch, Nolan et al. 2006). Multiplexed PCRs can be utilized to assess multiple alleles.

It is important to note that the *HLA-B*1502* allele does not predispose to carbamazepine-induced DIHS, maculopapular eruptions or other adverse reactions and continued vigilance for the symptoms of SCAR needs to be maintained if treatment is commenced (Hung, Chung et al. 2006). Currently, there is no recommendation for genetic screening prior to the commencement of allopurinol therapy. Although such a strategy is plausible, studies are required to determine the benefits of screening for the *HLA*5801* allele in at risk populations.

2.6.2 Diseases

The EuroSCAR study showed that HIV infection conferred the highest risk of SJS/TEN; multivariate relative risk (mvRR) 12 [2.4-59]. Other disease associations included collagen vascular disease mvRR 2.2 [0.9-5.0], recent malignancy mvRR 2.7 [1.3-5.7], recent radiotherapy mvRR 2.1 [0.5-9.0], or acute infection in the past 4 weeks [1.2-2.3] (Mockenhaupt, Viboud et al. 2008).

2.6.3 Pharmacokinetics

The EuroSCAR study revealed an increased risk of SJS/TEN at higher doses of allopurinol; adjusted odds ratio (OR) 36 [17-76] for doses ≥200 mg daily compared with an adjusted OR 3.0 [1.1-8.4] for doses <200 mg daily (Halevy, Ghislain et al. 2008). This study also revealed that the risk was mostly confined to short-term use (≤8 weeks, unadjusted OR 261 [36-∞]). Allopurinol is ideally commenced at a dose of 100 mg daily and increased by 100 mg increments until the desired serum uric acid level is attained. Previous reports have shown that allopurinol is often commenced at inappropriate doses (Stamp, Gow et al. 2000) and that higher doses are associated with an increased incidence of acute events (McInnes, Lawson et al. 1981). It is likely that the rapid accumulation of the chemically reactive metabolite oxypurinol when higher doses of allopurinol are commenced increases the risk of SJS/TEN (Kumar, Edward et al. 1996). This drug accumulation hypothesis is further supported by the 4.7 fold increased incidence of allopurinol-induced SCAR in renal insufficiency (Vazquez-Mellado, Morales et al. 2001). The established indications for allopurinol are treatment of hyperuricemia associated with chronic gout, acute uric acid nephropathy, recurrent uric acid stone formation, enzyme disorders of purine metabolism, and in the management of tumour lysis. Allopurinol is not indicated in the majority of patients with asymptomatic hyperuricemia (Dincer, Dincer et al. 2002). However, allopurinol is inappropriately prescribed in up to 86% of cases (Khoo and Leow 2000). A comparison of allopurinol exposure between the SCAR (1989-1993) and EuroSCAR (1997-2001) studies showed a 2-3 fold increase in exposure for both patients and control subjects, which may be attributed to the increased prescribing of the drug for the treatment of asymptomatic hyperuricemia. The authors of the EuroSCAR study postulate that up to 48 of the 56 cases of allopurinol-induced SJS/TEN could have been prevented if the treatment guidelines for prescribing allopurinol were followed.

Lamotrigine when commenced at high doses can also overwhelm the detoxifying capacity resulting in an increased risk of SJS/TEN and DIHS (Schlienger, Shapiro et al. 1998). The incidence has reduced significantly as a result of the now conventional practice of gradually titrating the dose (Mockenhaupt, Messenheimer et al. 2005). Coadministration of certain drugs can predispose to SCAR by competition for the same enzyme-binding site. Reactions to lamotrigine are more common when given in combination with valproic acid as the addition of valproic acid inhibits the clearance of lamotrigine by competing for glucoronic acid conjugation (Yalcin and Karaduman 2000). The role of slow acetylation phenotypes of N-acetyltransferase was thought to confer susceptibility of sulphonamide-induced SJS/TEN in two small studies (Dietrich, Kawakubo et al. 1995; Wolkenstein, Carriere et al. 1995) but this needs confirmation in larger studies.

2.7 Diagnosis

2.7.1 Skin biopsy

A presumptive diagnosis of SJS/TEN is made clinically and is confirmed with a skin biopsy (Figs. 7 & 8). Early lesions demonstrate scattered necrotic keratinocytes in the epidermal layers at the level of the stratum spinosum and the basal cell layer. Later, full thickness epidermal necrosis is evident, which eventuates in the formation of subepidermal bullae. The mononuclear predominantly T cell dermal infiltrate is generally sparse but dense infiltrates can also be present. Quinn et al, has shown an extensive infiltrate was associated with a 71% mortality rate, a moderate infiltrate with a 53% mortality, and a sparse infiltrate with a 27% mortality, respectively (Quinn, Brown et al. 2005). A fresh sample for direct immunofluoresence (DIF) reveals an absence of immunoglobulin and complement deposition. Cultures on blood, wounds and mucosal lesions should be performed to evaluate for superinfection. Serology may be performed for *Mycoplasma pneumoniae* if indicated.

A recent pilot study showed that serum granulysin levels may be raised early in the course of disease but rapidly wanes with progression of disease (Abe, Yoshioka et al. 2009). Further studies are required to determine whether this assay will prove to be a useful early diagnostic test for SJS/TEN.

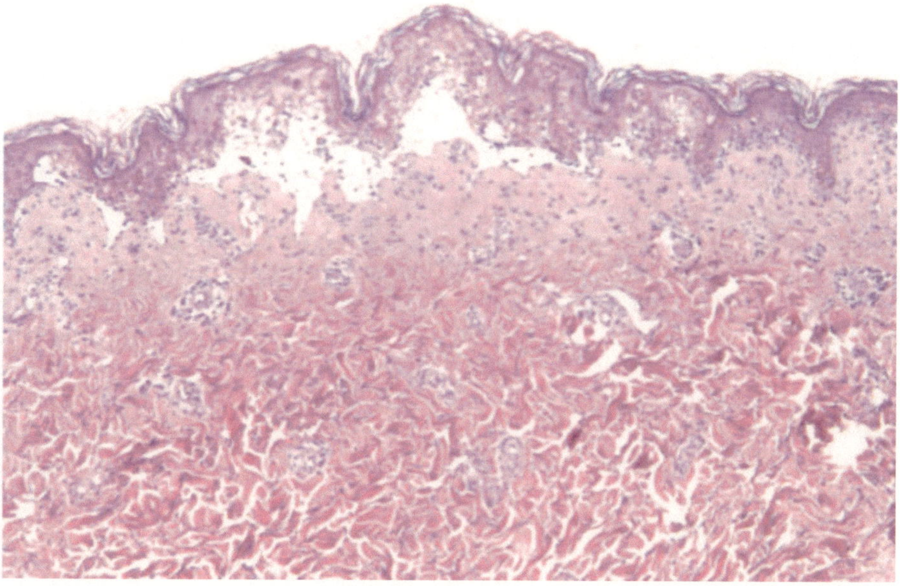

Fig. 7. Low power view of a skin biopsy from a patient with SJS demonstrates separation of the epidermis from the dermis at the level of the stratum spinosum and basal cell layer resulting in the formation of subepidermal bullae (Hematoxylin-eosin, original magnification x40).

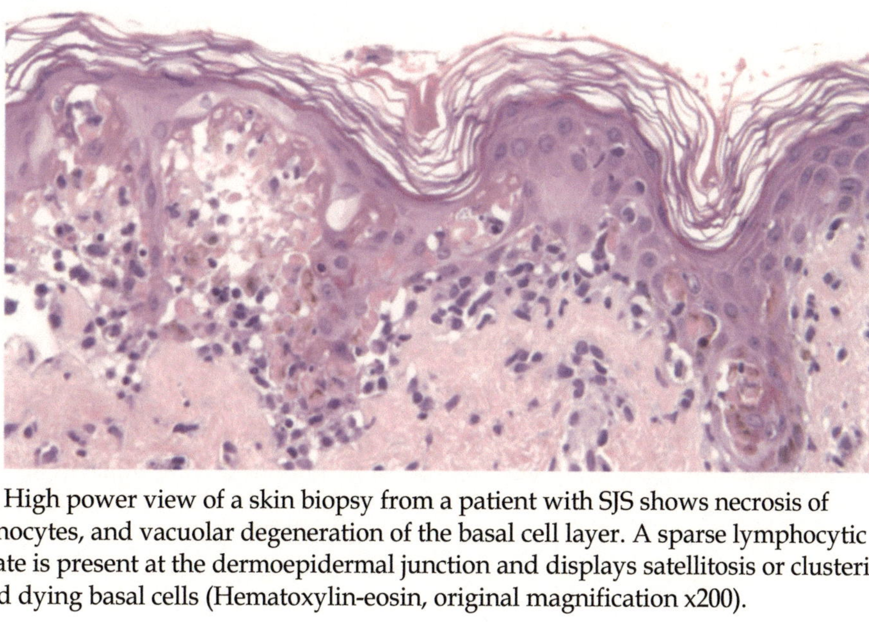

Fig. 8. High power view of a skin biopsy from a patient with SJS shows necrosis of keratinocytes, and vacuolar degeneration of the basal cell layer. A sparse lymphocytic infiltrate is present at the dermoepidermal junction and displays satellitosis or clustering around dying basal cells (Hematoxylin-eosin, original magnification x200).

2.7.2 Allergy testing

Skin tests and oral challenges are contraindicated in SJS/TEN because of the risk of inducing a recurrence of disease. Patch testing has not been investigated extensively. The biggest cohort comprised 22 patients and showed a poor sensitivity of only 9% (Wolkenstein, Chosidow et al. 1996). Lymphocyte transformation tests (LTTs) assess the proliferation of the patient's peripheral blood T cells cultured in the presence of a suspected drug for 6 days by measuring the incorporation of ^{3}H-thymidine during DNA synthesis. The result is expressed as a stimulation index, which is the ratio of cell proliferation with antigen and without antigen. The sensitivity of LTTs in SJS/TEN is greatly improved if the test is performed within 1 week of the onset of disease but becomes negative by 6 weeks (Kano, Hirahara et al. 2007). This may be attributed to loss of regulatory T cell function in the acute phase, which is then restored upon recovery (Takahashi, Kano et al. 2009). Recently, a new cytotoxicity assay combining the measurement of expression of the degranulation marker, CD107a, using flow cytometry and the release of the serine protease, granzyme B by Elispot after incubating the patient's peripheral blood mononuclear cells with the suspected drug for 3 days (Zawodniak, Lochmatter et al. 2010). The test has very good specificity with all of the 16 controls having a negative test and good sensitivity with 10 of the 12 patients having a positive result. One role of these in vitro tests is to determine the culprit drug when more than one drug is suspected.

2.8 Differential diagnosis

SJS/TEN is differentiated from other conditions on the basis of the acute onset of disease, the presence of targetoid and vesiculobullous lesions, sloughing of the epidermis, severe mucosal involvement, the histologic finding of full thickness epidermal necrosis, and a negative DIF. In EM major, erosive mucous membrane involvement is present but in contrast to SJS, the patient has typical target lesions mainly affecting the extremities and it is often induced by acute or recurrent HSV infection. The clinical manifestations of drug-induced maculopapular exanthems (MPE) are variable and often polymorphic and lesions may have a target-like appearance. Fever may be present but mucosal involvement is absent. The histopathology typically shows an interface dermatitis with hydropic degeneration of the basal cell layer. Some exanthems may progress to more severe reactions such as SJS/TEN or DIHS. Generalized bullous fixed drug eruption (GBFDE) features large brownish violaceous patches upon which flaccid blisters arise. These blisters affect only a small percentage of the TBSA. Mucosal involvement is rare and fever is absent. Most patients report a history of a similar local reaction or fixed drug eruption.

Staphylococcal scalded skin syndrome (SSSS) usually affects children under the age of 5 years and patients present with fever, erythema and painful skin, followed by blistering, which is typically accentuated in areas of friction and around orifices. SSSS is caused by the systemic distribution of epidermolytic toxins produced by certain strains of Staphylococci. These toxins cause separation at the level of the stratum granulosum, the upper layer of the epidermis, resulting in very superficial detachment of the skin and blistering. Mucous membrane involvement is rare. The condition usually but not always follows local or systemic staphylococcal infection. Adults are less susceptible as improved renal function allows for better clearance of the toxins. However SSSS has been described in adults who are immunosuppressed or in renal failure. Toxic shock syndrome (TSS) is caused by elaboration of toxins produced by *Staphylococcus aureus* and *Streptococcus pyogenes* that act as superantigens, which bind to the variable regions of β chains of antigen receptors on subsets of T cells and cross-link them to the MHC molecules of antigen-presenting cells. This results in activation of large numbers of T cells (5-30%) and the massive release of cytokines including IL-2, TNF, lymphotoxin and IL-1β. TSS is characterised by fever, diffuse red macular rash, hypotension and involvement of ≥3 organs: renal failure, hepatitis, thrombocytopenia, encephalopathy, mucous membrane hyperemia, gastrointestinal involvement with vomiting and diarrhoea.

Bullous disease	Fever	Mucositis	Rash	DIF	Onset	Other notable features
SJS/TEN	+	+	Erythroderma Targetoid lesions Vesicles, bullae Erosions, detachment	-	Acute	Starts on trunk, proximal upper limbs and face and then spreads
EM Major	+	+	Acral Target lesions	-	Acute	HSV-induced recurrences
Drug-induced MPE	+/-	-	Variable Pleomorphic	-	Acute	May progress to SJS or DIHS
GBFDE	-	-	Brown patches Large bullae	-	Acute	Antecedent local reaction Small % TBSA
SSSS	+	-	Erythroderma Skin tenderness Periorificial crusting	-	Acute	Children under 5 Adults with chronic renal failure and on immunosuppressive therapy
TSS	+	+	Diffuse red macular rash Desquamation of palms and soles	-	Acute	Hypotension Multiple organ failure
Drug-induced linear IgA dermatosis	-	-	Tense bullae	+	Acute	Vancomycin Pruritus
PNP	-	+	Polymorphous Bullae	+	Gradual	
Drug-induced Pemphigus	-	-	Erosions Crusts	+	Gradual	Thiol drugs
Drug-triggered pemphigus	-	+	Mucosal erosions Flaccid bullae	+	Gradual	Non-thiol drugs
AGVHD	+	+	Morbilliform rash Bullae Erosions, detachment	-	Acute	Starts acrally and then spreads
AGEP	+	+/-	Small nonfollicular pustules Erythroderma	-	Acute	

SJS/TEN, Stevens-Johnson syndrome/toxic epidermal necrolysis; EM, erythema multiforme; MPE, maculopapular exanthem; GBFDE, generalized bullous fixed drug eruption; SSSS, staphylococcal scalded skin syndrome; TSS, toxic shock syndrome; PNP, paraneoplastic pemphigus; AGVHD, acute graft versus host disease; AGEP, acute generalized exanthematous pustulosis

Table 2. The differential diagnosis of SJS/TEN

Desquamation occurs after 1-2 weeks and predominantly affects the palms and soles. Approximately 50% of cases are menstrually related due to the prolonged application of absorbent tampons. Notably, 50% of cases of TSS are not associated with menstruation. Non-menstrual cases of TSS usually complicate the use of barrier contraceptives, surgical and postpartum wound infections, burns, cutaneous lesions, osteomyelitis, and arthritis. Although most cases of TSS occur in women, about 25% of non-menstrual cases occur in men.

Autoimmune bullous diseases such as drug-induced linear IgA bullous dermatosis, drug-induced pemphigus, and paraneoplastic pemphigus need to be considered in the differential diagnosis of SJS/TEN. These conditions, in contrast to SJS/TEN, usually have a chronic course and are characterized by acantholysis on histopathology and immunoglobulin deposition on DIF. Bullous pemphigoid (BP) is a chronic disease that is typified by a tense bullous eruption that primarily affects individuals in the fifth through seventh decades of life.

Acute graft versus host disease (AGVHD) shares many of the same clinical, pathologic and immunologic features as SJS/TEN. Both conditions are mediated by cytotoxic T cells, which results in epidermal necrosis and keratinolysis (Schulz and Sheridan 2006). Furthermore, bone marrow transplantation patients receive medications that can trigger SJS/TEN. AGVHD generally occurs 4 weeks after stem cell transplantation. Patients describe a sensation of skin pain and itching followed by a morbilliform rash that in severe cases becomes generalized with diffuse areas of epidermal necrosis. Mucositis is usually present. AGVHD frequently begins acrally and spreads proximally in contrast to TEN, which begins on the trunk and spreads distally. Also, the early exanthem of AGVHD has a folliculocentric distribution.

AGEP is characterized by fever and as the disease progresses, widespread erosions mimicking SJS/TEN may be evident. Mucous membrane involvement is unusual and if present is mild.

2.9 Treatment

2.9.1 Supportive care

Immediate discontinuation of the culprit drug is mandatory to reduce mortality. As the management of TEN is similar to that of extensive burns, a transfer to a burns unit reduces morbidity and mortality. The unit has expertise in providing analgesia, ensuring adequate enteral or parenteral nutrition, maintaining fluid and electrolyte balance, and managing wounds. Ophthalmologic consultation is important in SJS/TEN and the combination of aggressive lubrication, topical antibiotics, topical corticosteroids, and lysis of adhesions may attenuate the acute ocular manifestations. However, these measures have only a modest effect on the long term ocular complications. Recently, the application of amniotic membranes has proved effective in preserving visual acuity and an intact ocular surface (Shammas, Lai et al. 2010). The benefit may be derived from creating a physical barrier between inflamed and denuded mucosal surfaces that minimizes the formation of adhesions. The membrane may also have antiinflammatory and antifibrotic effects.

Other supportive measures include hygienic mouthwashes and topical oral anaesthetics, and monitoring for urinary retention.

2.9.2 Corticosteroids

The role of corticosteroids in the treatment of SJS/TEN is controversial. Corticosteroids given 48 hours or more prior to admission are associated with an increase incidence of infection, length of hospital admission, and mortality in children and adults (Rasmussen 1976; Ginsburg 1982; Engelhardt, Schurr et al. 1997). A study in 1986 of 30 patients with TEN with an average TBSA involvement > 80% were equally divided into those receiving supportive care alone and those receiving dexamethasone at varying doses (Halebian, Corder et al. 1986). Although the incidence of sepsis was not significant different between the groups, the survival following onset of sepsis was less in the corticosteroid treated group. The use of corticosteroids doubled the rate of mortality (66% versus 33%). Corticosteroids do not prevent SJS/TEN from occurring and have no effect on arresting disease progression (Samimi and Siegfried 2002). A retrospective analysis of 379 patients from the EuroSCAR study found no benefit from corticosteroids or IVIg compared to supportive care alone (Schneck, Fagot et al. 2008).

The poor outcomes may have resulted from inadequate doses and the delay in the initiation of corticosteroid therapy. In a prospective study of 16 children with SJS in 1997, 10 received methylprednisolone (4 mg/kg/daily) within 3 days of the onset of rash whilst 6 received supportive care only; corticosteroids were associated with decreased length of fever and duration of skin eruption (Kakourou, Klontza et al. 1997). The use of pulsed IV corticosteroids has also been shown in retrospective analyses to reduce mortality. The initiation of IV methylprednisolone 500-1000 mg/daily for 3-4 days may also prevent ocular complications of cicatrization and preservation of visual acuity (Araki, Sotozono et al. 2009). The benefits of early pulsed therapy with IV corticosteroids need to be further evaluated in randomised control trials.

The current level of evidence suggests that high dose corticosteroids may be beneficial if commenced early in the course of disease with vigilant monitoring for emergence of infection. However, further evaluation in randomised control trials are required to confirm these benefits

2.9.3 Intravenous immunoglobulin (IVIg)

The rationale for the use of IVIg is based on its ability in vitro to block Fas and subsequently FasL-mediated apoptosis of keratinocytes. The beneficial role of IVIg in SJS/TEN has been demonstrated in retrospective studies. The largest such study to date comprised 48 patients with TEN recruited from centres across Europe and the United States. Treatment with IVIg resulted in a more rapid cessation of epidermal detachment and a survival rate of 88%. The authors subsequently recommended a dose of 1 g/kg/daily for 3 days (Prins, Vittorio et al. 2003). Studies have also demonstrated benefit when investigators have compared the rates of mortality following the use of IVIg with the pre-treatment estimate using SCORTEN (Campione, Marulli et al. 2003; Metry, Jung et al. 2003; Yang, Xu et al. 2009).

Despite the initial preponderance of evidence favouring the use of IVIg in SJS/TEN, a few published reports have not demonstrated any benefit. Most of these studies comparing the use of IVIg with supportive care alone used doses less than the recommended 2-3 g/kg. The largest restrospective analysis on the use of IVIg derived from the EuroSCAR study found no additional benefit from IVIg administered at a dose of 1.9 g/kg when compared to the use of supportive measures alone. This study involved the use of lower than recommended doses of IVIg and the patients from the IVIg group tended to have a greater TBSA involvement (Schneck, Fagot et al. 2008).

Randomized control studies are required using sufficient doses of IVIg to characterize its benefit in not only reducing mortality but also arresting the rate of progression and hastening the rate of re-epithelialization. However, the evidence thus far, would suggest that it should be at least considered as part of the adjunctive therapy in the treatment of SJS/TEN.

2.9.4 Cyclosporine

Cyclosporine inhibits CD8 activation and subsequent release of granulysin, granzyme and perforin as well as inhibiting the proapoptotic effect of NF-κB. Several case and case series reports have shown arrest of disease progression and shorter time to re-epithelialization with doses varying from 3-10 mg/kg/daily for a period ranging from 8 days to several weeks. One study showed that outcomes for 10 patients treated with cyclosporine was superior to 6 patients treated with cyclophosphamide and corticosteroids with respect to re-epithelialization, disease progression and death (Arevalo, Lorente et al. 2000). However, randomised control studies are required to better define its benefits, the appropriate dose and duration of therapy. Furthermore, no studies have been published to date evaluating the efficacy of using both IVIg and cyclosporine but may be worthwhile considering as different pathways involved in the pathogenesis of SJS/TEN are targeted.

2.9.5 Other pharmacotherapies

Plasmapheresis and N-acetylcysteine-induced detoxification of drugs have demonstrated benefit in a small number of studies but larger randomized control studies are required to elucidate their role in the management of SJS/TEN. However, thalidomide, a potent inhibitor of TNF, was found in a double blinded randomised placebo controlled to be lethal in 10 of 12 patients as compared with 3 of 10 control subjects (Wolkenstein, Latarjet et al. 1998). The exact mechanism underlying these fatalities is unknown but the drug is firmly contraindicated in SJS/TEN.

2.9.6 Restricted use of related medications

In addition to the restricted use of the same medication, structurally similar drugs should also be avoided. The aromatic anticonvulsants carbamazepine, phenytoin and phenobarbitol cross react with one another. Cross reactivity resulting in SJS/TEN can also occur across different classes of beta-lactam antibiotics, such as penicillins, cephalosporins and carbapenems. Administration of a structurally related drug can also result in different reactions. One case report described a patient with ceftriaxone-induced TEN who developed immediate anaphylaxis following the administration of piperacillin/tazobactam (Lam, Randhawa et al. 2008). The risk of SJS/TEN with structurally distinct agents within the same class of drug is less clear. For example, the cross reactivity between a priopionic acid NSAID and an enolic acid NSAID is unknown. The safest practice is to restrict all NSAIDs following NSAID-induced SJS/TEN.

3. Drug induced hypersensitivity syndrome

3.1 Nosology

The term hypersensitivity syndrome has been used for decades to describe a cutaneous drug reaction accompanied by involvement of internal organs. In 1938, Merritt and Putnam described a toxic reaction to phenytoin characterized by exfoliative dermatitis, fever and eosinophilia (Merritt and Putnam 1938). This was distinguished from those patients who developed a mild, morbilliform rash. The anticonvulsant hypersensitivity syndrome was named in 1988 by Shear and Spielberg to refer the similar cutaneous and systemic manifestations of idiosyncratic reactions to a range of anticonvulsant medications including phenytoin, phenobarbitol and carbamazepine (Shear and Spielberg 1988). In 1996, Bocquet et al introduced the term drug reaction with eosinophilia and systemic symptoms (DRESS) to distinguish it from drug-induced pseudolymphoma and other drug reactions that are not associated with eosinophilia (Bocquet, Bagot et al. 1996). Finally, Shiohara et al proposed the term drug induced hypersensitivity syndrome (DIHS) to include patients who may not have marked eosinophilia but have other evidence of leukocyte abnormalities, internal organ involvement and evidence of HHV-6 reactivation (Suzuki, Inagi et al. 1998; Shiohara, Inaoka et al. 2006).

3.2 Epidemiology

The incidence of DIHS is estimated to be between 1 in 1000 and 1 in 10000 to phenytoin (Gennis, Vemuri et al. 1991). The true incidence remains to be determined because of the variable presentations and the lack of universally accepted criteria. The JSCAR and RegiSCAR studies will provide more accurate reporting on the basis of stringent criteria. Preliminary data from the RegiSCAR study suggests that it affects males and females equally with a mean age of 47.4 years (range 3-84 years) (Mockenhaupt 2007).

3.3 Etiology and clinical features

Various diagnostic criteria have been proposed. Bocquet et al stipulated the presence of (1) cutaneous drug eruption; (2) hematologic abnormalities including eosinophilia greater than 1.5 $\times 10^9$/L or the presence of atypical lymphocytes; and (3) systemic involvement including adenopathy greater than 2 cm in diameter, hepatitis (liver transaminase values >2 normal), interstitial nephritis, interstitial pneumonia, or carditis.

Kardaun et al developed a scoring system to validate the diagnosis using fever $\geq$38.5°C, lymphadenopathy, eosinophilia $\geq$ 700/μL, atypical lymphocytosis, extensive skin rash (>50%), visceral organ involvement (liver, kidney, lung, heart, pancreas), prolonged resolution of the rash ($\geq$15 days), and the absence of infectious diseases serology (hepatitis A, B and C, Epstein Barr virus, cytomegalovirus, mycoplasma and chlamydia), negative autoimmune serology (ANA) and negative blood cultures as supportive criteria (Kardaun, Sidoroff et al. 2007).

The potential role of HHV-6 in the pathogenesis of DIHS was incorporated into the criteria for DIHS by the JSCAR group (Shiohara, Iijima et al. 2007): (1) maculopapular rash developing more than 3 weeks after starting a limited number of drugs; (2) prolonged clinical symptoms 2 weeks after discontinuation of the causative drug; (3) fever greater than 38° C; (4) liver abnormalities (eg, ALT levels >100 U/L); (5) leukocyte abnormalities such as leukocytosis (>11 x 10^9/L), atypical lymphocytosis (>5%), and/or eosinophilia (>1.5 x 10^9/L); (6) lymphadenopathy; and (7) HHV-6 reactivation. Diagnosis of typical DIHS requires the presence of all 7 criteria. If criteria 1-5 are present only, then a diagnosis of atypical DIHS is made.

The syndrome typically begins 3 weeks to 3 months after commencing therapy with a limited number of drugs of which the most prominent ones are listed below.

Carbamazepine
Phenytoin
Phenobarbitol
Zonisamide
Lamotrigine
Allopurinol
Dapsone
Sulphasalazine
Mexiletine
Minocycline
Strontium ranelate
Abacavir

Table 3. The main causative drugs of DIHS

High-grade fever (38-40°C) is usually the first symptom followed by a pruritic maculopapular rash. Patients have facial oedema (Fig. 9), often with pinhead-sized pustules. The rash evolves, especially if the causative drug is not withdrawn into a severe exfoliative dermatitis (Fig. 10) or erythroderma with edematous, follicular and purpuric lesions. Cheilitis (Fig. 9), pharyngeal erythema and oral ulceration may occur but severe stomatitis is not present. Tender lymphadenopathy in more than two sites and bilateral swelling of salivary glands with xerostomia is evident early in the course of disease. Hepatosplenomegaly is a common finding. Leukocytosis with atypical lymphocytes and eosinophilia (60-70% of cases) is a prominent feature of this syndrome although the eosinophilia may not be observed for 1-2 weeks. Thrombocytopenia and anemia may also be present. Hypogammaglobulinema is noted at the onset of disease with the nadir occurring several days after the withdrawal of the causative drug (Kano, Inaoka et al. 2004). An overshoot in the IgG level occurs 1-2 weeks after the nadir before returning to normal on full recovery. Internal organ involvement is summarised in table 4.

Manifestation	Comments
Hepatitis (mixed hepatocellular and cholestatic)	71%
Interstitial nephritis	11%, frequent with Allopurinol-induced DIHS
Pneumonitis/pleuritis	Common in minocycline and abacavir induced DIHS
Myocarditis	Occurs at onset or 40 days after onset of DIHS
Limbic encephalitis	2-4 weeks after onset of DIHS, HHV-6 reactivation in CSF May be assoiciated with SiADH
CMV Gastrointestinal ulceration with bleeding	4-5 weeks after onset of DIHS
Haemaophagocytic syndrome	Rare, occurs 2 weeks after onset of DIHS
Parotid gland enlargement	Rare
Pancreatitis	Rare

Table 4. Internal organ involvement in DIHS

The onset of symptoms is variable with patients developing 2-3 symptomatic features followed by stepwise development of other manifestations. In most cases, withdrawal of the drug is not followed by rapid resolution of symptoms. Many patients may continue to deteriorate and show periodic relapses for weeks after the withdrawal of the causative drug.

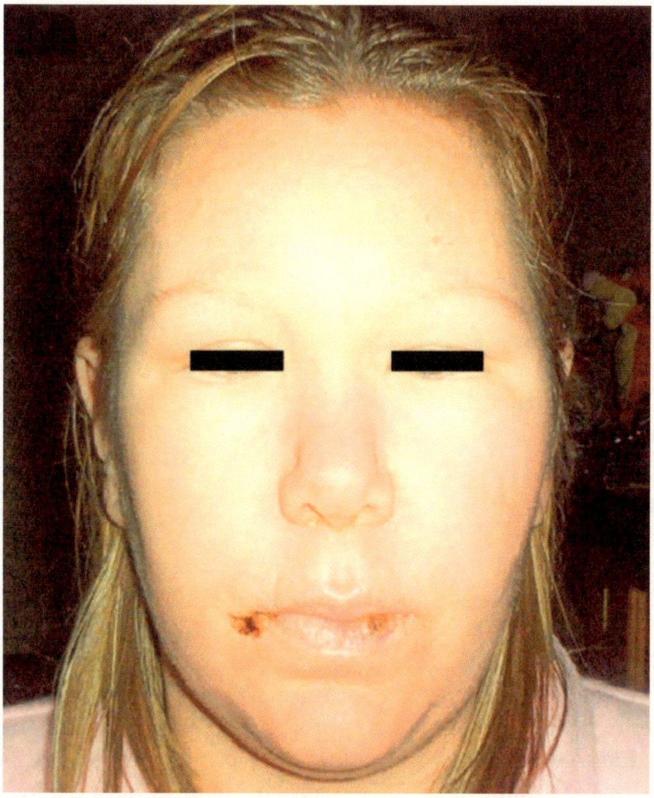

Fig. 9. Facial erythema and edema with labial ulceration in a young woman with DIHS/DRESS.

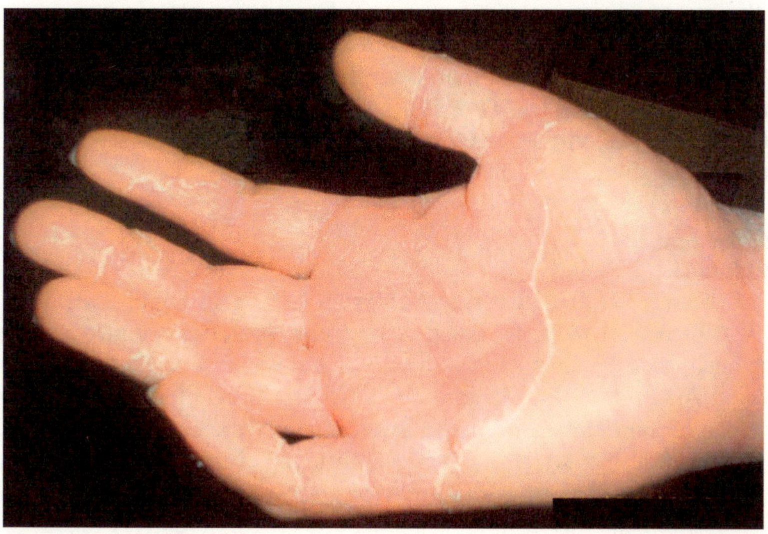

Fig. 10. Exfoliative dermatitis involving the hand in a young woman with DIHS/DRESS who had continued to ingest the culprit drug for 4 weeks when this image was taken.

Several reports have described the occurrence of autoantibody formation and autoimmune diseases up to 4 years after the acute resolution of DRESS (Aota and Shiohara 2009) and these include type 1 diabetes mellitus, autoimmune thyroid disease, scleroderma GVHD, SLE, and bullous pemphigoid. One of the likely explanations for the occurrence of autoimmune disease is the depletion of regulatory T cells upon recovery of disease.
Abacavir, an HIV nucleoside analogue reverse transcriptase inhibitor causes a potentially life-threatening hypersensitivity syndrome in approximately 5-8% of recipients within 6 weeks of therapy. The clinical and laboratory features of this syndrome differs from typical cases of DIHS/DRESS in that there is a predilection for the gastrointestinal system with nausea, abdominal pain, diarrhoea, and the respiratory tract with cough, pharyngitis and shortness of breath. Headache, myalgia and/or arthralgia may also be present. Eosinophilia is present in < 10% of cases and liver function test abnormalities are detected in < 20% of cases (Peyriere, Dereure et al. 2006). Also, the manifestations resolve within 72 hours rather than having a protracted relapsing course and the role of herpetic viruses in this condition is unknown.

3.4 Differential diagnosis

Viral infections such as EBV, CMV, and measles can be distinguished by the absence of eosinophilia, hypogammaglobulinemia, and supportive serology. In children, DIHS is differentiated from Kawasaki's disease by the absence of a bulbar conjunctivitis, strawberry tongue, coronary aneurysms, hypoalbuminemia and thrombocytosis. Serum sickness is characterized by urticarial lesions and the absence of internal organ involvement. Atopic erythroderma with bacterial infection does not usually involve hepatitis or nephritis. Drug-induced pseudolymphoma from carbamazepine or phenytoin is distinguished from DIHS by the absence of internal organ involvement and the prompt resolution of symptoms when the drug is withdrawn. Cutaneous B and T cell lymphomas have an indolent course and characteristic histopathology.

3.5 Pathology

The histopathology of DIHS is relatively non-specific and consists of a lymphocytic infiltrate that is superficial, perivascular, dense and diffuse. Eosinophils may be present but is often absent. The presence of loose rather than discrete granulomatous aggregates of histiocytes have been recently reported (Figs. 11 & 12) (Fernando, Henderson et al. 2009). HHV-6 and DNA from other herpes viruses may be detected in skin lesions by PCR or in situ hybridization (Suzuki, Inagi et al. 1998).

3.6 Drug allergy testing

3.6.1 Patch tests

Santiago et al recently studied the utility of patch testing in DIHS and found a positive reaction in 32% of the 56 patients. Patch testing was performed between 6 weeks and 6 months after healing of the lesion and at least one month after corticosteroids were ceased. They found that 76% of the 17 patients with carbamazepine-induced DIHS were patch test positive but none of the 19 allopurinol-sensitive patients were positive to allopurinol and its metabolite, oxypurinol. No systemic reactions occurred during or after testing (Santiago, Goncalo et al. 2010). Hence patch testing may prove useful once the reagent and timing of such testing is optimized. Patch testing has, however, proven to be very useful in confirming suspected cases for abacavir hypersensitivity with a higher degree of specificity than can be confirmed clinically (Phillips, Wong et al. 2005).

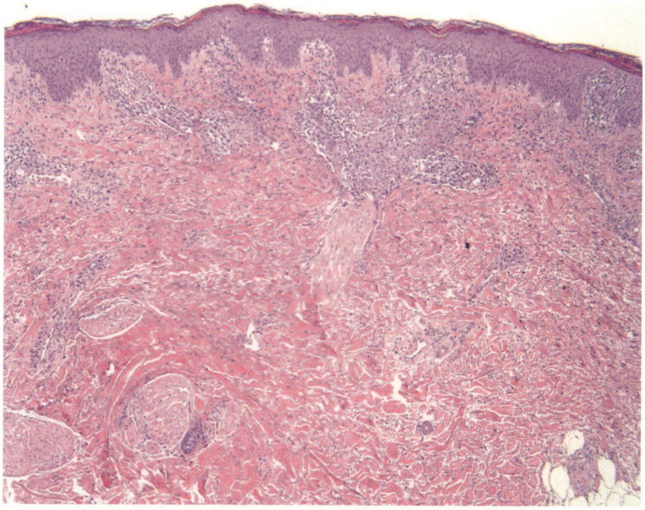

Fig. 11. Low power view of a skin biopsy from a patient with DIHS demonstrating the superficial dermal nature and perivascular distribution of the inflammatory infiltrate with acanthosis and hyperkeratosis of the epidermis (Hematoxylin-eosin, original magnification x40).

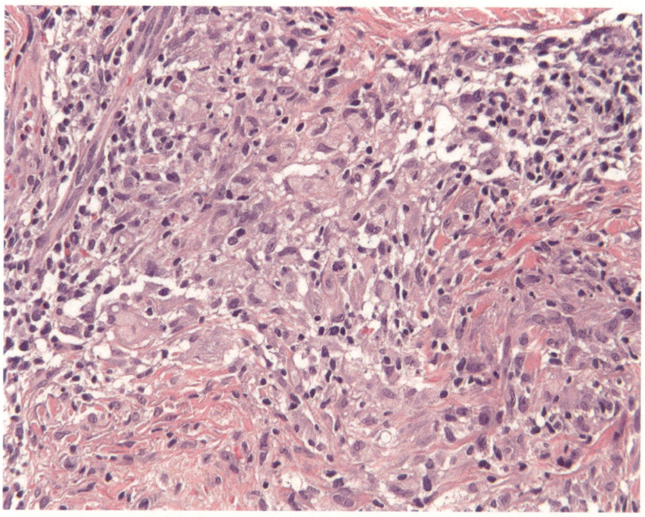

Fig. 12. High power view of a skin biopsy from a patient with DIHS demonstrates granulomatous inflammation with prominent, but relatively loosely aggregated histiocytes, mixed with lymphocytes. Eosinophils are absent (Hematoxylin-eosin, original magnification x200).

3.6.2 Lymphocyte transformation tests (LTTs)

LTTs are usually negative up to 3 weeks after the onset of DIHS but most patients are positive at 5-7 weeks and have persistent responses even at 1 year. Treatment with corticosteroids did not affect the results (Kano, Hirahara et al. 2007). One possible explanation for the negative LTT result during the acute phase of DIHS is the expansion T regulatory cells with a naïve phenotype (CD4CD25FoxP3), which then are depleted by apoptosis during the recovery phase. These regulatory T cells are capable of suppressing proliferation of memory T cells in LTTs (Takahashi, Kano et al. 2009).

3.7 Pathogenesis

The pathogenesis of DIHS is still to be fully elucidated. The precise role of HHV-6 in DIHS is unclear. The initiating event may be the reactivation of one or more herpetic viruses, which is clinically unapparent (Fig. 13). Virus-stimulated T cells may then cross react with drug-derived hapten-protein conjugates that are presented by dendritic cells to naïve antigen-specific CD4 T-cells with the subsequent differentiation into effector/memory CD4 cells. These dendritic cells may also activate CD8 T-cells by cross-presentation. The expansion of effector CD4 T-cells with their production of IFN-γ and other cytokines results in recruitment and activation of macrophages. Failure to eradicate the antigenic stimulus, in this instance due to the continued ingestion of the drug, causes persistent cytokine release and promotes differentiation of macrophages into epithelioid cells, which secrete large amounts of TNF promoting their fusion to form multinucleate giant cells (Fernando, Henderson et al. 2009). Analogous to that observed in GVHD, longitudinal real-time PCR analyses of viral loads in blood samples drawn from patients with DIHS show that various herpetic viruses are sequentially activated as a result of massive T cell stimulation, B cell loss and hypogammaglobulinemia (Hirahara, Kano et al. 2010); Activation of Epstein-Barr virus or HHV-6 extends to the sequential activation of HHV-7, cytomegalovirus and varicella-zoster virus (Kano, Inaoka et al. 2004). The frequent deterioration or several exacerbations that occur despite continuation of the drug may at least be partly explained by sequential reactivation of herpetic viruses and the immune response to viral replication. An alternative explanation is that drug specific T cells are activated resulting in reactivation of the viral genome and sequential reactivation of herpes viruses (Fig. 14).

Genetic susceptibility may also play a role as all patients with allopurinol-induced DIHS in a Han Chinese population harboured the *HLA-B*5801* allele compared with 15% of control subjects (Hung, Chung et al. 2005b). Recently, an association was described between *HLA-A*3101* and DIHS in Northern Europeans; OR 12.41 [1.27-121.03] (McCormack, Alfirevic et al. 2011) and in the Japanese; OR 9.5 [4.6–19.5] (Ozeki, Mushiroda et al. 2011). In a Western Australian HIV Cohort Study, *HLA-B*5701* was present in 14 (78%) of the 18 patients with abacavir hypersensitivity, and in four (2%) of the 167 abacavir tolerant patients; OR 117 [29-481] (Mallal, Nolan et al. 2002). There is a discrepancy in the association of *HLA-B*5701* and abacavir hypersensitivity across various racial groups The association was confirmed in a separate cohort of HIV-infected white Americans and was also found to confer susceptibility in Hispanics but not in blacks (Hughes, Mosteller et al. 2004). No association was found in a cohort of Korean patients (Park, Choe et al. 2009). The racial variation may be partly explained by the differences in MHC haplotypes across different racial groups. The Caucasian 57.1 ancestral haplotype, which confers susceptibility to abacavir hypersensitivity possibly as a result of strong linkage disequilibrium with other candidate genetic factors such as cellular chaperones (e.g. heat shock proteins), inflammatory cytokines (e.g. TNF), and proteins involved in the stress response (e.g. MHC class I chain-related genes, MIC-A and MIC-B). African populations do not demonstrate this haplotype (Cao, Hollenbach et al. 2001). However, in a recent study by Saag et al, all 42 white patients with immunologically confirmed (i.e. positive patch tests) hypersensitivity to abacavir reactions were *HLA-B*5701* positive (sensitivity 100%, OR 1945 [110-34,352]) but in addition all 5 black patients with immunologically confirmed hypersensitivity reactions were *HLA-B*5701* positive (sensitivity 100%, OR 900 [38-21,045]. Screening for the *HLA-B*5701* has eliminated immunologically confirmed cases of abacavir hypersensitivity (Mallal, Phillips et al. 2008).

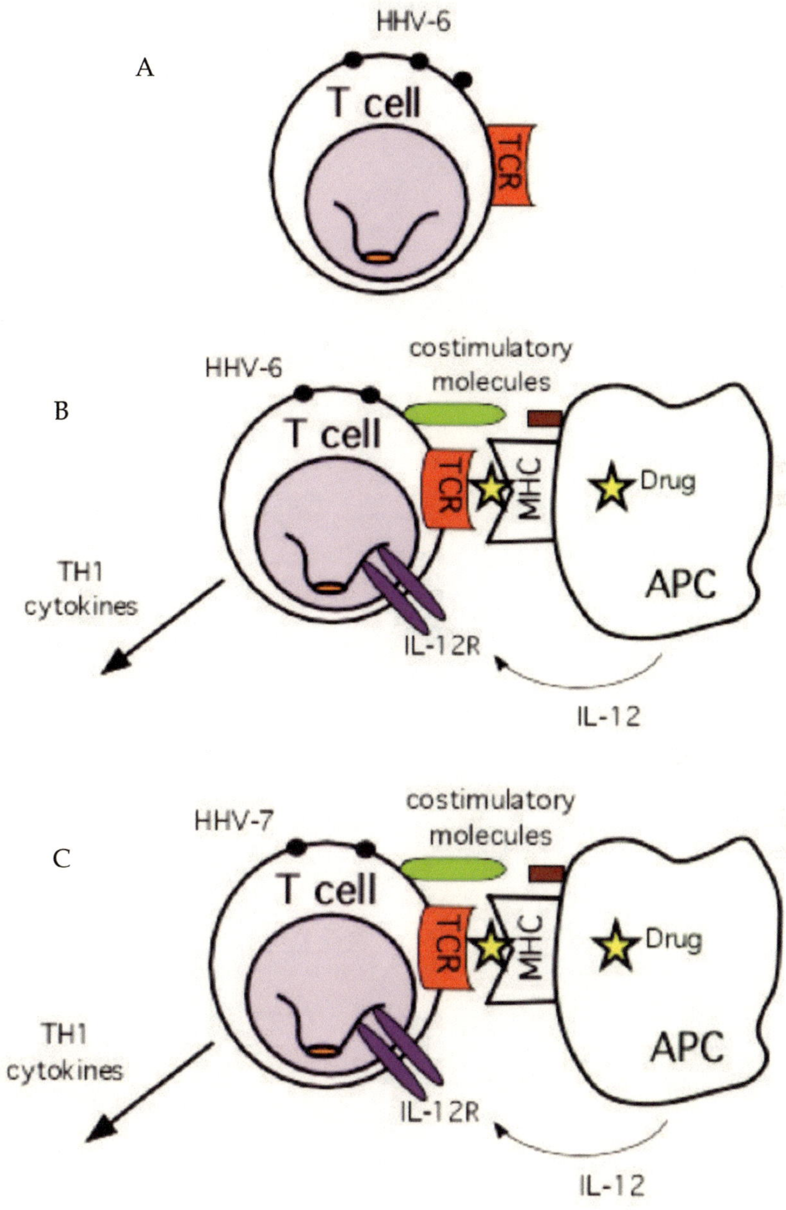

Fig. 13. One theory of the role of herpetic viruses in the pathogenesis of DIHS is the reactivation of HHV-6 within the T cell genome (A), which cross react with the culprit drug (B) resulting in the sequential activation of heterologous herpetic viruses (C).

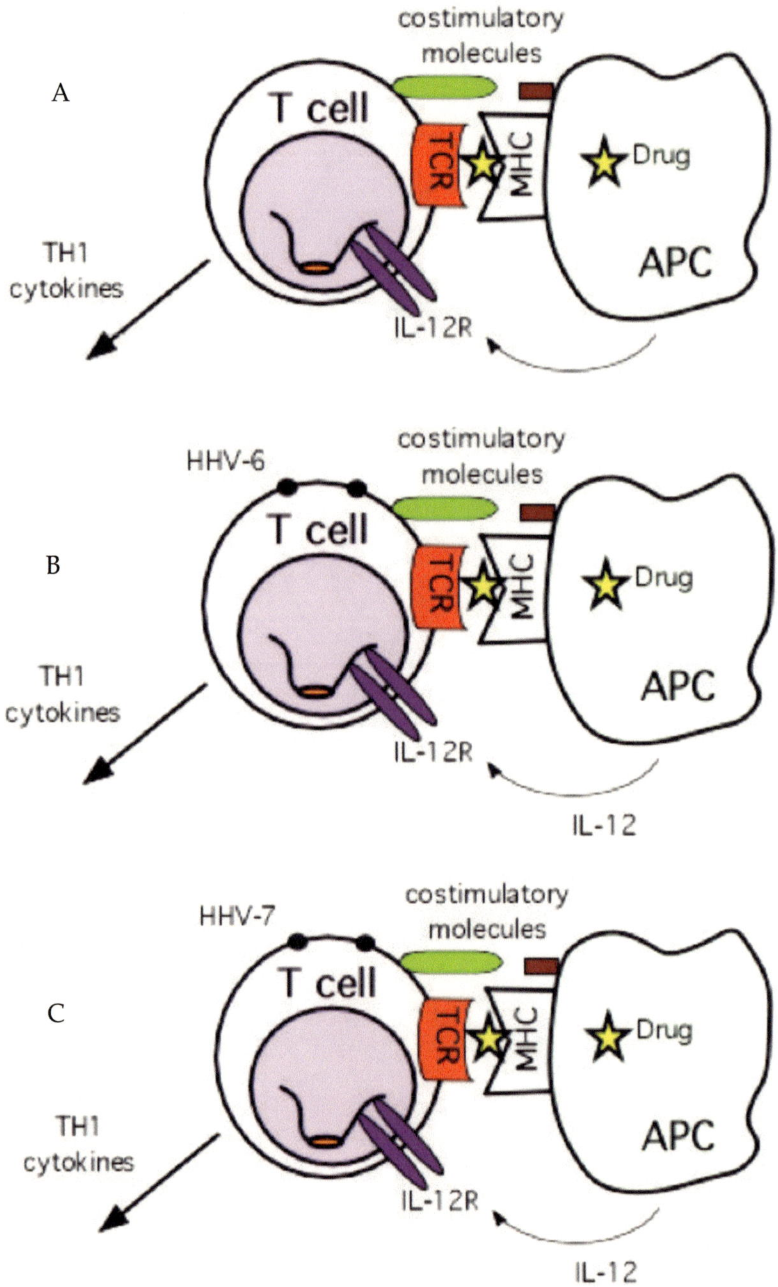

Fig. 14. An alternative theory proposes that drug-specific T cells are activated (A) resulting in reactivation of HHV-6 from within the T cell genome (B) with subsequent sequential reactivation of heterologous herpetic viruses (C).

3.8 Treatment

Early recognition of the syndrome with cessation of the causative drug is essential in improving patient outcomes. No randomized controlled trials have been conducted to determine the appropriate adjunctive therapy for DIHS. Oral corticosteroids at 1 mg/kg/daily is commenced and tapered over at least 6-8 weeks to prevent relapse of various cutaneous and visceral manifestations of the syndrome. If symptoms deteriorate despite corticosteroid therapy then IVIg, plasma exchange (Higuchi, Agatsuma et al. 2005), rituximab or a combination of these modalities could be considered although the evidence for their use is currently scant.

4. Acute generalized exanthematous pustulosis

4.1 Nosology

In 1980, Beylot et al introduced the term acute generalized exanthematous pustulosis (AGEP) to describe acute pustular reactions with distinct clinical and histological features thereby differentiating it from pustular psoriasis (Beylot, Bioulac et al. 1980).

4.2 Demography

AGEP is rare with an incidence of 1-5 cases per million per year (Sidoroff, Halevy et al. 2001). The EuroSCAR study comprising 97 validated cases of AGEP recruited from Austria, France, Israel, Italy and the Netherlands, revealed a mean age (±SD) of 56 (±21) years and a female preponderance with a male/female ratio of 0.8 (Sidoroff, Dunant et al. 2007). The predominance in women was shown to be even greater in case series reports from Taiwan (68.7% of 16 cases) (Chang, Huang et al. 2008), and Israel (76.9% of 13 cases) (Davidovici, Dodiuk-Gad et al. 2008). AGEP has been reported in children, with the largest pediatric series of 20 cases from China (Zhang, Chen et al. 2008).

4.3 Clinical features

The clinical manifestations are characterized by fever and a pruritic or burning edematous erythema followed by the rapid appearance of dozens of small (< 5 mm) non-follicular sterile pustules (Fig. 15). The skin lesions are often accentuated in the intertriginous areas.

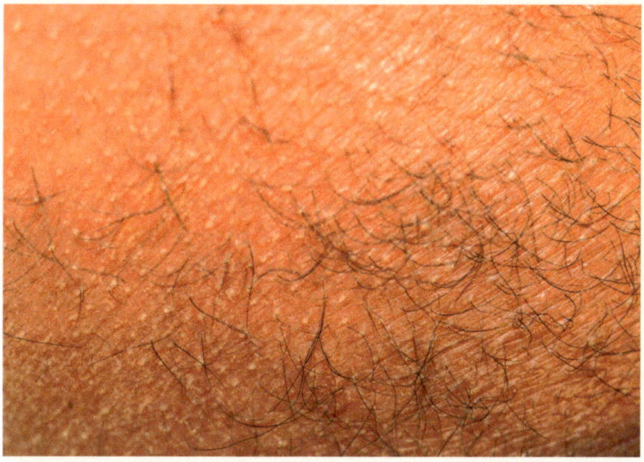

Fig. 15. The lesions of AGEP occur rapidly and are characterized by dozens of small (< 5 mm) non-follicular sterile pustules.

There is usually an accompanying marked neutrophilia (7 x 10^9/L) and in a third of cases, a mild eosinophilia. A mild non-erosive mucous membrane involvement occurs in 20% of cases. Internal organ involvement is uncommon and usually is confined to a slight reduction in creatinine clearance and mild elevation of aminotransferases. The clinical course is characterized by spontaneous resolution of skin and systemic manifestations over a period of up to 15 days once the offending agent is withdrawn. AGEP has a favourable prognosis; the reported mortality rate is up to 5% and poor outcomes usually result from secondary infection in the elderly or those patients with significant comorbidities.

4.4 Etiology

AGEP is caused by drugs in at least 90% of cases. According to the EuroSCAR study, the agents conferring the highest risk are pristinamycin, aminopenicillins, hydroxychloroquine, antibacterial sulphonamides, terbinafine and diltiazem (Sidoroff, Dunant et al. 2007). The latent period is short (usually 1-5 days) with the EuroScar study demonstrating that it may vary for different drugs. For antibiotics, including sulphonamides, the median latent period was 1 day, and for other drugs it was 11 days (Sidoroff, Dunant et al. 2007).
Contact sensitivity has been implicated in a few case reports. Causative agents include mercury, and bufexemac, a potent topical NSAID. Neither of these agents was implicated in the 97 cases of AGEP in the EuroScar study. The role of infectious agents in AGEP has been suggested in various case reports due to the absence of an inciting drug. The organisms include coxsackie B4, cytomegalovirus, parvovirus B19, *Chlamydia pneumoniae,* and *Escherichia coli.* No significant risk for infection was found in the EuroScar study although the study was not designed to identify potential causative organisms. Spider bites were suggested as a cause AGEP in a series of three cases from Israel, presumably as a result of the venom's ability to induce IL-8 and GM-CSF (Davidovici, Pavel et al. 2006). Finally, as illustrated in two recent cases, AGEP may develop without preceding medication or disease (Birnie and Litlewood 2008).

4.5 Pathogenesis

The pathogenesis of AGEP has been elucidated by patch (Schaerli, Britschgi et al. 2004) and in vitro tests (Girardi, Duncan et al. 2005) and initially involves activation, expansion and subsequent migration of drug-specific CD4 and CD8 cells to the skin. The initial influx of CD8 cytotoxic T cells results in apoptosis of keratinocytes and the formation of subcorneal vesicles. The infiltrating CD4 cells release CXCL-8, which results in recruitment of neutrophils, and granulocyte macrophage-colony stimulating factor (GM-CSF), which prevents apoptosis of neutrophils. This results in the conversion of vesicles into pustules. CD4 cells also release IFN-γ, which stimulates keratinocytes to secrete CXCL-8, as well as RANTES and IL-5, which contributes to the eosinophilia observed in some patients (Britschgi, Steiner et al. 2001). Resident Langerhans' cells may present drug antigens to CD4 cells and keratinocytes may act as antigen presenting cells to CD8 cells thereby augmenting the neutrophil-mediated inflammatory response. Genetic susceptibility to AGEP has not been robustly examined and therefore remains largely unknown.

4.6 Diagnostic tests

A pustular smear should be performed to exclude an infectious aetiology. A full blood count will reveal a neutrophilia. A skin biopsy may show (spongiform or non-spongiform) subcorneal and/or intradermal pustules, edema of the papillary dermis, perivascular infiltrates with neutrophils and exocytosis of some eosinophils and focal necrotic keratinocytes (Fig. 16). The typical changes of psoriasis such as acanthosis and papillomatosis are usually absent. Patch testing may be useful in confirming the association between AGEP and the culprit drugs. In a controlled study, patch tests were positive in half of the 14 cases of AGEP (Wolkenstein, Chosidow et al. 1996). Readings should not be restricted to 24 and 48 hours after the application of the drug but should also be determined at 96 and 120 hours to maximise sensitivity. Pustule formation is often observed in positive patch tests in cases of AGEP. The test can be conducted one month after resolution of the disease. The risk of AGEP with patch testing is considered to be low but not negligible (Mashiah and Brenner 2003). A small number of studies have supported a role for LTT, IFN-γ release, lymphokine macrophage migration inhibition factor release assays but these in vitro tests are not widely available and its value remains to be determined in large cohorts.

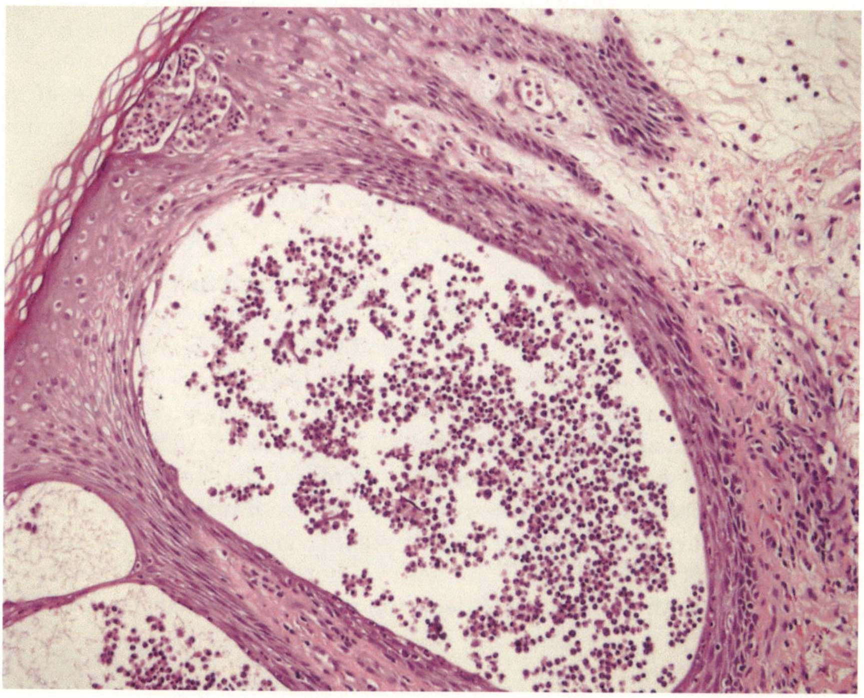

Fig. 16. A moderate power view of a skin biopsy from a patient with AGEP shows spongiform subcorneal pustules, edema of the papillary dermis and perivascular infiltrates with neutrophils and exocytosis of some eosinophils.

4.7 Differential diagnosis

AGEP, which is characterized by non-follicular pustules can be readily distinguished from diseases with follicular pustulosis such as bacterial folliculitis, furunculosis, acneiform eruptions, pustular contact dermatitis, dermatophyte infection, viral exanthema with primary vesiculation and secondary postulation, impetigo, Sweet syndrome and SSSS. Other diseases are not as easily differentiated from AGEP. Generalized pustular psoriasis

(Zumbusch psoriasis) is characterized by pustules that slowly develop on areas of psoriasis accompanied by the histological changes of psoriasis on skin biopsy. There is also usually a family history of psoriasis. Sneddon-Wilkinson disease (subcorneal pustulosis) and subcorneal IgA dermatosis are characterized by the subacute development of larger pustules than those that erupt in AGEP and maybe associated with hyopyon formation. A diagnostic score was devised to validate the diagnosis of AGEP based on the morphology, course of disease, and histology, and assist in the differentiation from similar diseases (Sidoroff, Halevy et al. 2001).

4.8 Treatment

As AGEP is a self-limiting disease with a favourable prognosis. Cessation of the causative agent and supportive treatment is usually all that his required. In the pustular phase, supportive measures consist of moist dressings with drying and disinfecting solutions to avoid superinfection. In the postpustular desquamation phase, emollients are used to optimise preservation of skin barrier function. In a study of nine cases from Israel, all of who made a full recovery, seven received supportive care alone and the other two received corticosteroids (Tamir, Wohl et al. 2006). It remains to be established whether oral or parenteral corticosteroids hasten the resolution of disease. A brief course of systemic corticosteroids may be considered in patients with severe and widespread inflammation of the skin.

5. Conclusion

SCARs such as SJS/TEN, DIHS/DRESS, and AGEP are idiosyncratic and specific types of reactions that have distinct clinical, laboratory and histological features. The definition of DIHS/DRESS has not been universally adopted and will need to be clarified once the role of herpetic viruses and characteristic histological features are known. The early identification of these reactions and the subsequent prompt withdrawal of therapy and the implementation of supportive and adjunctive therapies are crucial in minimising morbidity and rates of mortality. Multicentre randomized studies are required to adopt the most suitable therapies for these potentially life-threatening conditions. The emergence in the understanding of HLA susceptibility genes will enable patients to be screened for the risk of developing a SCAR and will hopefully be more widely performed once cost effective and rapid methods of detection are widely available to the prescribing doctor.

6. References

Abe, R., Shimizu, T., Shibaki, A., Nakamura, H., Watanabe, H. and Shimizu, H. (2003). Toxic epidermal necrolysis and Stevens-Johnson syndrome are induced by soluble Fas ligand. Am J Pathol 162(5): 1515-1520

Abe, R., Yoshioka, N., Murata, J., Fujita, Y. and Shimizu, H. (2009). Granulysin as a marker for early diagnosis of the Stevens-Johnson syndrome. Ann Intern Med 151(7): 514-515

Abood, G. J., Nickoloff, B. J. and Gamelli, R. L. (2008). Treatment strategies in toxic epidermal necrolysis syndrome: where are we at? J Burn Care Res 29(1): 269-276

Aota, N. and Shiohara, T. (2009). Viral connection between drug rashes and autoimmune diseases: how autoimmune responses are generated after resolution of drug rashes. Autoimmun Rev 8(6): 488-494

Araki, Y., Sotozono, C., Inatomi, T., Ueta, M., Yokoi, N., Ueda, E., Kishimoto, S. and Kinoshita, S. (2009). Successful treatment of Stevens-Johnson syndrome with steroid pulse therapy at disease onset. Am J Ophthalmol 147(6): 1004-1011, 1011 e1001

Arevalo, J. M., Lorente, J. A., Gonzalez-Herrada, C. and Jimenez-Reyes, J. (2000). Treatment of toxic epidermal necrolysis with cyclosporin A. J Trauma 48(3): 473-478

Atiyeh, B. S., Dham, R., Yassin, M. F. and El-Musa, K. A. (2003). Treatment of toxic epidermal necrolysis with moisture-retentive ointment: a case report and review of the literature. Dermatol Surg 29(2): 185-188

Ball, R., Ball, L. K., Wise, R. P., Braun, M. M., Beeler, J. A. and Salive, M. E. (2001). Stevens-Johnson syndrome and toxic epidermal necrolysis after vaccination: reports to the vaccine adverse event reporting system. Pediatr Infect Dis J 20(2): 219-223

Bastuji-Garin, S., Fouchard, N., Bertocchi, M., Roujeau, J. C., Revuz, J. and Wolkenstein, P. (2000). SCORTEN: a severity-of-illness score for toxic epidermal necrolysis. J Invest Dermatol 115(2): 149-153

Bastuji-Garin, S., Rzany, B., Stern, R. S., Shear, N. H., Naldi, L. and Roujeau, J. C. (1993). Clinical classification of cases of toxic epidermal necrolysis, Stevens-Johnson syndrome, and erythema multiforme. Arch Dermatol 129(1): 92-96

Beylot, C., Bioulac, P. and Doutre, M. S. (1980). [Acute generalized exanthematic pustuloses (four cases) (author's transl)]. Ann Dermatol Venereol 107(1-2): 37-48

Birnie, A. J. and Litlewood, S. M. (2008). Acute generalized exanthematous pustulosis does not always have a drug-related cause. Br J Dermatol 159(2): 492-493

Bocquet, H., Bagot, M. and Roujeau, J. C. (1996). Drug-induced pseudolymphoma and drug hypersensitivity syndrome (Drug Rash with Eosinophilia and Systemic Symptoms: DRESS). Semin Cutan Med Surg 15(4): 250-257

Britschgi, M., Steiner, U. C., Schmid, S., Depta, J. P., Senti, G., Bircher, A., Burkhart, C., Yawalkar, N. and Pichler, W. J. (2001). T-cell involvement in drug-induced acute generalized exanthematous pustulosis. J Clin Invest 107(11): 1433-1441

Campione, E., Marulli, G. C., Carrozzo, A. M., Chimenti, M. S., Costanzo, A. and Bianchi, L. (2003). High-dose intravenous immunoglobulin for severe drug reactions: efficacy in toxic epidermal necrolysis. Acta Derm Venereol 83(6): 430-432

Cao, K., Hollenbach, J., Shi, X., Shi, W., Chopek, M. and Fernandez-Vina, M. A. (2001). Analysis of the frequencies of HLA-A, B, and C alleles and haplotypes in the five major ethnic groups of the United States reveals high levels of diversity in these loci and contrasting distribution patterns in these populations. Hum Immunol 62(9): 1009-1030

Chang, S. L., Huang, Y. H., Yang, C. H., Hu, S. and Hong, H. S. (2008). Clinical manifestations and characteristics of patients with acute generalized exanthematous pustulosis in Asia. Acta Derm Venereol 88(4): 363-365

Chen, P., Lin, J. J., Lu, C. S., Ong, C. T., Hsieh, P. F., Yang, C. C., Tai, C. T., Wu, S. L., Lu, C. H., Hsu, Y. C., Yu, H. Y., Ro, L. S., Lu, C. T., Chu, C. C., Tsai, J. J., Su, Y. H., Lan, S. H., Sung, S. F., Lin, S. Y., Chuang, H. P., Huang, L. C., Chen, Y. J., Tsai, P. J., Liao, H. T., Lin, Y. H., Chen, C. H., Chung, W. H., Hung, S. I., Wu, J. Y., Chang, C. F., Chen, L., Chen, Y. T. and Shen, C. Y. (2011). Carbamazepine-induced toxic effects and HLA-B*1502 screening in Taiwan. N Engl J Med 364(12): 1126-1133

Chung, W. H., Hung, S. I., Hong, H. S., Hsih, M. S., Yang, L. C., Ho, H. C., Wu, J. Y. and Chen, Y. T. (2004). Medical genetics: a marker for Stevens-Johnson syndrome. Nature 428(6982): 486

Chung, W. H., Hung, S. I., Yang, J. Y., Su, S. C., Huang, S. P., Wei, C. Y., Chin, S. W., Chiou, C. C., Chu, S. C., Ho, H. C., Yang, C. H., Lu, C. F., Wu, J. Y., Liao, Y. D. and Chen, Y. T. (2008). Granulysin is a key mediator for disseminated keratinocyte death in Stevens-Johnson syndrome and toxic epidermal necrolysis. Nat Med 14(12): 1343-1350

Cote, B., Wechsler, J., Bastuji-Garin, S., Assier, H., Revuz, J. and Roujeau, J. C. (1995). Clinicopathologic correlation in erythema multiforme and Stevens-Johnson syndrome. Arch Dermatol 131(11): 1268-1272

Davidovici, B., Dodiuk-Gad, R., Rozenman, D. and Halevy, S. (2008). Profile of acute generalized exanthematous pustulosis in Israel during 2002-2005: results of the RegiSCAR Study. Isr Med Assoc J 10(6): 410-412

Davidovici, B. B., Pavel, D., Cagnano, E., Rozenman, D. and Halevy, S. (2006). Acute generalized exanthematous pustulosis following a spider bite: report of 3 cases. J Am Acad Dermatol 55(3): 525-529

Deng, A., Chen, S., Li, Q., Lyu, S. C., Clayberger, C. and Krensky, A. M. (2005). Granulysin, a cytolytic molecule, is also a chemoattractant and proinflammatory activator. J Immunol 174(9): 5243-5248

Dietrich, A., Kawakubo, Y., Rzany, B., Mockenhaupt, M., Simon, J. C. and Schopf, E. (1995). Low N-acetylating capacity in patients with Stevens-Johnson syndrome and toxic epidermal necrolysis. Exp Dermatol 4(5): 313-316

Dincer, H. E., Dincer, A. P. and Levinson, D. J. (2002). Asymptomatic hyperuricemia: to treat or not to treat. Cleve Clin J Med 69(8): 594, 597, 600-592 passim

Engelhardt, S. L., Schurr, M. J. and Helgerson, R. B. (1997). Toxic epidermal necrolysis: an analysis of referral patterns and steroid usage. J Burn Care Rehabil 18(6): 520-524

Fernando, S. L. and Broadfoot, A. J. (2010). Prevention of severe cutaneous adverse drug reactions: the emerging value of pharmacogenetic screening. Cmaj 182(5): 476-480

Fernando, S. L., Henderson, C. J. and O'Connor, K. S. (2009). Drug-induced hypersensitivity syndrome with superficial granulomatous dermatitis--a novel finding. Am J Dermatopathol 31(6): 611-613

Gamen, S., Hanson, D. A., Kaspar, A., Naval, J., Krensky, A. M. and Anel, A. (1998). Granulysin-induced apoptosis. I. Involvement of at least two distinct pathways. J Immunol 161(4): 1758-1764

Gennis, M. A., Vemuri, R., Burns, E. A., Hill, J. V., Miller, M. A. and Spielberg, S. P. (1991). Familial occurrence of hypersensitivity to phenytoin. Am J Med 91(6): 631-634

Ginsburg, C. M. (1982). Stevens-Johnson syndrome in children. Pediatr Infect Dis 1(3): 155-158

Girardi, M., Duncan, K. O., Tigelaar, R. E., Imaeda, S., Watsky, K. L. and McNiff, J. M. (2005). Cross-comparison of patch test and lymphocyte proliferation responses in patients with a history of acute generalized exanthematous pustulosis. Am J Dermatopathol 27(4): 343-346

Guegan, S., Bastuji-Garin, S., Poszepczynska-Guigne, E., Roujeau, J. C. and Revuz, J. (2006). Performance of the SCORTEN during the first five days of hospitalization to predict the prognosis of epidermal necrolysis. J Invest Dermatol 126(2): 272-276

Halebian, P. H., Corder, V. J., Madden, M. R., Finklestein, J. L. and Shires, G. T. (1986). Improved burn center survival of patients with toxic epidermal necrolysis managed without corticosteroids. Ann Surg 204(5): 503-512

Halevy, S., Ghislain, P. D., Mockenhaupt, M., Fagot, J. P., Bouwes Bavinck, J. N., Sidoroff, A., Naldi, L., Dunant, A., Viboud, C. and Roujeau, J. C. (2008). Allopurinol is the most common cause of Stevens-Johnson syndrome and toxic epidermal necrolysis in Europe and Israel. J Am Acad Dermatol 58(1): 25-32

Higuchi, M., Agatsuma, T., Iizima, M., Yamazaki, Y., Saita, T., Ichikawa, T., Kamijo, Y., Arakura, H., Hora, K. and Kiyosawa, K. (2005). A case of drug-induced hypersensitivity syndrome with multiple organ involvement treated with plasma exchange. Ther Apher Dial 9(5): 412-416

Hirahara, K., Kano, Y., Mitsuyama, Y., Takahashi, R., Kimishima, M. and Shiohara, T. (2010). Differences in immunological alterations and underlying viral infections in two well-defined severe drug eruptions. Clin Exp Dermatol 35(8): 863-868

House, R. A., Jakubovic, H., Wong, L. and Holness, D. L. (1992). Work-related toxic epidermal necrolysis? J Occup Med 34(2): 135-139

Hughes, A. R., Mosteller, M., Bansal, A. T., Davies, K., Haneline, S. A., Lai, E. H., Nangle, K., Scott, T., Spreen, W. R., Warren, L. L. and Roses, A. D. (2004). Association of genetic variations in HLA-B region with hypersensitivity to abacavir in some, but not all, populations. Pharmacogenomics 5(2): 203-211

Hung, S. I., Chung, W. H. and Chen, Y. T. (2005a). HLA-B genotyping to detect carbamazepine induced Stevens-Johnson syndrome: implications for personalizing medicine. Personalized Med. 2: 225-237

Hung, S. I., Chung, W. H. and Chen, Y. T. (2007). Genetics of severe drug hypersensitivity reactions in Han Chinese. Drug Hypersensitivity. Pichler, W. J. Basel., Karger.: 105-114.

Hung, S. I., Chung, W. H., Jee, S. H., Chen, W. C., Chang, Y. T., Lee, W. R., Hu, S. L., Wu, M. T., Chen, G. S., Wong, T. W., Hsiao, P. F., Chen, W. H., Shih, H. Y., Fang, W. H.,

Wei, C. Y., Lou, Y. H., Huang, Y. L., Lin, J. J. and Chen, Y. T. (2006). Genetic susceptibility to carbamazepine-induced cutaneous adverse drug reactions. Pharmacogenet Genomics 16(4): 297-306

Hung, S. I., Chung, W. H., Liou, L. B., Chu, C. C., Lin, M., Huang, H. P., Lin, Y. L., Lan, J. L., Yang, L. C., Hong, H. S., Chen, M. J., Lai, P. C., Wu, M. S., Chu, C. Y., Wang, K. H., Chen, C. H., Fann, C. S., Wu, J. Y. and Chen, Y. T. (2005b). HLA-B*5801 allele as a genetic marker for severe cutaneous adverse reactions caused by allopurinol. Proc Natl Acad Sci U S A 102(11): 4134-4139

Kakourou, T., Klontza, D., Soteropoulou, F. and Kattamis, C. (1997). Corticosteroid treatment of erythema multiforme major (Stevens-Johnson syndrome) in children. Eur J Pediatr 156(2): 90-93

Kaniwa, N., Saito, Y., Aihara, M., Matsunaga, K., Tohkin, M., Kurose, K., Sawada, J., Furuya, H., Takahashi, Y., Muramatsu, M., Kinoshita, S., Abe, M., Ikeda, H., Kashiwagi, M., Song, Y., Ueta, M., Sotozono, C., Ikezawa, Z. and Hasegawa, R. (2008). HLA-B locus in Japanese patients with anti-epileptics and allopurinol-related Stevens-Johnson syndrome and toxic epidermal necrolysis. Pharmacogenomics 9(11): 1617-1622

Kano, Y., Hirahara, K., Mitsuyama, Y., Takahashi, R. and Shiohara, T. (2007). Utility of the lymphocyte transformation test in the diagnosis of drug sensitivity: dependence on its timing and the type of drug eruption. Allergy 62(12): 1439-1444

Kano, Y., Inaoka, M. and Shiohara, T. (2004). Association between anticonvulsant hypersensitivity syndrome and human herpesvirus 6 reactivation and hypogammaglobulinemia. Arch Dermatol 140(2): 183-188

Kardaun, S. H., Sidoroff, A., Valeyrie-Allanore, L., Halevy, S., Davidovici, B. B., Mockenhaupt, M. and Roujeau, J. C. (2007). Variability in the clinical pattern of cutaneous side-effects of drugs with systemic symptoms: does a DRESS syndrome really exist? Br J Dermatol 156(3): 609-611

Khoo, B. P. and Leow, Y. H. (2000). A review of inpatients with adverse drug reactions to allopurinol. Singapore Med J 41(4): 156-160

Kumar, A., Edward, N., White, M. I., Johnston, P. W. and Catto, G. R. (1996). Allopurinol, erythema multiforme, and renal insufficiency. Bmj 312(7024): 173-174

Lam, A., Randhawa, I. and Klaustermeyer, W. (2008). Cephalosporin induced toxic epidermal necrolysis and subsequent penicillin drug exanthem. Allergol Int 57(3): 281-284

Lam, N. S., Yang, Y. H., Wang, L. C., Lin, Y. T. and Chiang, B. L. (2004). Clinical characteristics of childhood erythema multiforme, Stevens-Johnson syndrome and toxic epidermal necrolysis in Taiwanese children. J Microbiol Immunol Infect 37(6): 366-370

Lebargy, F., Wolkenstein, P., Gisselbrecht, M., Lange, F., Fleury-Feith, J., Delclaux, C., Roupie, E., Revuz, J. and Roujeau, J. C. (1997). Pulmonary complications in toxic epidermal necrolysis: a prospective clinical study. Intensive Care Med 23(12): 1237-1244

Letko, E., Papaliodis, D. N., Papaliodis, G. N., Daoud, Y. J., Ahmed, A. R. and Foster, C. S. (2005). Stevens-Johnson syndrome and toxic epidermal necrolysis: a review of the literature. Ann Allergy Asthma Immunol 94(4): 419-436; quiz 436-418, 456

Levi, N., Bastuji-Garin, S., Mockenhaupt, M., Roujeau, J. C., Flahault, A., Kelly, J. P., Martin, E., Kaufman, D. W. and Maison, P. (2009). Medications as risk factors of Stevens-Johnson syndrome and toxic epidermal necrolysis in children: a pooled analysis. Pediatrics 123(2): e297-304

Lonjou, C., Borot, N., Sekula, P., Ledger, N., Thomas, L., Halevy, S., Naldi, L., Bouwes-Bavinck, J. N., Sidoroff, A., de Toma, C., Schumacher, M., Roujeau, J. C., Hovnanian, A. and Mockenhaupt, M. (2008). A European study of HLA-B in Stevens-Johnson syndrome and toxic epidermal necrolysis related to five high-risk drugs. Pharmacogenet Genomics 18(2): 99-107

Lonjou, C., Thomas, L., Borot, N., Ledger, N., de Toma, C., LeLouet, H., Graf, E., Schumacher, M., Hovnanian, A., Mockenhaupt, M. and Roujeau, J. C. (2006). A marker for Stevens-Johnson syndrome ...: ethnicity matters. Pharmacogenomics J 6(4): 265-268

Lyell, A. (1956). Toxic epidermal necrolysis: an eruption resembling scalding of the skin. Br J Dermatol 68(11): 355-361

Mallal, S., Nolan, D., Witt, C., Masel, G., Martin, A. M., Moore, C., Sayer, D., Castley, A., Mamotte, C., Maxwell, D., James, I. and Christiansen, F. T. (2002). Association between presence of HLA-B*5701, HLA-DR7, and HLA-DQ3 and hypersensitivity to HIV-1 reverse-transcriptase inhibitor abacavir. Lancet 359(9308): 727-732

Mallal, S., Phillips, E., Carosi, G., Molina, J. M., Workman, C., Tomazic, J., Jagel-Guedes, E., Rugina, S., Kozyrev, O., Cid, J. F., Hay, P., Nolan, D., Hughes, S., Hughes, A., Ryan, S., Fitch, N., Thorborn, D. and Benbow, A. (2008). HLA-B*5701 screening for hypersensitivity to abacavir. N Engl J Med 358(6): 568-579

Mashiah, J. and Brenner, S. (2003). A systemic reaction to patch testing for the evaluationof acute generalized exanthematous pustulosis. Arch Dermatol 139(9): 1181-1183

McCormack, M., Alfirevic, A., Bourgeois, S., Farrell, J. J., Kasperaviciute, D., Carrington, M., Sills, G. J., Marson, T., Jia, X., de Bakker, P. I., Chinthapalli, K., Molokhia, M., Johnson, M. R., O'Connor, G. D., Chaila, E., Alhusaini, S., Shianna, K. V., Radtke, R. A., Heinzen, E. L., Walley, N., Pandolfo, M., Pichler, W., Park, B. K., Depondt, C., Sisodiya, S. M., Goldstein, D. B., Deloukas, P., Delanty, N., Cavalleri, G. L. and Pirmohamed, M. (2011). HLA-A*3101 and carbamazepine-induced hypersensitivity reactions in Europeans. N Engl J Med 364(12): 1134-1143

McInnes, G. T., Lawson, D. H. and Jick, H. (1981). Acute adverse reactions attributed to allopurinol in hospitalised patients. Ann Rheum Dis 40(3): 245-249

Merritt, H. H. and Putnam, T. J. (1938). Sodium diphenylhydantoinate in the treatment of convulsive disorders. JAMA 111: 1068-1073

Metry, D. W., Jung, P. and Levy, M. L. (2003). Use of intravenous immunoglobulin in children with stevens-johnson syndrome and toxic epidermal necrolysis: seven cases and review of the literature. Pediatrics 112(6 Pt 1): 1430-1436

Mockenhaupt, M. (2007). Epidemiology and causes of severe cutaneous adverse drug reactions. Drug hypersensitivity. Pichler, W. J. Basel, Karger: 18-31.

Mockenhaupt, M., Messenheimer, J., Tennis, P. and Schlingmann, J. (2005). Risk of Stevens-Johnson syndrome and toxic epidermal necrolysis in new users of antiepileptics. Neurology 64(7): 1134-1138

Mockenhaupt, M., Viboud, C., Dunant, A., Naldi, L., Halevy, S., Bouwes Bavinck, J. N., Sidoroff, A., Schneck, J., Roujeau, J. C. and Flahault, A. (2008). Stevens-Johnson syndrome and toxic epidermal necrolysis: assessment of medication risks with emphasis on recently marketed drugs. The EuroSCAR-study. J Invest Dermatol 128(1): 35-44

Nassif, A., Bensussan, A., Boumsell, L., Deniaud, A., Moslehi, H., Wolkenstein, P., Bagot, M. and Roujeau, J. C. (2004). Toxic epidermal necrolysis: effector cells are drug-specific cytotoxic T cells. J Allergy Clin Immunol 114(5): 1209-1215

Nassif, A., Bensussan, A., Dorothee, G., Mami-Chouaib, F., Bachot, N., Bagot, M., Boumsell, L. and Roujeau, J. C. (2002). Drug specific cytotoxic T-cells in the skin lesions of a patient with toxic epidermal necrolysis. J Invest Dermatol 118(4): 728-733

Ng, P. P., Sun, Y. J., Tan, H. H. and Tan, S. H. (2003). Detection of herpes simplex virus genomic DNA in various subsets of Erythema multiforme by polymerase chain reaction. Dermatology 207(4): 349-353

Ozeki, T., Mushiroda, T., Yowang, A., Takahashi, A., Kubo, M., Shirakata, Y., Ikezawa, Z., Iijima, M., Shiohara, T., Hashimoto, K., Kamatani, N. and Nakamura, Y. (2011). Genome-wide association study identifies HLA-A*3101 allele as a genetic risk factor for carbamazepine-induced cutaneous adverse drug reactions in Japanese population. Hum Mol Genet 20(5): 1034-1041

Park, W. B., Choe, P. G., Song, K. H., Lee, S., Jang, H. C., Jeon, J. H., Park, S. W., Park, M. H., Oh, M. D. and Choe, K. W. (2009). Should HLA-B*5701 screening be performed in every ethnic group before starting abacavir? Clin Infect Dis 48(3): 365-367

Peyriere, H., Dereure, O., Breton, H., Demoly, P., Cociglio, M., Blayac, J. P. and Hillaire-Buys, D. (2006). Variability in the clinical pattern of cutaneous side-effects of drugs with systemic symptoms: does a DRESS syndrome really exist? Br J Dermatol 155(2): 422-428

Phillips, E. J., Wong, G. A., Kaul, R., Shahabi, K., Nolan, D. A., Knowles, S. R., Martin, A. M., Mallal, S. A. and Shear, N. H. (2005). Clinical and immunogenetic correlates of abacavir hypersensitivity. Aids 19(9): 979-981

Pichler, W. J. (2005). Direct T-cell stimulations by drugs--bypassing the innate immune system. Toxicology 209(2): 95-100

Pichler, W. J., Adam, J., Daubner, B., Gentinetta, T., Keller, M. and Yerly, D. (2010). Drug hypersensitivity reactions: pathomechanism and clinical symptoms. Med Clin North Am 94(4): 645-664, xv

Posadas, S. J., Padial, A., Torres, M. J., Mayorga, C., Leyva, L., Sanchez, E., Alvarez, J., Romano, A., Juarez, C. and Blanca, M. (2002). Delayed reactions to drugs show levels of perforin, granzyme B, and Fas-L to be related to disease severity. J Allergy Clin Immunol 109(1): 155-161

Prins, C., Vittorio, C., Padilla, R. S., Hunziker, T., Itin, P., Forster, J., Brocker, E. B., Saurat, J. H. and French, L. E. (2003). Effect of high-dose intravenous immunoglobulin therapy in Stevens-Johnson syndrome: a retrospective, multicenter study. Dermatology 207(1): 96-99

Quinn, A. M., Brown, K., Bonish, B. K., Curry, J., Gordon, K. B., Sinacore, J., Gamelli, R. and Nickoloff, B. J. (2005). Uncovering histologic criteria with prognostic significance in toxic epidermal necrolysis. Arch Dermatol 141(6): 683-687

Rasmussen, J. E. (1976). Erythema multiforme in children. Response to treatment with systemic corticosteroids. Br J Dermatol 95(2): 181-186

Rauch, A., Nolan, D., Martin, A., McKinnon, E., Almeida, C. and Mallal, S. (2006). Prospective genetic screening decreases the incidence of abacavir hypersensitivity reactions in the Western Australian HIV cohort study. Clin Infect Dis 43(1): 99-102

Roujeau, J. C. (2005). Clinical heterogeneity of drug hypersensitivity. Toxicology 209(2): 123-129

Roujeau, J. C., Kelly, J. P., Naldi, L., Rzany, B., Stern, R. S., Anderson, T., Auquier, A., Bastuji-Garin, S., Correia, O., Locati, F. and et al. (1995). Medication use and the risk of Stevens-Johnson syndrome or toxic epidermal necrolysis. N Engl J Med 333(24): 1600-1607

Rzany, B., Correia, O., Kelly, J. P., Naldi, L., Auquier, A. and Stern, R. (1999). Risk of Stevens-Johnson syndrome and toxic epidermal necrolysis during first weeks of antiepileptic therapy: a case-control study. Study Group of the International Case Control Study on Severe Cutaneous Adverse Reactions. Lancet 353(9171): 2190-2194

Rzany, B., Mockenhaupt, M., Baur, S., Schroder, W., Stocker, U., Mueller, J., Hollander, N., Bruppacher, R. and Schopf, E. (1996). Epidemiology of erythema exsudativum multiforme majus, Stevens-Johnson syndrome, and toxic epidermal necrolysis in Germany (1990-1992): structure and results of a population-based registry. J Clin Epidemiol 49(7): 769-773

Samimi, S. S. and Siegfried, E. (2002). Stevens-Johnson syndrome developing in a girl with systemic lupus erythematosus on high-dose corticosteroid therapy. Pediatr Dermatol 19(1): 52-55

Sanderson, J. P., Naisbitt, D. J., Farrell, J., Ashby, C. A., Tucker, M. J., Rieder, M. J., Pirmohamed, M., Clarke, S. E. and Park, B. K. (2007). Sulfamethoxazole and its metabolite nitroso sulfamethoxazole stimulate dendritic cell costimulatory signaling. J Immunol 178(9): 5533-5542

Santiago, F., Goncalo, M., Vieira, R., Coelho, S. and Figueiredo, A. (2010). Epicutaneous patch testing in drug hypersensitivity syndrome (DRESS). Contact Dermatitis 62(1): 47-53

Schaerli, P., Britschgi, M., Keller, M., Steiner, U. C., Steinmann, L. S., Moser, B. and Pichler, W. J. (2004). Characterization of human T cells that regulate neutrophilic skin inflammation. J Immunol 173(3): 2151-2158

Schlienger, R. G., Shapiro, L. E. and Shear, N. H. (1998). Lamotrigine-induced severe cutaneous adverse reactions. Epilepsia 39 Suppl 7: S22-26

Schneck, J., Fagot, J. P., Sekula, P., Sassolas, B., Roujeau, J. C. and Mockenhaupt, M. (2008). Effects of treatments on the mortality of Stevens-Johnson syndrome and toxic epidermal necrolysis: A retrospective study on patients included in the prospective EuroSCAR Study. J Am Acad Dermatol 58(1): 33-40

Schulz, J. T., Sheridan, R. L. (2006). Severe desquamating disorder after liver transplant: toxic epidermal necrolysis or graft versus host disease? J Burns Wounds 5(e1).

Shammas, M. C., Lai, E. C., Sarkar, J. S., Yang, J., Starr, C. E. and Sippel, K. C. (2010). Management of acute Stevens-Johnson syndrome and toxic epidermal necrolysis utilizing amniotic membrane and topical corticosteroids. Am J Ophthalmol 149(2): 203-213 e202

Shear, N. H. and Spielberg, S. P. (1988). Anticonvulsant hypersensitivity syndrome. In vitro assessment of risk. J Clin Invest 82(6): 1826-1832

Shiohara, T., Iijima, M., Ikezawa, Z., Hashimoto, K. (2007). The diagnosis of a DRESS syndrome has been sufficiently established on the basis of typical clinical features and viral reactivations. Br J Dermatol 156(5): 1083-1804

Shiohara, T., Inaoka, M. and Kano, Y. (2006). Drug-induced hypersensitivity syndrome (DIHS): a reaction induced by a complex interplay among herpesviruses and antiviral and antidrug immune responses. Allergol Int 55(1): 1-8

Sidoroff, A., Dunant, A., Viboud, C., Halevy, S., Bavinck, J. N., Naldi, L., Mockenhaupt, M., Fagot, J. P. and Roujeau, J. C. (2007). Risk factors for acute generalized exanthematous pustulosis (AGEP)-results of a multinational case-control study (EuroSCAR). Br J Dermatol 157(5): 989-996

Sidoroff, A., Halevy, S., Bavinck, J. N., Vaillant, L. and Roujeau, J. C. (2001). Acute generalized exanthematous pustulosis (AGEP)--a clinical reaction pattern. J Cutan Pathol 28(3): 113-119

Stamp, L., Gow, P., Sharples, K. and Raill, B. (2000). The optimal use of allopurinol: an audit of allopurinol use in South Auckland. Aust N Z J Med 30(5): 567-572

Stevens, A. M. and Johnson, F. C. (1922). A new eruptive fever associated with stomatitis and ophthalmia: report of two cases in children. Am J Dis Child 24: 526-533

Sugimoto, Y., Mizutani, H., Sato, T., Kawamura, N., Ohkouchi, K. and Shimizu, M. (1998). Toxic epidermal necrolysis with severe gastrointestinal mucosal cell death: a patient who excreted long tubes of dead intestinal epithelium. J Dermatol 25(8): 533-538

Suzuki, Y., Inagi, R., Aono, T., Yamanishi, K. and Shiohara, T. (1998). Human herpesvirus 6 infection as a risk factor for the development of severe drug-induced hypersensitivity syndrome. Arch Dermatol 134(9): 1108-1112

Takahashi, R., Kano, Y., Yamazaki, Y., Kimishima, M., Mizukawa, Y. and Shiohara, T. (2009). Defective regulatory T cells in patients with severe drug eruptions: timing of the dysfunction is associated with the pathological phenotype and outcome. J Immunol 182(12): 8071-8079

Tamir, E., Wohl, Y., Mashiah, J. and Brenner, S. (2006). Acute generalized exanthematous pustulosis: a retrospective analysis showing a clear predilection for women. Skinmed 5(4): 186-188

Thomas, B. A. (1950). The so-called Stevens-Johnson syndrome. Br Med J 1(4667): 1393-1397

Ueta, M., Sotozono, C., Inatomi, T., Kojima, K., Hamuro, J. and Kinoshita, S. (2008). Association of combined IL-13/IL-4R signaling pathway gene polymorphism with Stevens-Johnson syndrome accompanied by ocular surface complications. Invest Ophthalmol Vis Sci 49(5): 1809-1813

Vazquez-Mellado, J., Morales, E. M., Pacheco-Tena, C. and Burgos-Vargas, R. (2001). Relation between adverse events associated with allopurinol and renal function in patients with gout. Ann Rheum Dis 60(10): 981-983

Viard, I., Wehrli, P., Bullani, R., Schneider, P., Holler, N., Salomon, D., Hunziker, T., Saurat, J. H., Tschopp, J. and French, L. E. (1998). Inhibition of toxic epidermal necrolysis by blockade of CD95 with human intravenous immunoglobulin. Science 282(5388): 490-493

Viard-Leveugle, I., Bullani, R. R., Meda, P., Micheau, O., Limat, A., Saurat, J. H., Tschopp, J. and French, L. E. (2003). Intracellular localization of keratinocyte Fas ligand explains lack of cytolytic activity under physiological conditions. J Biol Chem 278(18): 16183-16188

Wen, S. H., Lai, M. J. and Yang, K. L. (2008). Human leukocyte antigen-A, -B, and -DRB1 haplotypes of cord blood units in the Tzu Chi Taiwan Cord Blood Bank. Hum Immunol 69(7): 430-436

Wolkenstein, P., Carriere, V., Charue, D., Bastuji-Garin, S., Revuz, J., Roujeau, J. C., Beaune, P. and Bagot, M. (1995). A slow acetylator genotype is a risk factor for sulphonamide-induced toxic epidermal necrolysis and Stevens-Johnson syndrome. Pharmacogenetics 5(4): 255-258

Wolkenstein, P., Chosidow, O., Flechet, M. L., Robbiola, O., Paul, M., Dume, L., Revuz, J. and Roujeau, J. C. (1996). Patch testing in severe cutaneous adverse drug reactions, including Stevens-Johnson syndrome and toxic epidermal necrolysis. Contact Dermatitis 35(4): 234-236

Wolkenstein, P., Latarjet, J., Roujeau, J. C., Duguet, C., Boudeau, S., Vaillant, L., Maignan, M., Schuhmacher, M. H., Milpied, B., Pilorget, A., Bocquet, H., Brun-Buisson, C. and Revuz, J. (1998). Randomised comparison of thalidomide versus placebo in toxic epidermal necrolysis. Lancet 352(9140): 1586-1589.0140-6736 (Print) 0140-6736 (Linking)

Wolkenstein, P. and Revuz, J. (2000). Toxic epidermal necrolysis. Dermatol Clin 18(3): 485-495, ix

Yalcin, B. and Karaduman, A. (2000). Stevens-Johnson syndrome associated with concomitant use of lamotrigine and valproic acid. J Am Acad Dermatol 43(5 Pt 2): 898-899

Yang, Y., Xu, J., Li, F. and Zhu, X. (2009). Combination therapy of intravenous immunoglobulin and corticosteroid in the treatment of toxic epidermal necrolysis and Stevens-Johnson syndrome: a retrospective comparative study in China. Int J Dermatol 48(10): 1122-1128

Zawodniak, A., Lochmatter, P., Yerly, D., Kawabata, T., Lerch, M., Yawalkar, N. and Pichler, W. J. (2010). In vitro detection of cytotoxic T and NK cells in peripheral blood of patients with various drug-induced skin diseases. Allergy 65(3): 376-384

Zhang, J. L., Chen, X., Li, J. and Xie, H. F. (2008). [Clinical analysis of childhood acute generalized exanthematous pustulosis]. Zhongguo Dang Dai Er Ke Za Zhi 10(4): 497-499

8

Mechanisms Regulating Epidermal Innervation in Pruritus of Atopic Dermatitis

Mitsutoshi Tominaga[1] and Kenji Takamori[1,2]
[1]*Institute for Environmental and Gender Specific Medicine, Juntendo University Graduate School of Medicine*
[2]*Department of Dermatology, Juntendo University Urayasu Hospital*
Japan

1. Introduction

Histamine, the best-known pruritogen in humans, is also regarded as an experimental itch-causing substance. Clinically, antihistamines, *i.e.*, H_1-receptor blockers, are used to treat all types of itch resulting from renal and liver diseases, as well as from serious skin diseases such as atopic dermatitis. Antihistamines, however, often lack efficacy in patients with chronic itch involving other agonists, including proteases, neuropeptides, cytokines, and opioids, as well as their cognate receptors, including thermoreceptors, PAR-2, and opioid receptors. Release of these pruritogenic mediators and modulators into the periphery may directly activate itch-sensitive C-fibers by binding to specific receptors on the nerve terminals (Ikoma et al., 2006; Paus et al., 2006). Nerve fibers can also be activated by exogenous mechanical, chemical, or biological stimuli, resulting in itch responses (Tominaga and Takamori, 2010). Histological examination has shown increased epidermal nerve densities in patients with atopic dermatitis (AD), suggesting that this higher density may be at least partly responsible for the intense itching in the skin. Such hyperinnervation is probably caused by an imbalance of nerve elongation factors (*e.g.* nerve growth factor, amphiregulin, and gelatinase) and nerve repulsion factors (*e.g.* semaphorin 3A and anosmin-1) produced by keratinocytes (Tominaga and Takamori, 2010; Tengara et al., 2010). Using a unique system of culturing rat dorsal root ganglion (DRG) neurons, consisting of Boyden chambers and extracellular matrix (ECM), we recently demonstrated that neuronal matrix metalloproteinase-2 (MMP-2) is involved in the penetration of sensory nerve fibers into basement membrane through modulation by axonal guidance molecules and/or ECM (Tominaga et al., 2009a). Clinically, psoralen-UVA (PUVA) therapy may reduce epidermal hyperinnervation in patients with AD by normalizing abnormal Sema3A and NGF expression in the epidermis, decreasing in visual analog scale (VAS) scores of pruritus severity (Tominaga et al., 2009c). Such anti-nerve growth effects have been observed in the dry skin of acetone-treated mice following exposure to narrowband-UVB and excimer lamps (Kamo et al., 2011a). These findings may help understand the mechanisms by which UV-based therapy modulate epidermal innervation. This chapter presents recent knowledge regarding the relationship between pruritus and epidermal nerve density, especially in AD.

2. Itch involving epidermal nerve fibers

Many pruritogenic mediators and modulators released into the periphery may directly activate itch-sensitive C-fibers by binding to specific receptors on the nerve terminal. Alternatively, these molecules may act indirectly by inducing other cells to release pruritogenic mediators and modulators. Nerve fibers are activated by exogenous mechanical, chemical, and biological stimuli, resulting in itch responses (Ikoma et al., 2006; Paus et al., 2006; Tominaga and Takamori, 2010).

Sensory nerve fibers are acceptors of itch and pain sensations in the skin. The neuronal mechanisms underlying intractable pruritus have been partially identified to date. Histological examination has shown that the density of epidermal nerve fibers is higher in the skin of patients with AD, contact dermatitis and xerosis than in control individuals (Figure 1) (Ikoma et al., 2006; Tominaga and Takamori, 2010), although the nerve density in patients with pruigo nodularis and psoriasis remain unclear (Stander et al., 2011; Taneda et al., 2011). Similar findings have been observed in animal models such as AD NC/Nga (Tominaga et al., 2007a) and dry skin (Tominaga et al., 2007b) mice, indicating increases in sensory receptors responsive to exogenous triggering factors and endogenous pruritogens from immune cells and keratinocytes and suggesting that hyperinnervation is at least partly responsible for intense itch sensations (Ikoma et al., 2006).

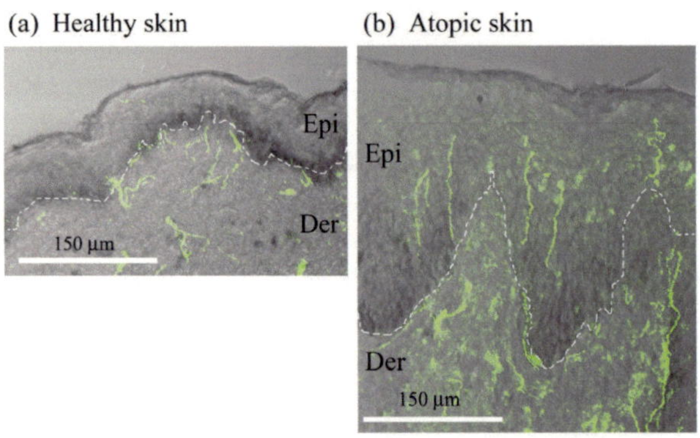

Fig. 1. Distribution of epidermal nerve fibers in healthy and atopic skin.
Staining of the skin of healthy volunteers and AD patients with antibody to protein gene product 9.5 (anti-PGP9.5). Nerve fibers images were overlapped with differential interference microscopic images. (a) PGP9.5-immunoreactive nerve fibers (green) were occasionally present in the epidermis of healthy volunteers. (b) Epidermal nerve fibers were observed at higher densities in AD patients. Scale bars = 150 μm.

In patients with lichen amyloidosis, itch has been associated with low densities of nerve fibers in the epidermis and dermoepidermal junctions (Maddison et al., 2008). Recently, a missense mutation in the OSMR gene, which encodes oncostatin M-specific receptor beta (OSMRb), was found in three families affected by familial primary localized cutaneous amyloidosis, an autosomal dominant disorder (Tanaka et al., 2009). OSMRb is a component of the interleukin (IL)-31 receptor, and IL-31 is an inducer of itch (Sonkoly et al., 2006). In addition, IL-31 receptor and OSMRb are expressed in afferent fibers in the spinal cord and the dermis of the skin (Bando et al., 2006). Therefore, cross-talk between cutaneous nerve fibers and IL-31 may induce itch in lichen amyloidosis, although further studies are required to determine the correlation between IL-31 receptor function and nerve degeneration in lichen amyloidosis.

In addition, diminished skin innervation has been observed in the skin of patients with neuropathic itch (Wallengren et al., 2002). This spontaneous itching may emanate from a central nervous system disorder, such as stroke, and continue in partly denervated skin. However, its mechanisms have not yet been elucidated.

3. Regulation of epidermal nerve fiber density by axonal guidance molecules

3.1 Nerve elongation factors

Nerve growth factor (NGF) is a neurotrophin that affects neurite outgrowth and neuronal survival (Lewin et al., 1993). Keratinocyte-derived NGF is a major mediator of skin innervation density, with higher local NGF concentrations in the lesional skin of patients with prurigo nodularis, AD, psoriasis, contact dermatitis and xerosis than in normal skin (Ikoma et al., 2006). In adult rat primary sensory neurons, NGF has been shown to upregulate neuropeptides, especially substance P (SP) and calcitonin-gene-related peptide (CGRP) (Verge et al., 1995), both of which are involved in the hypersensitivity of itch sensation and neurogenic inflammation (Steinhoff et al., 2003). Several studies using NC/Nga mice have demonstrated that anti-NGF approaches significantly inhibited both epidermal nerve growth and scratching behavior, but did not ameliorate scratching that had already developed (Takano et al., 2005; Takano et al., 2007). These anti-NGF approaches, however, did not completely inhibit itch responses, indicating that other mechanisms may also regulate epidermal innervation.

Amphiregulin (AR), a protein belonging to the epidermal growth factor (EGF) family, has been found to affect nerve fiber elongation (Kimura et al., 1992; Nilsson and Kanje, 2005). AR expression was also shown to be upregulated in the epidermis of NC/Nga mice with AD (Tominaga et al., 2007a), suggesting that AR is a regulator of epidermal nerve density in the skin.

Matrix metalloproteinases (MMPs) have been reported to catalyze the release of AR from transmembrane precursors, a release blocked by GM6001, a broad-spectrum MMP inhibitor, and by MMP-2/MMP-9 (i.e. gelatinase A/B) inhibitors (Kansra et al., 2004). Gelatinase activities were found to be higher in the suprabasal layer of atopic NC/Nga mice than in controls (Tominaga et al., 2007a). In addition, transmembrane-type AR was found to localize on the cell surface of basal cells, whereas AR was diffused in the suprabasal layer. Thus, gelatinase in suprabasal cells may be involved in AR elaboration into the intercellular space between keratinocytes.

TNF-α is a pivotal proinflammatory cytokine in the innate immune response and a key molecule for skin inflammation. Mast cells have been identified as important sources of TNF-α (Steinhoff et al., 2003). Plasma TNF-α concentration is increased in AD (Sumimoto et al., 1992), and both TNF-α and its receptors are upregulated in dermal blood vessels from patients with psoriasis (Kristensen et al., 1993). A study using mast cell- and TNF-deficient mice demonstrated that TNF produced by mast cells promotes the elongation of epidermal and dermal nerve fibers in a mouse model of contact dermatitis (Kakurai et al., 2006). Partly because of their close anatomical association, it has been suggested that cutaneous sensory nerves and mast cells may represent a functional unit, whereby stimulated nerve fibers may activate local mast cells, which in turn can control local nerve function (Steinhoff et al., 2003). Thus, mast cell-derived TNF may act as a nerve elongation factor in inflamed skin. TNF receptors are also expressed on peripheral nerves (Shubayev et al., 2004). TNF may also directly affect sensory nerves, but the details are still uncertain. More recently, TNF-α was reported to enhance NGF production in human keratinocytes (Takaoka A., 2009), suggesting a close relationship between mast cells and keratinocytes in nerve fiber elongation.

3.2 Nerve repulsion factors

During neural development, nerve fibers are regulated by both attraction and repulsion factors to reach its targets (e.g. skin and muscle). Semaphorin 3A (Sema3A) is a diffusible molecule that induces growth cone collapse and axonal repulsion of several neuronal populations through its interaction with a neuropilin-1 (Nrp-1)/plexin-A receptor complex (Fujisawa, 2004). Sema3A acts by selectively repelling axons from a subset of embryonic dorsal root ganglion (DRG) neurons, which are small in diameter and responsive to NGF (Messersmith et al., 1995; Shepherd et al., 1997). Sema3A has been found to induce the retraction of NGF-responsive sensory afferents in adult mammalian spinal cord (Dontchev and Letourneau, 2002).

Sema3A transcripts are also expressed in cultured normal human epidermal keratinocytes, and Sema3A proteins are mainly distributed in the suprabasal layer of normal human skin (Tominaga et al., 2008) (Figure 2).

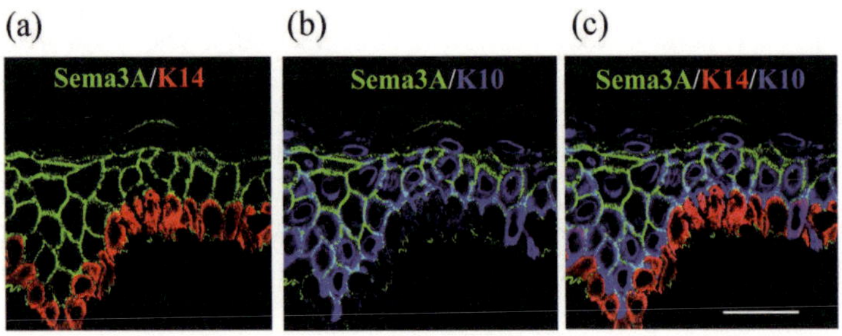

Fig. 2. Distribution of Sema3A in human healthy skin.
Normal human skin was triply stained for Sema3A (green), keratin 14 (K14; red) and K10 (blue). (a) A merged image of Sema3A (green) and K14 (red). (b) A merged image of Sema3A (green) and K10 (blue). (c) A merged image of Sema3A (green), K14 (red) and K10 (blue). Immunoreactivity for Sema3A was slight in the K14-positive cell layer but stronger in the K10-positive cell layer. Scale bars = 30 μm.

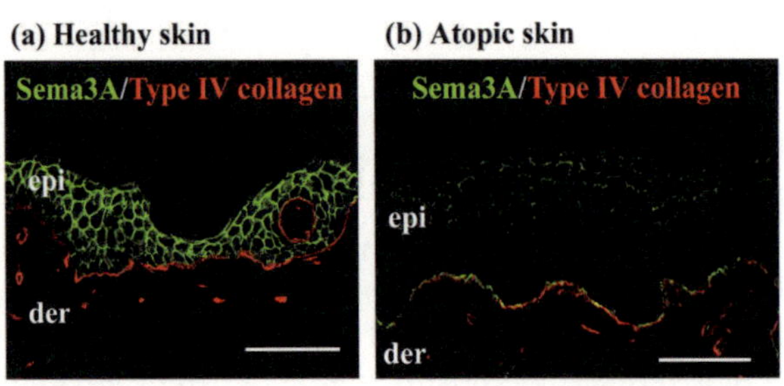

Fig. 3. Decreased production of Sema3A in the epidermis of AD patients.
Skins of healthy volunteers (a) and AD patients (b) were doubly stained for Sema3A (green) and type IV collagen (red). Sema3A expression was lower in the epidermis of AD patients than in healthy volunteers. Scale bars = 75 μm. epi: epidermis, der: dermis.

Recently, epidermal Sema3A levels were reported to be lower in patients with AD than in healthy volunteers, concomitant with an increase in epidermal nerve density (Tominaga et al., 2008), indicating a good correlation between epidermal innervation and Sema3A levels (Figure 3). Moreover, Sema3A has been found to inhibit NGF-induced sprouting of sensory afferents in adult rat spinal cord (Tang et al., 2004), whereas elevated levels of NGF reduced the Sema3A-induced collapse of sensory growth cones (Dontchev and Letourneau, 2002). These findings suggest that decreasing the expression of Sema3A can accelerate epidermal nerve growth in individuals with AD. Thus, epidermal innervation may be regulated by a fine balance between nerve elongation and repulsion factors (Figure 4). These findings may also provide new potential therapeutic targets for ameliorating pruritus associated with epidermal nerve density, including AD. The role of Sema3A in abnormal itch perception has been confirmed by recombinant Sema3A replacement approaches in atopic NC/Nga mice (Yamaguchi et al., 2008).

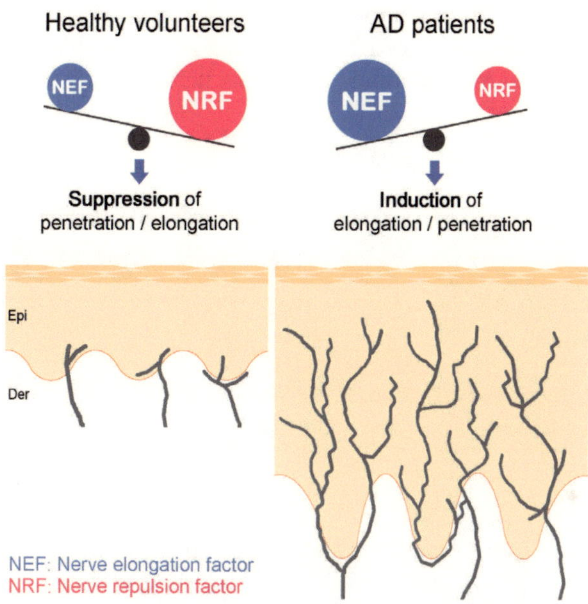

Fig. 4. A regulatory model of sensory nerve fiber penetration into the epidermis by a balance of nerve elongation and repulsion factors.
Epidermal NEF levels were lower and epidermal NRF levels were higher in healthy than in atopic skin, suggesting the suppression of penetration and/or elongation into the normal epidermis. In contrast, epidermal NEF levels were higher and epidermal NRF levels were lower in atopic than in healthy skin. Epidermal nerve density may be regulated by a fine balance between NEF and NRF. Epi, epidermis; Der, dermis; NEF, nerve elongation factors; NRF, nerve repulsion factors.

Anosmin-1, an extracellular matrix glycoprotein anosmin-1 encoded by *KAL1* (Kallmann syndrome 1 sequence), the gene responsible for the X chromosome-linked recessive form of Kallmann syndrome (Soussi-Yanicostas et al., 1996; Kim et al., 2008), was recently shown to be involved in epidermal innervations in AD (Tengara et al., 2010). Anosmin-1 has been shown to play several roles during neural development. For example, it was found to promote the migration of gonadotropin-releasing hormone-producing neurons, to guide the navigation of axons from mitral cells and to participate in the formation of their collaterals, and to stimulate the outgrowth and branching of Purkinje axons *in vitro* (Soussi-Yanicostas et al., 1998; Kim et al., 2008). Interestingly, coculturing of cerebellar granular neurons with anosmin-1-overexpressing CHO cells showed that anosmin-1 also has an inhibitory effect on neurite outgrowth (Soussi-Yanicostas et al., 1998) and further indicates the importance of anosmin-1 in regulating neurons.

We recently reported that conditioned medium from *KAL1*-overexpressing cells inhibited neurite outgrowth in cultured DRG neurons (Tengara et al., 2010). *KAL1* transcripts are expressed in cultured keratinocytes and in normal human skin. Anosmin-1 is strongly expressed in the basal cell layer of normal skin, but its expression is lower in atopic skin, concomitant with increases of epidermal nerve fibers (Figure 5). Moreover, *KAL1* expression is downregulated during keratinocyte differentiation in a high-calcium medium but is upregulated by IL-4, IL-13 or transforming growth factor (TGF)-β1. TGF-β1 was found to act synergistically with IL-13 to enhance *KAL1* expression, whereas IFN-γ inhibited its expression. Thus, anosmin-1 produced by epidermal keratinocytes in response to calcium concentrations or cytokines may modulate epidermal nerve density in individuals with AD.

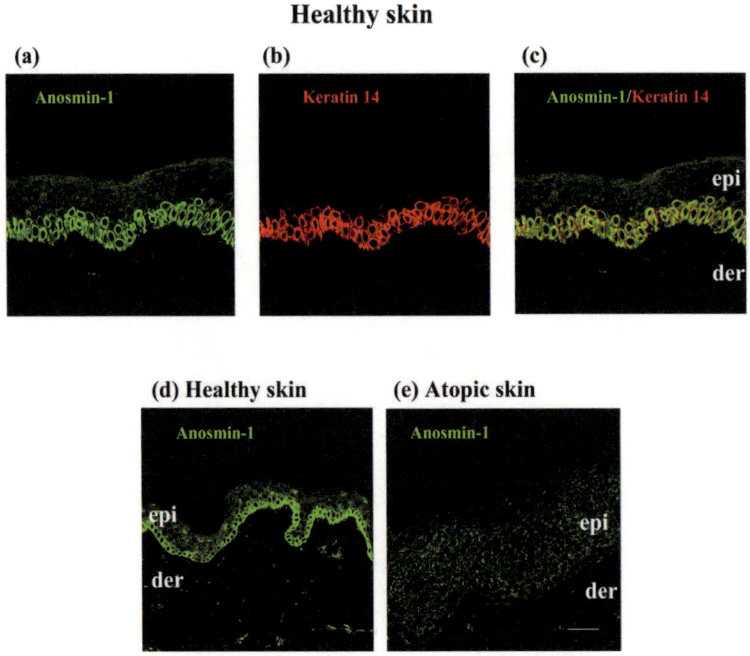

Fig. 5. Patterns of anosmin-1 expression in healthy and atopic skin.
(a,b) Cryosections of normal human skin were doubly labelled for anosmin-1 (a; green) and keratin-14 (b; red). Strong anosmin-1 immunoreactivity was detected in keratin-14-positive cells and in some dermal cells. (c) Superimposition of (a) and (b); the yellow areas were those doubly labelled. (d,e) Immunolabelling with anti-anosmin-1 antibody (green) of healthy (d) and atopic (e) skin. Anosmin-1 was strongly expressed in the basal cell layer of normal skin, but its expression was decreased in the basal cell layer of atopic skin. Scale bar: 50 μm. epi, epidermis; der, dermis.

Epidermal innervation in atopic skin is probably regulated by skin concentrations of both nerve elongation and nerve repulsion factors. A more recent study in psoriasis patients with pruritus reported no close relationship between the number of epidermal nerve fibers and Sema3A levels (Taneda et al., 2011). Although patients with Kallmann syndrome do not express anosmin-1 due to the lack of the *KAL1* gene (Soussi-Yanicostas et al., 1996; Kim et al., 2008), there have been no reports of itchy skin in these patients (Sato et al., 2004). Thus, in many individuals who have skin diseases with pruritus, epidermal innervation may be regulated by combinations of axonal guidance molecules. Further research should involve the altered balance of expression of these molecules in skin diseases with pruritus.

4. Skin barrier disruption and epidermal nerve fibers

Seasonal changes affect the condition of normal skin and trigger various cutaneous disorders. In common dermatoses, such as xerosis, AD and psoriasis, a decline in skin barrier function often parallels an increased severity of clinical symptomatology, including pruritus. These conditions all tend to worsen during the winter season, when humidity is lower (Yosipovitch et al., 2004; Loden and Maibach, 2006). Other indirect evidence suggests that decreased humidity precipitates these disorders (Rycroft and Smith, 1980), whereas increased skin hydration appears to ameliorate these conditions (Chernosky, 1976; Rawlings et al., 1994). Moreover, histological studies have shown that xerotic and AD patients have a higher density of nerve fibers and higher levels of NGF expression than normal individuals (Tominaga and Takamori, 2010). Basal transepidermal water loss (TEWL) is also higher in individuals with AD, including in clinically uninvolved skin, than in normal individuals (Yosipovitch et al., 2004).

Skin barrier disruption causes changes in epidermal innervation, making the skin more susceptible to any stimulation and more sensitive to itching. This has been demonstrated in studies using acetone and acetone/ether/water (AEW)-treated mice, models of acute and chronic dry skin, respectively (Grubauer et al., 1989; Miyamoto et al., 2002; Tominaga et al., 2007b). In acetone-treated mice, the number of epidermal nerve fibers is increased (Tominaga et al., 2007b), suggesting that barrier disruption causes nerve fibers located at the epidermal-dermal border to penetrate into the epidermis. Moreover, acetone treatment led to immediate increases in epidermal NGF and AR mRNA levels, followed by increased expression of the respective proteins (Grubauer et al., 1989; Tominaga et al., 2007b), as well as decreased levels of Sema3A in the epidermis (Kamo et al., 2011a). All of these changes occurred before the nerve fibers penetrated into the epidermis. Artificial restoration of the barrier by latex occlusion immediately after acetone-induced barrier disruption inhibited the increases in epidermal NGF and AR mRNAs (Grubauer et al., 1989; Liou et al., 1997). Thus, alterations in cutaneous barrier permeability induced the abnormal expression of nerve elongation and repulsion factors (Figure 4), suggesting that topically applied emollient may work by normalizing the expression of these genes.

Recently, application of petrolatum or heparinoid cream was found to attenuate dry skin-inducible intraepidermal nerve growth (Kamo et al., 2011b). Immediate application of these emollients after acetone treatment significantly inhibited the acetone-induced increase in epidermal nerve density. Both emollients also attenuated the acetone-induced increase in epidermal NGF levels, but had no effects on epidermal Sema3A levels. These anti-nerve growth effects were also observed when petrolatum or heparinoid cream, especially the latter, was applied 24 hours after acetone treatment, although immediate-type application seemed to

be more effective. Therefore, prompt application of emollients after skin barrier disruption may be therapeutically effective for pruritus involving epidermal hyperinnervation.
A close relationship between skin barrier disruption and itch sensation has been demonstrated using AEW-treated mice (Miyamoto et al., 2002). AEW treatment elicited spontaneous scratching, concomitant with an increase in TEWL and a reduction in stratum corneum (SC) hydration. Treatment also induced spontaneous scratching in mast cell-deficient mice, indicating that mast cells may not be involved in the AEW-inducible scratching behavior. Although the mechanisms are unclear, scratching behaviors in mast cell-deficient mice may be caused, at least in part, by increases in epidermal nerve fibers or pruritogens from other dermal cells and keratinocytes. This idea is partly supported by a recent study using this model (Akiyama et al., 2010).
Alternatively, spontaneous scratching may be induced by water treatment following AE, but not by organic solvents alone. Water can remove natural moisturizing factors important for skin hydration, impairing SC hydration and flexibility (Yosipovitch et al., 2004). Water may also induce transient swelling of the SC followed by a drying out of the surface layers. Physical swelling and shrinking may act as a mechanical stimulus of C-fibers in the upper epidermis, where it is perceived as itch. This hypothesis is supported by findings showing that mechanical stimuli were associated with enhanced neurogenic inflammation (Yamaoka et al., 2007).

5. Relationship between epidermal nerve fibers and abnormal expression of cell-cell junction molecules

Adherens junctions and tight junctions are critical for skin barrier function and have been shown to be altered in individuals with psoriasis (Pummi et al., 2001; Perez-Moreno et al., 2003; Zhou et al., 2003; Harhaj et al., 2004) and AD (Tominaga et al., 2007a). Epidermally targeted amphiregulin (AR)-transgenic mouse strains develop many features of psoriasis spontaneously (Cook et al., 1997; Cook et al., 2004). The levels of expression of the adherins junction protein E-cadherin (Chung et al., 2005) and the tight junction proteins zona occludens 1 (ZO-1) and ZO-2, are decreased in the epidermis of these transgenic mice. In addition, the levels of expression of E-cadherin and ZO-1 are decreased in the epidermis of atopic NC/Nga mice, while the expression of AR is increased (Tominaga et al., 2007a). These findings suggest that AR downregulates epithelial junctional molecules in atopic and psoriatic skin and that AR affects the integrity of cell-cell junctions. Moreover, skin barrier function against external mechanical, chemical, and biological stimuli may be attenuated or abrogated in inflammatory skin diseases.
In cocultures of human corneal fibroblasts and epithelial cells, overexpression of Sema3A by corneal fibroblasts increased the expression of E- and N-cadherin mRNA and protein by corneal epithelial cells (Ko et al., 2010), suggesting that Sema3A may modulate the expression of cell-cell junctional molecules in epidermal keratinocytes.
Desmosomes are complex intercellular junctions that link the keratin filaments of adjacent cells, providing mechanical strength to epithelial tissues such as the epidermis. Desmoglein 3 (Dsg3) is a desmosomal cadherin highly expressed in the basal layer of mammalian skin (Wheelock and Johnson, 2003). Following differentiation, however, the expression of Dsg3 decreases (Wheelock and Johnson, 2003). Electron microscopic analysis has shown that a keratin 1 promoter increases intercellular spaces in the basal and spinous layers of Dsg3-transgenic mice (Merritt et al., 2002). Dsg3 is also aberrantly expressed in the epidermis of atopic NC/Nga mice (Tominaga et al., 2007a).

Taken together, these findings suggest that widening of intercellular spaces in the epidermis is required for the penetration and/or elongation of nerve fibers into the epidermis (Figure 6), as well as for inflammatory cell infiltration into the dermatitis (Wittmann and Werfel, 2006). Thus, epidermal hyperinnervation is enhanced by the abnormal expression of cell-cell junctional molecules, and thereby may induce and/or enhance itch in skin diseases associated with barrier disruption.

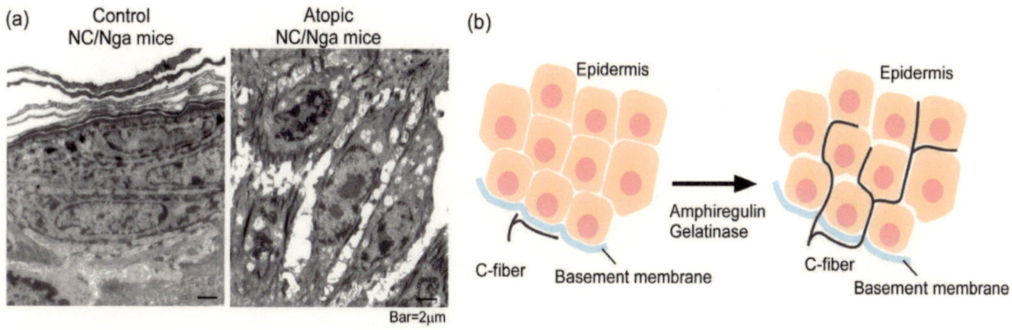

Fig. 6. Relationship between widening of intercellular spaces in the epidermis and nerve fiber density.
(a) Electron micrographs of the skins of NC/Nga mice. Intercellular spaces between keratinocytes were tight in the skin of control, specific pathogen-free (SPF)-NC/Nga mice, but were wider in the skins of conventional (Cnv)-NC/Nga mice, which developed AD-like symptoms. (b) Increased AR downregulates epithelial junctional molecules in atopic skin, suggesting that AR affects the integrity of cell-cell junctions. Gelatinase activities were also high in atopic skin, suggesting that gelatinase may be involved in the activation of transmembrane-type AR. Moreover, desmoglein 3 (Dsg3) is aberrantly expressed in the epidermis of atopic NC/Nga mice, suggesting that Dsg3 may be involved in widening intercellular spaces in the epidermis. Increased spaces may be required for the penetration and/or elongation of nerve fibers into the epidermis.

6. Mechanism of penetration of nerve fibers into basement membrane

Although epidermal innervation was found closely related to itch in AD, the mechanisms by which dermal nerve fibers pass through the basement membrane (BM) at the epidermal-dermal border remain unclear.

Matrix metalloproteinases (MMPs) are a family of zinc-dependent endopeptidases capable of degrading extracellular matrix (ECM) components, including BM proteins. The MMP family is divided into two major groups according to their cellular localization, secreted and membrane-type (MT) MMPs. Breakdown of ECM by MMPs is important in cell migration, tissue remodelling, inflammatory diseases and tumor cell invasion and metastasis (Page-McCaw et al., 2007). Interestingly, studies using DRG neurons showed that MMPs promote neurite extension (Muir et al., 1994; Hayashita-Kinoh et al., 2001), suggesting that MMPs may be involved in the penetration of nerve fibres into the BM and that axonal guidance molecules modulate the expression and enzymatic activity of MMPs that degrade BM components.

We have developed an *in vitro* model of BM, in which DRG neurons are cultured in a unique system, consisting of Boyden chambers and Matrigel (MG) (Figure 7). This system mimics the pathological skin condition of intractable pruritus because nerve fiber penetration into the MG was induced by the NGF concentration gradient (Tominaga et al., 2009a). We found that MMP-2 is localized on the growth cone in the penetration mechanism and that it may be involved in intractable pruritus (Tominaga et al., 2009a).

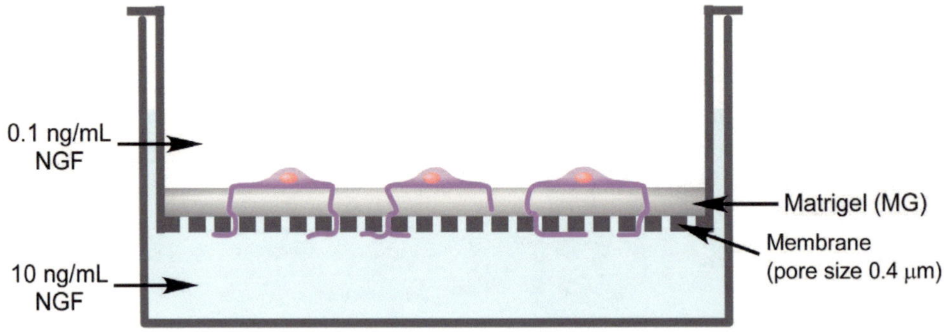

Fig. 7. Schematic representation of the Boyden chamber culture system.
The chamber used to assess the mechanism by which nerve fibers penetrate into the BM is shown schematically. The upper surface of the 0.4-μm pore size polyester insert of a 24-well Boyden chamber was coated with Matrigel (MG). DRG neurons, in 200 μL culture medium containing 0.1 ng/mL NGF, were placed on the MG, and 1 mL of culture medium containing 10 ng/mL NGF was added to the lower chamber. After culture for 24 hours, the cells were fixed with 4% paraformaldehyde in 0.1 mol/L phosphate buffer (pH 7.4). The MG-coated membrane was removed from the Boyden chamber and stained with an antibody against Tau, a protein enriched in axons. Immunofluorescence staining of the underside of the membrane was assessed using a confocal laser-scanning microscope, which revealed nerve fibers that had crossed the MG-coated membrane.

In the DRG neuron cultures, NGF induced expression of *MMP-2*, whereas MMP-2 blockers inhibited the penetration of nerve fibers across the membrane, suggesting that NGF-inducible MMP-2 is involved in the process of nerve fiber penetration into MG, similar to findings using chick DRG neurons (Muir et al., 1994). Pruritogens and cytokines have been found to upregulate keratinocyte MMP-9 production (Gschwandtner et al., 2008; Purwar et al., 2008), and gelatinase activities were found to be higher in the epidermis of atopic NC/Nga mice than in control mice (Tominaga et al., 2007a). Thus, non-neuronal cell-derived gelatinases may contribute indirectly to nerve fiber penetration *in vivo*.
Growth cones are subject to multiple environmental cues as they navigate (Goodman, 1996). MMP-2 was shown present within the cell bodies, neurites and growth cones of permeabilized DRG neurons (Zuo et al., 1998). In the absence of permeabilization, however, MMP-2 localized to the growth cones of NGF-responsive fibers, and zymographic analyses showed type IV collagenase activity on the cell surface of growth cones, including filopodia, in NGF-responsive fibers (Tominaga et al., 2009a). These results suggest that nerve fiber penetration is caused by activated MMP-2 on the cell surface of growth cones (Figure 8).

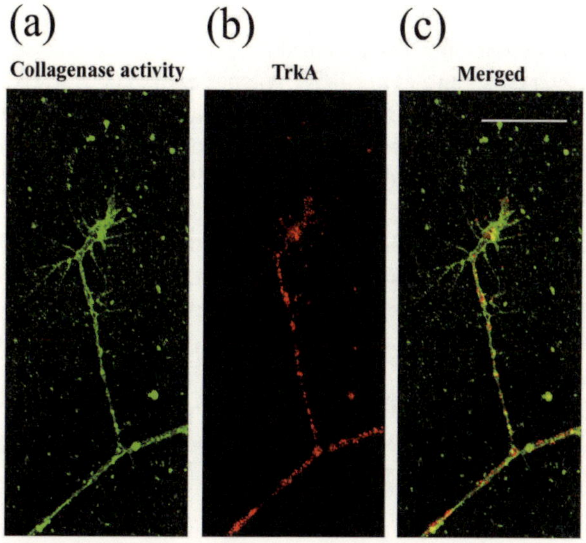

Fig. 8. Type-IV collagenase activities on DRG growth cone.
(a) DRG neurons were cultured for 48 hours in serum-free medium supplemented with 10 ng/mL NGF, followed by *in situ* zymography using FITC-labelled DQ-type IV collagen (green). (b) Following *in situ* zymography, the cells were stained with anti-TrkA (red) antibody. (c) Merged image of (a) FITC-labelled DQ-type IV collagen (green) and (b) TrkA (red). Type IV collagenase activity was detected primarily on the cell membrane of growth cones including the filopodia of TrkA$^+$ fibers. Scale bars, 23.81 μm.

MMP-2 is produced as pro-MMP-2, an inactive zymogen, which is activated by MT-MMPs rather than serine proteases. During the activation process, the MT-MMPs form a complex with pro-MMP-2 through interaction with tissue inhibitor of metalloproteinase-2 (TIMP-2) (Seiki, 1999; Wang et a., 1999). Immunocytochemical analyses of unpermeabilized DRG neurons indicated that MT5-MMP partially colocalized with MMP-2 and/or TIMP-2 in NGF-responsive growth cones. Nerve fiber penetration into the MG was also inhibited by anti-TIMP-2 neutralizing antibody (Tominaga et al., 2009a), suggesting that MT5-MMP also functions as an adaptor when complexed and that MT5-MMP may be involved in MMP-2 activity on the cell surface of growth cones. Moreover, NGF may enhance the ability of MMP-2 to degrade BM components through the upregulation of pro-MMP-2 activation molecules in cultured neurons (Tominaga et al., 2009a). Accordingly, activated MMP-2 on the cell surface may be more effective than its free form in degrading BM components during the nerve fiber penetration process (Figure 9).

In addition to NGF, *MMP-2* expression in cultured neurons is modulated by other factors, including Sema3A, which induces growth cone collapse and axonal repulsion (Fujisawa, 2004). Sema3A molecule inhibits nerve fiber penetration due to the NGF concentration gradient, concomitant with the downregulation of *MMP-2* and *MT5-MMP*, suggesting that these two molecules have reciprocal mechanisms in the regulation of nerve fiber penetration.

MMP-2 is also modulated by its ECM substrates. *In vitro* studies of neurite outgrowth on different ECM components has suggested the involvement of integrins in growth cone movement during neural development and repair (Reichardt and Tomaselli, 1991). In addition, neurotrophins and ECM together induce robust axon outgrowth (Goldberg et al.,

2002; Liu et al., 2002), suggesting that coordinated activation of neurotrophin and ECM-integrin signalling is necessary for efficient and long-distance axon extension (Rossino et al., 1990; Lefcort et al., 1992; Grabham et al., 1997; Werner et al., 2000; Danker et al., 2001). Thus, NGF stimulated elongation of nerve fibers, either in experimental culture systems or *in vivo*, will result in the accumulation of integrins at the growth cone, enabling them to interact with a variety of ECM components (Grabham et al., 1997). During this process, MMPs are required for growth cones to abrogate the three-dimensional ECM barriers. This process involves the selection and upregulation of MMPs corresponding to surrounding ECM components of the growing nerve fiber, resulting in efficient nerve fiber penetration. The expression of genes encoding molecules involved in pro-MMP activation may also be affected. In contrast, Sema3A stimulation of growing nerve fibers may constitute a reverse signalling pathway because class 3 semaphorin signalling inhibits integrin-mediated adhesion signalling (Zhou et al., 2008). Therefore, although the integrin-mediated regulatory system remains unclear in our culture system, this mechanism may be applicable to pruritic skin diseases involving epidermal hyperinnervation.

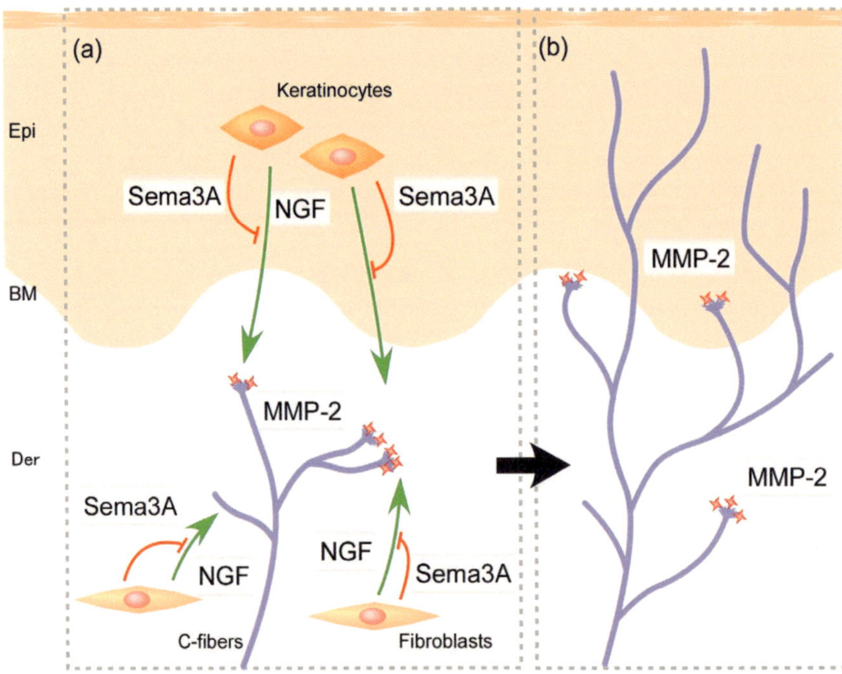

Fig. 9. A model of nerve fiber penetration into the BM.
(a) NGF, which is produced by cutaneous cells such as epidermal keratinocytes, immune cells and fibroblasts, promotes MMP-2 production in sensory nerve fibers and activates pro-MMP-2 on the growth cone. Sema3A produced by keratinocytes and fibroblasts may have opposite effects on these NGF-dependent events. NGF induced expression of *MMP-2* in nerve fibers may be also modulated by the extracellular matrix (ECM) substrates of this enzyme. (b) Activated MMP-2 on the growth cone may contribute to penetration of nerve fibers into the basement membrane.

7. Characterization of nerve fibers containing gastrin-releasing peptide in the skin

It has been difficult to histologically identify itch-specific fibers in the skin because no itch-specific markers have been identified. However, using gastrin-releasing peptide receptor (GRPR)-mutant mice or saporin-conjugating bombesin, the GRP/GRPR system was shown to be involved specifically in itch perception via the spinal cord (Sun and Chen, 2007; Sun et al., 2009). Recently, GRP^+ fibers were histologically shown to be present in mouse skin, with the percentage of $PGP9.5^+$ fibers that are GRP^+ being exceptionally high only in the epidermis of NC/Nga mice with AD (Figure 10) (Tominaga et al., 2009b). Small- to medium-sized adult DRG neurons expressed GRP, and its receptor was present in the superficial dorsal horn. Intrathecal injection of $GRP_{18\text{-}27}$ into wild-type mice induced scratching behavior but did not affect pain sensitivity (Sun and Chen, 2007), suggesting that GRP^+ fibers in the skin are itch- but not pain-specific.

Moreover, GRP^+ fibers have been found to contain SP or CGRP and to express itch-related molecules such as TRPV1, PAR-2, mu-opioid receptor (MOR) and TrkA, a receptor for NGF (Tominaga et al., 2009b). Although additional research is required to determine whether GRP^+ fibers in human and animal skin express histamine receptors or whether different types of itch-mediating fibers coexist in the periphery, GRP^+ fiber density may become an objective indicator of itching.

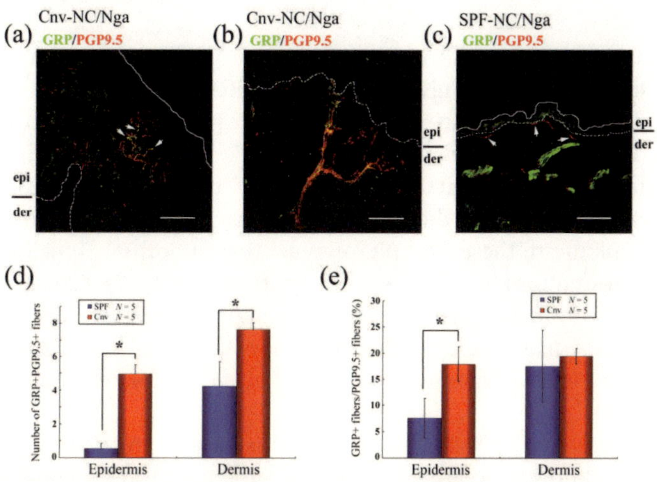

Fig. 10. Distribution of GRP^+ fibers in the skin of NC/Nga mice.
a-c, Double-labeling of GRP (green) and PGP9.5 (red) in the skin of NC/Nga mice. A small proportion of $PGP9.5^+$ fibers expressed GRP in the epidermis (arrows in a) and dermis (b) of conventional (Cnv)-NC/Nga mice. $GRP^+PGP9.5^+$ fibers were mainly observed in the dermis of specific pathogen-free (SPF)-NC/Nga mice (arrows), but they were occasionally present in the epidermis (c). d, The number of $GRP^+PGP9.5^+$ fibers was significantly higher in the epidermis and dermis of Cnv-NC/Nga than of SPF-NC/Nga mice. $^*P < 0.05$. e, The percentage of $PGP9.5^+$ fibers that were GRP^+ was significantly higher in the epidermis of Cnv-NC/Nga than of SPF-NC/Nga mice, but was similar in the dermis of these mice. Yellow areas are double-labeled, and white and broken lines indicate the skin surface and the border between the epidermis (epi) and dermis (der), respectively. Scale bars = 47.62 μm.

8. UV-based therapy of AD pruritus involving epidermal hyperinnervation

Various types of UV-based therapy, including oral and topical PUVA and narrow-band UVB, are widely used to treat AD (Krutmann, 2000). Interestingly, UV-based therapy was shown to reduce the number of cutaneous nerve fibers, especially in the epidermis, in patients with AD and psoriasis (Wallengren and Sundler, 2004). The intense itch associated with these dermatoses can also be controlled by UV-based therapy. Excimer laser treatment has been shown to ameliorate dermatitis in psoriasis patients and pruritus in AD patients (Baltas et al., 2006). Therefore, these findings suggest a relationship between the antipruritic effects of UV-based therapy and the reduction of epidermal nerve density in atopic skin. The mechanisms underlying UV-induced changes in epidermal nerve density are being assessed.

8.1 Effects of PUVA therapy on epidermal nerve fibers

NGF levels are higher, and Sema3A levels are lower, in the epidermis of patients with AD than in controls, suggesting that abnormal levels of axonal guidance molecules are involved in epidermal hyperinnervation in AD (Tominaga et al., 2008; Tominaga et al., 2009c). We hypothesized that epidermal Sema3A and NGF levels in AD patients are influenced by PUVA therapy, resulting in decreased epidermal nerve density in atopic skin. Using skin biopsies, we recently showed that PUVA therapy reduces epidermal hyperinnervation in AD patients by normalizing abnormal epidermal Sema3A and NGF expression (Tominaga et al., 2009c).

Following PUVA treatment, Sema3A upregulation and NGF downregulation were observed in the epidermis of AD patients (Figure 11). These patients also showed decreases in VAS for itching and clinical severity scores, concomitant with decreases in epidermal nerve densities (Figure 12) (Tominaga et al., 2009c). Sema3A inhibits NGF-induced sprouting of sensory afferents in the adult rat spinal cord (Dontchev and Letourneau, 2002). Although the signaling pathways that mediate the regulation of expression of these axonal guidance molecules remain unknown, these findings suggest that abnormal Sema3A and NGF levels in atopic skin are normalized by PUVA therapy, resulting in decreased epidermal nerve density. These PUVA-induced changes in epidermal innervation also have antipruritic effects, as shown by the use of anti-NGF or recombinant Sema3A replacement approaches against pruritus in atopic NC/Nga mice (Takano et al., 2005; Takano et al., 2007; Yamaguchi et al., 2008).

Although the mechanisms by which PUVA influences expression of axonal guidance molecules remain unknown, treatment may affect chromatin remodeling and various transcription factors, such as activator protein-1 (AP-1) and poly(C) binding protein (Borner et al., 2002; Kim et al., 2004; Kim et al., 2005; Park et al., 2005). The NGF promoter contains an AP-1 element important for NGF transcriptional activity (Hengerer et al., 1990; D'Mello et al., 1991). Psoralen functions by interfering with AP-1 in murine keratinocytes, thereby inhibiting DNA binding by AP-1 (Martey et al., 2005). In addition, chromatin structure in human epithelial cells is affected by PUVA (Ree et al., 1981; Gasparro et al., 1997), and changes in chromatin structure influence DNA binding by transcription factors (Park et al., 2005). Although the Sema3A promoter has not yet been investigated, this type of mechanism may occur during the PUVA-induced normalization of Sema3A expression. Therefore, these studies may explain the mechanism of by which PUVA regulates gene expression in epidermal keratinocytes.

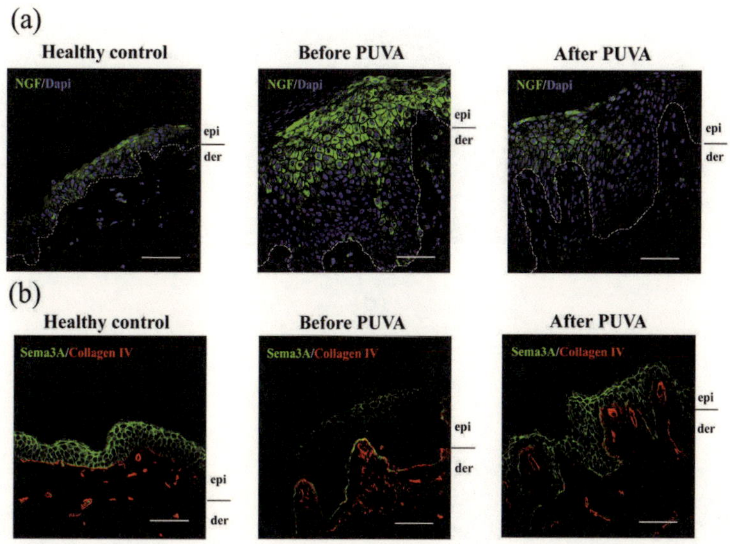

Fig. 11. Epidermal NGF and Sema3A levels in AD patients before and after PUVA therapy. (a) Skin biopsies from healthy volunteers and AD patients before and after PUVA treatment were stained with anti-NGF antibody. Epidermal NGF levels (green) were higher in AD patients than in healthy controls. Nuclei were counterstained with DAPI (blue). NGF expression was reduced in PUVA-treated than in untreated individuals. The white dotted line in each panel indicates the border between the epidermis and dermis (basement membrane). (b) Double labeling for Sema3A (green) and type IV collagen (red) in the skin of AD patients before and after PUVA therapy. Epidermal Sema3A levels were lower in AD patients than in healthy volunteers, but were higher in PUVA-treated than in untreated individuals. Scale bars = 75 μm. epi, epidermis; der, dermis.

Alternatively, genes encoding axonal guidance molecules may be regulated by inflammatory cytokines produced by cutaneous cells, such as keratinocytes and immune cells. TNF-α was recently shown to enhance NGF production *via* the Raf-1/MEK/ERK pathway in cultured normal human epidermal keratinocytes (Takaoka et al., 2009). Although UV irradiation induces cytokine secretion from cultured keratinocytes, successful UV-based therapy of AD has been associated with downregulation of cytokine production in inflamed skin (Krutmann and Morita, 1999). Therefore, PUVA may regulate the expression of axonal guidance molecules by reducing cytokine levels in the skin.

NGF is produced not only by epidermal keratinocytes but by mast cells, eosinophils, and fibroblasts in inflamed skin (Ikoma et al., 2006; Leon et al., 1994). Several semaphorins are also produced by fibroblasts and immune cells (Suzuki et al., 2008; Fukamachi et al., 2011). UV radiation has been shown to affect dermal fibroblasts, dermal dendritic cells, endothelial cells, and skin-infiltrating inflammatory cells, such as T lymphocytes and mast cells (Krutmann and Morita, 1999). UV-based therapy has been shown to affect the production of soluble factors (cytokines, neuropeptides, and prostanoids) and the expression of cell-surface receptors (adhesion molecules, cytokine and growth factor receptors), and to induce apoptosis in these cells (Krutmann and Morita, 1999). Thus, PUVA treatment may modulate the production of axonal guidance molecules in dermal cells and/or inflammatory cells of the atopic skin, as well as in epidermal keratinocytes.

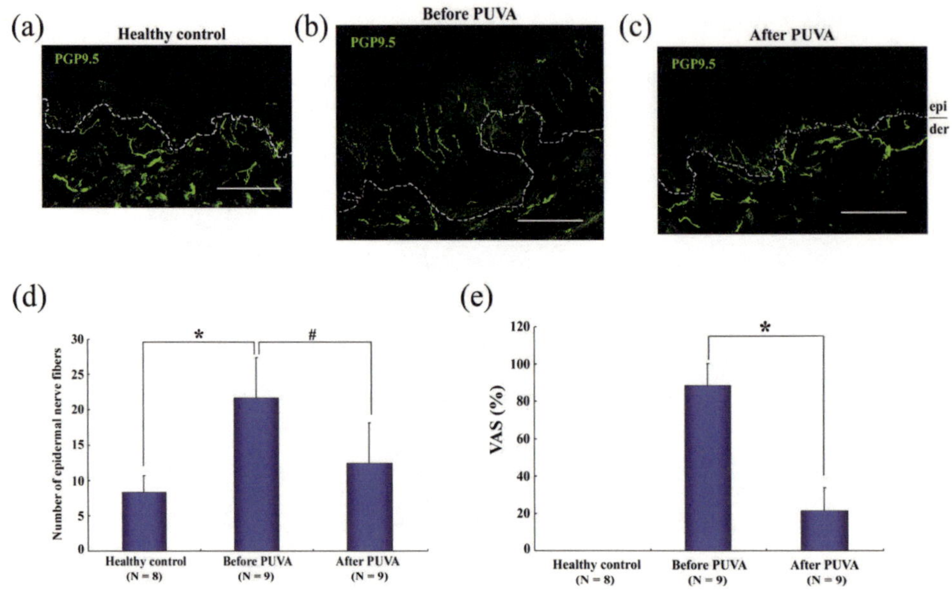

Fig. 12. Epidermal nerve densities in AD patients before and after PUVA therapy. Skin biopsies from healthy volunteers and AD patients before and after PUVA therapy were stained with anti-PGP9.5 antibody. PGP9.5-immunoreactive fibers (green) were mainly located in the dermis and at the epidermal- dermal border of normal skin, but some nerve fibers penetrated into the epidermis (a). Higher nerve densities were observed in the epidermis of AD patients (b). Reduced nerve densities were observed in the epidermis after PUVA therapy (c). The white dotted line in each panel indicates the border between the epidermis and dermis (basement membrane). Scale bars = 150 µm. epi, epidermis; der, dermis. The number of epidermal nerve fibers was significantly higher in AD patients than in healthy controls, while the number was significantly decreased in AD patients after PUVA treatment (d). Values are the means ± SD ($^*P < 0.01$; $^\#P < 0.05$). Visual analog scale (VAS) scores were significantly lower after than before PUVA therapy in AD patients ($^*P < 0.01$), and there was no itch in healthy controls (e).

8.2 Effects of NB-UVB and excimer lamp on epidermal nerve fibers

Narrowband 311-nm ultraviolet B (NB-UVB) is widely recognized as an effective treatment modality for patients with chronic AD (Der-Petrossian et al., 2000). More recently, the 308-nm XeCl excimer laser and lamp was introduced as a new type of UV-based therapy for some dermatoses including AD (Wolkerstorfer and Brenninkmeijer, 2011). Excimer laser treatment has been shown to ameliorate pruritus in AD patients and dermatitis in psoriatic patients (Baltas et al., 2006). The 308-nm excimer lamp and laser has demonstrated similar efficacy in treating vitiligo, although the lamp induced more erythema than the laser (Le Duff et al., 2010). The anti-nerve growth effects of these UV-based therapies have not been fully characterized to date. Using acetone-treated mice as a model of acute dry skin model, we assessed the effects of NB-UVB and excimer lamps on nerve growth (Kamo et al., 2011a). We previously showed that nerve fibers penetrate into the epidermis 24 h after acetone treatment, with nerve growth peaking 48 h after acetone treatment (Tominaga et al., 2007b). We therefore treated the mice with NB-UVB and excimer lamps 24 h after acetone treatment and obtained skin samples 48 h later.

Interestingly, we found that the anti-nerve growth effects of NB-UVB and excimer lamp treatments were more effective than PUVA treatment (Figure 13). UVA penetrates into the dermis, whereas UVB is limited almost exclusively to the epidermis (Meinhardt et al., 2008). Thus, UVB irradiation, which is restricted to the epidermal region, had greater efficacy, and may explain the different anti-nerve growth effects of UV-based therapies. Our findings are supported by clinical studies using PUVA, NB-UVB, and excimer lamp therapies (Van Weelden et al., 1990; Ortel et al., 1993).

Photobiologically, the wavelengths of the NB-UVB and excimer lamp are close to each other, and their therapeutic effects are similar (Asawanonda et al., 2008), with both showing strong inhibition of epidermal nerve growth. Although NB-UVB normalized the abnormal expression of NGF and Sema3A in the epidermis, no such normalization was observed with excimer lamp treatment. Thus, excimer lamp treatment, the most effective form of therapy for intraepidermal nerve fibers, did not alter the epidermal expression of axonal guidance molecules. Experimentally, keratinocytes are more resistant than lymphocytes to UVB-induced apoptosis (Krueger et al., 1995). Therefore, the anti-nerve growth effects may depend on the sensitivity of cutaneous cells to different UV wavelengths.

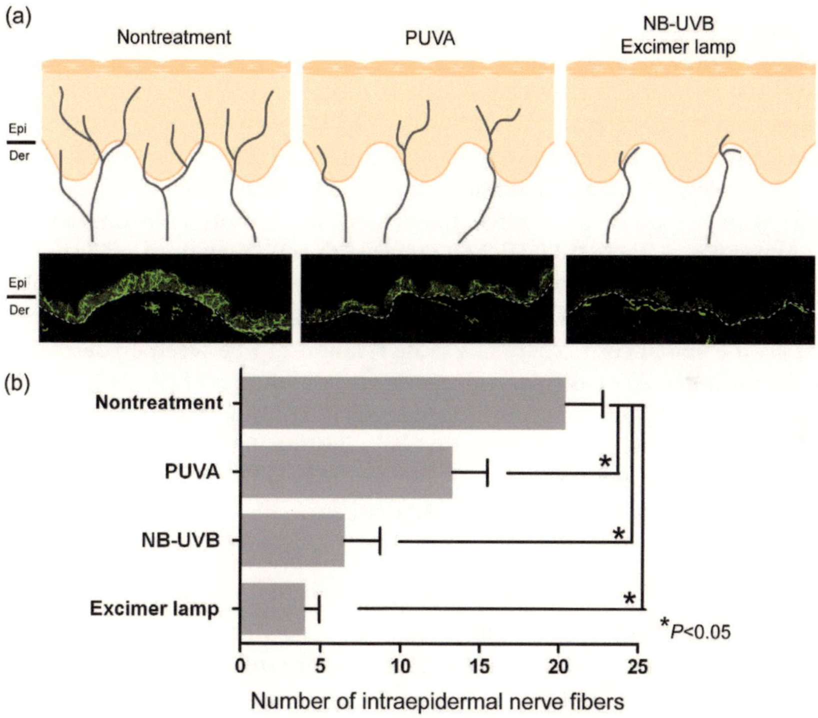

Fig. 13. Effects of UV-based therapy on intraepidermal nerve fibers in acetone-treated mice. (a) Distributions of intraepidermal PGP9.5+ fibers after a single topical application of PUVA, NB-UVB and excimer lamp in acetone-treated mice. White broken lines indicate the border between the epidermis and dermis. Scale bars, 50 μm. (b) A marked decrease in the number of intraepidermal PGP9.5+ fibers was observed in the group of mice treated with PUVA, NB-UVB and excimer lamp (*$P < 0.05$). All values represent the means ± SD of 6 animals.

Short-wave radiation, such as UVB, also excites DNA directly and generates photoproducts, such as cyclobutane pyrimidine dimers and (6-4) photoproducts, resulting in considerable bending of DNA (Kielbassa et al., 1997). A recent study demonstrated that 311 - 313-nm UVB radiation (dose: 750 mJ/cm^2) induced AP-1 binding to DNA (Hopper et al., 2009), suggesting that NB-UVB can modulate the expression of NGF in keratinocytes. UV irradiation may also induce ligand-independent activation of cell-surface receptors, such as epidermal growth factor receptor (Fisher et al., 1998; Wang et al., 2003), suggesting that NB-UVB may modulate the expression of Sema3A in keratinocytes. Epidermal growth factor was found to increase the expression of Sema3A mRNA and protein in human corneal epithelial cells (Ko et al., 2008). However, as photoproducts are among the factors involved in skin carcinogenesis, further studies are needed to determine therapeutically effective irradiation doses that also have low DNA damage potential.

9. Conclusion

Considerable progress has been made in clarifying the complex pathophysiology of itch. Histamine-independent itch occurs in both humans and animals, with amines, proteases, neuropeptides, cytokines, cannabinoids and opioids, as well as their cognate receptors, acting as mediators and/or modulators of itch. The itch response in the periphery is modulated by interactions among immune cells, keratinocytes and sensory nerve fibers. Epidermal nerve density is partly responsible for abnormal itch perception in several skin diseases, and hyperinnervation is regulated by a fine balance between nerve elongation and repulsion factors. Skin barrier disruption induces the abnormal expression of axonal guidance molecules, thereby increasing epidermal nerve density. There may be a relationship between epidermal nerve fibers and the abnormal expression of cell-cell junctional molecules. Activated MMP-2 on the growth cone may function as a micro-drill to facilitate efficient nerve penetration through the BM, under the control of axonal guidance molecules and/or ECM components. The GRP/GRPR system is specifically involved in itch perception *via* the spinal cord. There is a close relationship between epidermal GRP$^+$ fiber density and pruritus in AD patients. A deeper understanding of these pathways is required for the development of novel antipruritic strategies. Clinically, UV-based therapies such as PUVA, NB-UVB and excimer lamps may be effective for AD patients with pruritus involving epidermal hyperinnervation. These findings will also expand our knowledge regarding effective treatments for pruritic skin diseases.

10. Acknowledgment

This work was supported by a Health Labor Sciences Research Grant for Research on Allergic Disease and Immunology from the Japanese Ministry of Health, Labor and Welfare, by a KAKENHI (20591354 and 2079081) and a "High-Tech Research Center" Project for Private Universities: matching fund subsidy from MEXT, and by a JSPS Research Fellow.

11. References

Akiyama, T., Carstens, M.I. & Carstens, E. (2010). Enhanced scratching evoked by PAR-2 agonist and 5-HT but not histamine in a mouse model of chronic dry skin itch. *Pain* 151:378–83.

Asawanonda, P., Kijluakiat, J., Korkij, W. & Sindhupak, W. (2008). Targeted broadband ultraviolet b phototherapy produces similar responses to targeted narrowband ultraviolet B phototherapy for vitiligo: a randomized, double-blind study. *Acta Derm Venereol* 88:376–81.

Baltas, E., Csoma, Z., Bodai, L., Ignacz, F., Dobozy, A. & Kemeny, L. (2006). Treatment of atopic dermatitis with the xenon chloride excimer laser. *J Eur Acad Dermatol Venereol* 20:657–60.

Bando, T., Morikawa, Y., Komori, T. & Senba, E. (2006). Complete overlap of interleukin-31 receptor A and oncostatin M receptor beta in the adult dorsal root ganglia with distinct developmental expression patterns. *Neuroscience* 142:1263–71.

Borner, C., Hollt, V. & Kraus, J. (2002). Involvement of activator protein-1 in transcriptional regulation of the human mu-opioid receptor gene. *Mol Pharmacol* 61:800–5.

Chernosky, M.E. (1976). Clinical aspects of dry skin. *J Soc Cosmet Chem* 27:365–6.

Chung, E., Cook, P.W., Parkos, C.A., Park, Y.K., Pittelkow, M.R. & Coffey, R.J. (2005). Amphiregulin causes functional downregulation of adherens junctions in psoriasis. *J Invest Dermatol* 124:1134–40.

Cook, P.W., Brown, J.R., Cornell, K.A. & Pittelkow, M.R. (2004). Suprabasal expression of human amphiregulin in the epidermis of transgenic mice induces a severe, early-onset, psoriasis-like skin pathology: expression of amphiregulin in the basal epidermis is also associated with synovitis. *Exp Dermatol* 13:347–56.

Cook, P.W., Piepkorn, M., Clegg, C.H., Plowman, G.D., DeMay, J.M., Brown, J.R. & Pittelkow, M.R. (1997). Transgenic expression of the human amphiregulin gene induces a psoriasis-like phenotype. *J Clin Invest* 100:2286–94.

Danker, K., Mechai, N., Lucka, L., Reutter, W. & Horstkorte, R. (2001). The small GTPase Ras is involved in growth factor-regulated expression of the α1 integrin subunit in PC12 cells. *Biol Chem* 382:969–72.

Der-Petrossian, M., Seeber, A., Hönigsmann, H. & Tanew, A. (2000). Half-side comparison study on the efficacy of 8-methoxypsoralen bath-PUVA versus narrow-band ultraviolet B phototherapy in patients with severe chronic atopic dermatitis. *Br J Dermatol* 142:39–43.

D'Mello, S.R. & Heinrich, G. (1991). Structural and functional identification of regulatory regions and cis elements surrounding the nerve growth factor gene promoter. *Brain Res Mol Brain Res* 11:255–64.

Dontchev, V.D. & Letourneau, P.C. (2002). Nerve growth factor and semaphorin 3A signaling pathways interact in regulating sensory neuronal growth cone motility. *J Neurosci* 22:6659–69.

Fisher, G.J., Talwar, H.S., Lin, J., Lin, P., McPhillips, F., Wang, Z., Li, X., Wan, Y., Kang, S. & Voorhees, J.J. (1998). Retinoic acid inhibits induction of c-Jun protein by ultraviolet radiation that occurs subsequent to activation of mitogen-activated protein kinase pathways in human skin in vivo. *J Clin Invest* 101:1432–40.

Fujisawa, H. (2004). Discovery of semaphorin receptors, neuropilin and plexin, and their functions in neural development. *J Neurobiol* 59:24–33.

Fukamachi, S., Bito, T., Shiraishi, N., Kobayashi, M., Kabashima, K., Nakamura, M. & Tokura, Y. (2011). Modulation of semaphorin 3A expression by calcium concentration and histamine in human keratinocytes and fibroblasts. *J Dermatol Sci* 61:118–23.

Gasparro, F.P., Felli, A. & Schmitt, I.M. (1997). Psoralen photobiology: the relationship between DNA damage, chromatin structure, transcription, and immunogenic effects. *Recent Results Cancer Res* 143:101–27.

Goldberg, J.L., Espinosa, J.S., Xu, Y., Davidson, N., Kovacs, G.T. & Barres, B.A. (2002). Retinal ganglion cells do not extend axons by default: promotion by neurotrophic signaling and electrical activity. *Neuron* 33:689–702.

Goodman, C.S. (1996). Mechanisms and molecules that control growth cone guidance. *Annu Rev Neurosci* 19:341–77.

Grabham, P.W. & Goldberg, D.J. (1997). Nerve growth factor stimulates the accumulation of beta1 integrin at the tips of filopodia in the growth cones of sympathetic neurons. *J Neurosci* 17:5455–65.

Grubauer, G., Elias, P.M. & Feingold, K.R. (1989). Transepidermal water loss: the signal for recovery of barrier structure and function. *J Lipid Res* 30:323–33.

Gschwandtner, M., Purwar, R., Wittmann, M., Bäumer, W., Kietzmann, M., Werfel, T. & Gutzmer, R. (2008). Histamine upregulates keratinocyte MMP-9 production via the histamine H1 receptor. *J Invest Dermatol* 128:2783–91.

Harhaj, N.S. & Antonetti, D.A. (2004). Regulation of tight junctions and loss of barrier function in pathophysiology. *Int J Biochem Cell Biol* 36:1206–37.

Hayashita-Kinoh, H., Kinoh, H., Okada, A., Komori, K., Itoh, Y., Chiba, T., Kajita, M., Yana, I. & Seiki, M. (2001). Membrane-type 5 matrix metalloproteinase is expressed in differentiated neurons and regulates axonal growth. *Cell Growth Differ* 12:573–80.

Hengerer, B., Lindholm, D., Heumann, R., Rüther, U., Wagner, E.F. & Thoenen, H. (1990). Lesion-induced increase in nerve growth factor mRNA is mediated by c-fos. *Proc Natl Acad Sci U S A* 87:3899–903.

Hopper, B.D., Przybyszewski, J., Chen, H.W., Hammer, K.D. & Birt, D.F. (2009). Effect of ultraviolet B radiation on activator protein 1 constituent proteins and modulation by dietary energy restriction in SKH-1 mouse skin. *Mol Carcinog* 48:843–52.

Ikoma, A., Steinhoff, M., Ständer, S.,Yosipovitch, G., Schmelz, M. (2006). The neurobiology of itch. *Nat Rev Neurosci* 7: 535–47.

Kakurai, M., Monteforte, R., Suto, H., Tsai, M., Nakae, S. & Galli, S.J. (2006). Mast cell-derived tumor necrosis factor can promote nerve fiber elongation in the skin during contact hypersensitivity in mice. *Am J Pathol* 169:1713–21.

Kamo, A., Tominaga, M., Tengara, S., Ogawa, H. & Takamori, K. (2011a). Inhibitory effects of UV-based therapy on dry skin-inducible nerve growth in acetone-treated mice. *J Dermatol Sci* J Dermatol Sci 62:91-7.

Kamo, A., Tominaga, M., Negi, O., Tengara, S., Ogawa, H. & Takamori, K. (2011b). Topical application of emollients prevents dry skin-inducible intraepidermal nerve growth in acetone-treated mice. *J Dermatol Sci* J Dermatol Sci 62:64-6.

Kansra, S., Stoll, S.W., Johnson, J.L. & Elder, J.T. (2004). Autocrine extracellular signal-regulated kinase (ERK) activation in normal human keratinocytes: metalloproteinase-mediated release of amphiregulin triggers signaling from ErbB1 to ERK. *Mol Biol Cell* 15: 4299–309.

Kielbassa, C., Roza, L. & Epe, B. (1997). Wavelength dependence of oxidative DNA damage induced by UV and visible light. *Carcinogenesis* 18:811–6.

Kim, C.S., Hwang, C.K., Choi, H.S., Song, K.Y., Law, P.Y., Wei, L.N. & Loh, H.H. (2004). Neuron-restrictive silencer factor (NRSF) functions as a repressor in neuronal cells to regulate the mu opioid receptor gene. *J Biol Chem* 279:46464–73.

Kim, S.H., Hu, Y., Cadman, S. & Bouloux, P. (2008). Diversity in fibroblast growth factor receptor 1 regulation: learning from the investigation of Kallmann syndrome. *J Neuroendocrinol* 20:141–63.

Kim, S.S., Pandey, K.K., Choi, H.S., Kim, S.Y., Law, P.Y., Wei, L.N. & Loh, H.H. (2005). Poly(C) binding protein family is a transcription factor in mu-opioid receptor gene expression. *Mol Pharmacol* 68:729–36.

Kimura, H. & Schubert, D. (1992). Schwannoma-derived growth factor promotes the neuronal differentiation and survival of PC12 cells. *J Cell Biol* 116:777–83.

Ko, J.A., Akamatsu, Y., Yanai, R. & Nishida, T. (2010). Effects of semaphorin 3A overexpression in corneal fibroblasts on the expression of adherens-junction proteins in corneal epithelial cells. *Biochem Biophys Res Commun* 396:781–6.

Ko, J.A., Morishige, N., Yanai, R. & Nishida, T. (2008). Up-regulation of semaphorin 3A in human corneal fibroblasts by epidermal growth factor released from cocultured human corneal epithelial cells. *Biochem Biophys Res Commun* 377:104–8.

Kristensen, M., Chu, C.Q., Eedy, D.J., Feldmann, M., Brennan, F.M. & Breathnach, S.M. (1993). Localization of tumour necrosis factor-alpha (TNF-alpha) and its receptors in normal and psoriatic skin: epidermal cells express the 55-kD but not the 75-kD TNF receptor. *Clin Exp Immunol* 94:354–62.

Krueger, J.G., Wolfe, J.T., Nabeya, R.T., Vallat, V.P., Gilleaudeau, P., Heftler, N.S., Austin, L.M. & Gottlieb, A.B. (1995). Successful ultraviolet B treatment of psoriasis is accompanied by a reversal of keratinocyte pathology and by selective depletion of intraepidermal T cells. *J Exp Med* 182:2057–68.

Krutmann, J. (2000). Phototherapy for atopic dermatitis. *Clin Exp Dermatol* 25:552–8.

Krutmann, J. & Morita, A. (1999). Mechanisms of ultraviolet (UV) B and UVA phototherapy. *J Investig Dermatol Symp Proc* 4:70–2.

Le Duff, F., Fontas, E., Giacchero, D., Sillard, L., Lacour, J.P., Ortonne, J.P. & Passeron, T. (2010). 308-nm excimer lamp vs. 308-nm excimer laser for treating vitiligo: a randomized study. *Br J Dermatol* 163:188-92.

Lefcort, F., Venstrom, K., McDonald, J.A. & Reichardt, L.F. (1992). Regulation of expression of fibronectin and its receptor, alpha 5 beta 1, during development and regeneration of peripheral nerve. *Development* 116:767–82.

Leon, A., Buriani, A., Dal Toso, R., Fabris, M., Romanello, S., Aloe, L. & Levi-Montalcini, R. (1994). Mast cells synthesize, store, and release nerve growth factor. *Proc Natl Acad Sci U S A* 91:3739–43.

Lewin, G.R. & Mendell, L.M. (1993). Nerve growth factor and nociception. *Trends Neurosci* 16:353–9.

Liou, A., Elias, P.M., Grunfeld, C., Feingold, K.R. & Wood, L.C. (1997). Amphiregulin and nerve growth factor expression are regulated by barrier status in murine epidermis. *J Invest Dermatol* 108:73–7.

Liu, R.Y., Schmid, R.S., Snider, W.D. & Maness, P.F. (2002). NGF enhances sensory axon growth induced by laminin but not by the L1 cell adhesion molecule. *Mol Cell Neurosci* 20:2–12.

Loden, M. & Maibach, H.I. (2006). *DRY SKIN and MOISTURIZERS: Chemistry and Function*, Taylor & Francis Group, Boca Raton.

Maddison, B., Namazi, M.R., Samuel, L.S., Sanchez, J., Pichardo, R., Stocks, J., Maruziva, D. & Yosipovitch, G. (2008). Unexpected diminished innervation of epidermis and dermoepidermal junction in lichen amyloidosus. *Br J Dermatol* 159:403–6.

Martey, C.A., Vetrano, A.M., Whittemore, M.S., Mariano, T.M., Heck, D.E., Laskin, D.L., Heindel, N.D. & Laskin, J.D. (2005). Inhibition of interferon-gamma signaling by a mercurio-substituted dihydropsoralen in murine keratinocytes. *Biochem Pharmacol* 70:1726–34.

Meinhardt, M., Krebs, R., Anders, A., Heinrich, U. & Tronnier, H. (2008). Wavelength-dependent penetration depths of ultraviolet radiation in human skin. *J Biomed Opt* 13:044030.

Merritt, A.J., Berika, M.Y., Zhai, W., Kirk, S.E., Ji, B., Hardman, M.J. & Garrod, D.R. (2002). Suprabasal desmoglein 3 expression in the epidermis of transgenic mice results in hyperproliferation and abnormal differentiation. Mol Cell Biol 22: 5846–58.

Messersmith, E.K., Leonardo, E.D., Shatz, C.J., Tessier-Lavigne, M., Goodman, C.S. & Kolodkin, A.L. (1995). Semaphorin III can function as a selective chemorepellent to pattern sensory projections in the spinal cord. *Neuron* 14:949–59.

Miyamoto, T., Nojima, H., Shinkado, T., Nakahashi, T. & Kuraishi, Y. (2002). Itch-associated response induced by experimental dry skin in mice. *Jpn J Pharmacol* 88:285–92.

Muir, D. (1994). Metalloproteinase-dependent neurite outgrowth within a synthetic extracellular matrix is induced by nerve growth factor. *Exp Cell Res* 210:243–52.

Nilsson, A. & Kanje, M. (2005). Amphiregulin acts as an autocrine survival factor for adult sensory neurons. *Neuroreport* 16:213–8.

Ortel, B., Perl, S., Kinaciyan, T., Calzavara-Pinton, P.G. & Honigsmann, H. (1993). Comparison of narrow-band (311 nm) UVB and broad-band UVA after oral or bath-water 8-methoxypsoralen in the treatment of psoriasis. *J Am Acad Dermatol* 29:736–40.

Page-McCaw, A., Ewald, A.J. & Werb, Z. (2007). Matrix metalloproteinases and the regulation of tissue remodelling. *Nat Rev Mol Cell Biol* 8:221–33.

Park, S.W., Huq, M.D., Loh, H.H. & Wei, L.N. (2005). Retinoic acid-induced chromatin remodeling of mouse kappa opioid receptor gene. *J Neurosci* 25:3350–7.

Paus, R., Schmelz, M., Bíró, T. & Steinhoff, M. (2006). Frontiers in pruritus research: scratching the brain for more effective itch therapy. *J Clin Invest* 116:1174–86.

Perez-Moreno, M., Jamora, C. & Fuchs, E. (2003). Sticky business: orchestrating cellular signals at adherens junctions. *Cell* 112:535–48.

Pummi, K., Malminen, M., Aho, H., Karvonen, S.L., Peltonen, J. & Peltonen, S. (2001). Epidermal tight junctions: ZO-1 and occludin are expressed in mature, developing, and affected skin and in vitro differentiating keratinocytes. *J Invest Dermatol* 117:1050–8.

Purwar, R., Kraus, M., Werfel, T. & Wittmann, M. (2008). Modulation of keratinocyte-derived MMP-9 by IL-13: a possible role for the pathogenesis of epidermal inflammation. *J Invest Dermatol* 128:59–66.

Rawlings, A.V., Scott, I.R., Harding, C.R. & Bowser, P.A. (1994). Stratum corneum moisturization at the molecular level. *J Invest Dermatol* 103:731–41.

Ree, K., Johnsen, A.S. & Hovig, T. (1981). Ultrastructural studies on the effect of photoactivated 8-methoxy psoralen. Nuclear changes in a human epithelial cell line. *Acta Pathol Microbiol Scand A* 89:81–90.

Reichardt, L.F. & Tomaselli, K.J. (1991) Extracellular matrix molecules and their receptors: functions in neural development. *Annu Rev Neurosci* 14:531–70.

Rossino, P., Gavazzi, I., Timpl, R., Aumailley, M., Abbadini, M., Giancotti, F., Silengo, L., Marchisio, P.C. & Tarone, G. (1990). Nerve growth factor induces increased expression of a laminin-binding integrin in rat pheochromocytoma PC12 cells. *Exp Cell Res* 189:100–8.

Rycroft, R.J.G. & Smith, W.D.L. (1980). Low humidity occupational dermatoses. *Contact Dermatitis* 6:488–92.

Sato, N., Katsumata, N., Kagami, M., Hasegawa, T., Hori, N., Kawakita, S., Minowada, S., Shimotsuka, A., Shishiba, Y., Yokozawa, M., Yasuda, T., Nagasaki, K., Hasegawa, D., Hasegawa, Y., Tachibana, K., Naiki, Y., Horikawa, R., Tanaka, T. & Ogata, T. (2004). Clinical assessment and mutation analysis of Kallmann syndrome 1 (KAL1) and fibroblast growth factor receptor 1 (FGFR1, or KAL2) in five families and 18 sporadic patients. J Clin Endocrinol *Metab* 89:1079–88.

Schuhknecht, B., Marziniak, M., Wissel, A., Phan, N.Q., Pappai, D,. Dangelmaier, J., Metze, D. & Ständer S. (2011). Reduced intraepidermal nerve fiber density in lesional and non-lesional prurigo nodularis skin as potential sign of subclinical cutaneous neuropathy. *Br J Dermatol* in press.

Seiki, M. (1999). Membrane-type matrix metalloproteinases. *APMIS* 107:137–43.

Shepherd, I.T., Luo, Y., Lefcort, F., Reichardt, L.F. & Raper, J.A. (1997). A sensory axon repellent secreted from ventral spinal cord explants is neutralized by antibodies raised against collapsin-1. *Development* 124:1377–85.

Shubayev, V.I. & Myers, R.R. (2004). Matrix metalloproteinase-9 promotes nerve growth factor-induced neurite elongation but not new sprout formation in vitro. *J Neurosci Res* 77:229–39.

Sonkoly, E., Muller, A., Lauerma, A.I., Pivarcsi, A., Soto, H., Kemeny, L., Alenius, H., Dieu-Nosjean, M.C., Meller, S., Rieker, J., Steinhoff, M., Hoffmann, T.K., Ruzicka, T., Zlotnik, A. & Homey, B. (2006). IL-31: a new link between T cells and pruritus in atopic skin inflammation. *J Allergy Clin Immunol* 117:411–7.

Soussi-Yanicostas, N., Faivre-Sarrailh, C., Hardelin, J.P., Levilliers, J., Rougon, G. & Petit, C. (1998). Anosmin-1 underlying the X chromosome-linked Kallmann syndrome is an adhesion molecule that can modulate neurite growth in a cell-type specific manner. *J Cell Sci* 111:2953–65.

Soussi-Yanicostas, N., Hardelin, J.P., Arroyo-Jimenez, M.M., Ardouin, O., Legouis, R., Levilliers, J., Traincard, F., Betton, J.M., Cabanié, L. & Petit, C. (1996). Initial characterization of anosmin-1, a putative extracellular matrix protein synthesized by definite neuronal cell populations in the central nervous system. *J Cell Sci* 109:1749–57.

Steinhoff, M., Ständer, S., Seeliger, S., Ansel, J,C., Schmelz, M. & Luger, T. (2003). Modern aspects of cutaneous neurogenic inflammation. *Arch Dermatol* 139:1479–88.

Sumimoto, S., Kawai, M., Kasajima, Y. & Hamamoto, T. (1992). Increased plasma tumour necrosis factor-alpha concentration in atopic dermatitis. *Arch Dis Child* 67:277–9.

Sun, Y.G. & Chen, Z.F. (2007). A gastrin-releasing peptide receptor mediates the itch sensation in the spinal cord. *Nature* 448:700–3.

Sun, Y.G., Zhao, Z.Q., Meng, X.L., Yin, J., Liu, X.Y. & Chen, Z.F. (2009). Cellular basis of itch sensation. *Science* 325:1531–4.

Suzuki, K., Kumanogoh, A. & Kikutani, H. (2008). Semaphorins and their receptors in immune cell interactions. *Nat Immunol* 9:17–23.

Takano, N., Sakurai, T. & Kurachi, M. (2005). Effects of anti-nerve growth factor antibody on symptoms in the NC/Nga mouse, an atopic dermatitis model. *J Pharmacol Sci* 99:277–86.

Takano, N., Sakurai, T., Ohashi, Y. & Kurachi, M. (2007). Effects of high-affinity nerve growth factor receptor inhibitors on symptoms in the NC/Nga mouse atopic dermatitis model. *Br J Dermatol* 156:241–6.

Takaoka, K., Shirai, Y. & Saito, N. (2009). Inflammatory cytokine tumor necrosis factor-alpha enhances nerve growth factor production in human keratinocytes, HaCaT cells. *J Pharmacol Sci* 111:381–91.

Tanaka, A., Arita, K., Lai-Cheong, J.E., Palisson, F., Hide, M. & McGrath, J.A. (2009). New insight into mechanisms of pruritus from molecular studies on familial primary localized cutaneous amyloidosis. *Br J Dermatol* 161:1217–24.

Taneda, K., Tominaga, M., Negi, O., Tengara, S., Kamo, A., Ogawa, H. & Takamori, K. (2011). Evaluation of epidermal nerve density and opioid receptor levels in psoriatic itch. *Br J Dermatol* doi: 10.1111/j.1365-2133.2011.

Tang, X.Q., Tanelian, D.L. & Smith, G.M. (2004). Semaphorin3A inhibits nerve growth factor-induced sprouting of nociceptive afferents in adult rat spinal cord. *J Neurosci* 24:819–27.

Tengara, S., Tominaga, M., Kamo, A., Taneda, K., Negi, O., Ogawa, H. & Takamori, K. (2010). Keratinocyte-derived anosmin-1, an extracellular glycoprotein encoded by the X-linked Kallmann syndrome gene, is involved in modulation of epidermal nerve density in atopic dermatitis. *J Dermatol Sci* 58:64–71.

Tominaga, M., Kamo, A., Tengara, S., Ogawa, H. & Takamori, K. (2009a). *In vitro* model for penetration of sensory nerve fibres on a Matrigel basement membrane: implications for possible application to intractable pruritus. *Br J Dermatol* 161:1028–37.

Tominaga, M. & Takamori, K. (2010). Recent advances in pathophysiological mechanisms of itch. *Expert Rev Dermatol* 5:197–212.

Tominaga, M., Tengara, S., Kamo, A., Ogawa, H. & Takamori, K. (2009c). Psoralen-ultraviolet A therapy alters epidermal Sema3A and NGF levels and modulates epidermal innervation in atopic dermatitis. *J Dermatol Sci* 55:40–6.

Tominaga, M., Ogawa, H. & Takamori, K. (2008). Decreased production of semaphorin 3A in the lesional skin of atopic dermatitis. *Br J Dermatol* 158:842–4.

Tominaga, M., Ogawa, H. & Takamori, K. (2009b). Histological characterization of cutaneous nerve fibers containing gastrin-releasing peptide in NC/Nga mice: an atopic dermatitis model. *J Invest Dermatol* 129:2901–5.

Tominaga, M., Ozawa, S., Ogawa, H. & Takamori, K. (2007a). A hypothetical mechanism of intraepidermal neurite formation in NC/Nga mice with atopic dermatitis. *J Dermatol Sci* 46:199–210.

Tominaga, M., Ozawa, S., Tengara, S., Ogawa, H. & Takamori, K. (2007b). Intraepidermal nerve fibers increase in dry skin of acetone-treated mice. *J Dermatol Sci* 48:103–11.

Van Weelden, H., Baart de la Faille, H., Young, E. & van der Leun, JC. (1990). Comparison of narrow-band UV-B phototherapy and PUVA photochemotherapy in the treatment of psoriasis. *Acta Derm Venereol* 70:212–5.

Verge, V,M., Richardson, P,M., Wiesenfeld-Hallin, Z. & Hokfelt, T. (1995). Differential influence of nerve growth factor on neuropeptide expression in vivo: a novel role in peptide suppression in adult sensory neurons. *J Neurosci* 15:2081–96.

Wallengren, J. & Sundler, F. (2004). Phototherapy reduces the number of epidermal and CGRP-positive dermal nerve fibres. *Acta Derm Venereol* 84:111–5.

Wallengren, J., Tegner, E. & Sundler, F. (2002). Cutaneous sensory nerve fibers are decreased in number after peripheral and central nerve damage. *J Am Acad Dermatol* 46:215–7.

Wang, H.Q., Quan, T., He, T., Franke, T.F., Voorhees, J.J. & Fisher, G.J. (2003). Epidermal growth factor receptor-dependent, NF-kappaB-independent activation of the phosphatidylinositol 3-kinase/Akt pathway inhibits ultraviolet irradiation-induced caspases-3, -8, and -9 in human keratinocytes. *J Biol Chem* 278:45737–45.

Wang, X., Yi, J., Lei, J. & Pei, D. (1999). Expression, purification and characterization of recombinant mouse MT5-MMP protein products. *FEBS Lett* 462:261–6.

Werner, A., Willem, M., Jones, L.L., Kreutzberg, G.W., Mayer, U. & Raivich, G. (2000). Impaired axonal regeneration in alpha7 integrin-deficient mice. *J Neurosci* 20:1822–30.

Wheelock, M.J. & Johnson, K.R. (2003). Cadherins as modulators of cellular phenotype. *Annu Rev Cell Dev Biol* 19:207–35.

Wittmann, M. & Werfel, T. (2006). Interaction of keratinocytes with infiltrating lymphocytes in allergic eczematous skin diseases. *Curr Opin Allergy Clin Immunol* 6:329–34.

Wolkerstorfer, A. & Brenninkmeijer, E.E.A, (2011). Excimer laser: a treatment option for the prurigo form of atopic dermatitis. *Expert Rev Dermatol* 6:1–3.

Yamaguchi, J., Nakamura, F., Aihara, M., Yamashita, N., Usui, H., Hida, T., Takei, K., Nagashima, Y., Ikezawa, Z. & Goshima, Y. (2008). Semaphorin3A alleviates skin lesions and scratching behavior in NC/Nga mice, an atopic dermatitis model. *J Invest Dermatol* 128:2842–49.

Yamaoka, J., Di, Z.H., Sun, W. & Kawana, S. (2007). Changes in cutaneous sensory nerve fibers induced by skin-scratching in mice. *J Dermatol Sci* 46:41–51.

Yosipovitch, G. (2004). Dry skin and impairment of barrier function associated with itch - new insights. *Int J Cosmet Sci* 26:1–7.

Zuo, J., Ferguson, T.A., Hernandez, Y.J., Stetler-Stevenson, W.G. & Muir, D. (1998). Neuronal matrix metalloproteinase-2 degrades and inactivates a neurite-inhibiting chondroitin sulfate proteoglycan. *J Neurosci* 18:5203–11.

Zhou, S., Matsuyoshi, N., Takeuchi, T., Ohtsuki, Y. & Miyachi, Y. (2003). Reciprocal altered expression of T-cadherin and P-cadherin in psoriasis vulgaris. *Br J Dermatol* 149:268–73.

Zhou, Y., Gunput, R,A. & Pasterkamp, R,J. (2008). Semaphorin signaling: progress made and promises ahead. *Trends Biochem Sci* 33:161–70.

Diagnosing Vascular Dementia by Skin Biopsy - Uniqueness of CADASIL

Saara Tikka[1], Kati Mykkänen[2], Maija Junna[2], Robert Bergholm[3], Minna Pöyhönen[3], Marc Baumann[3], Matti Viitanen[2] and Hannu Kalimo[3]

[1]Harvard Medical School,
[2]University of Turku,
[3]University of Helsinki,
[1]USA
[2,3]Finland

1. Introduction

Cerebral autosomal dominant arteriopathy with subcortical infarcts and leukoencephalopathy (CADASIL) is the most common hereditary subcortical vascular dementia. CADASIL is caused by mutations in *NOTCH3* gene, which encodes a large transmembrane receptor NOTCH3. The key pathological finding is the accumulation of granular osmiophilic material (GOM), which contains extracellular domains of NOTCH3, on degenerating vascular smooth muscle cells (VSMCs). CADASIL is usually suspected on the basis of patient's clinical picture, relatively characteristic findings in brain MRI and information on family history. Definite diagnosis can be established by molecular genetic detection of a pathogenic mutation in *NOTCH3* gene. The gene analysis may, however, be laborious, due to the high number of different pathogenic mutations (over 200 at present) and besides, comprehensive genetic analyses are available only in few genetic laboratories. However, CADASIL is a unique dementing disorder, because it is also possible to diagnose it at a high level of certainty by a skin biopsy using electron microscopic (EM) or immunohistochemical (IHC) analysis of dermal arteries.

2. CADASIL

2.1 Epidemiology

CADASIL, the most common hereditary vascular dementia, is characterized by migraineous headache with aura, recurrent ischemic attacks, cognitive decline and psychiatric symptoms as the four main features. Migraneous headache with aura occurs in about one third of patients and it may begin already before the age of 10 years (Kalimo et al., 2008). The age at first ever stroke varies widely, usually from 25 to 65 years [yet, the youngest patient who has suffered from a stroke was 11 years-of-age (Granild-Jensen et al., 2009)].

2.2 Etiology

CADASIL is caused by mutations in *NOTCH3* gene encoding a transmembrane receptor NOTCH3 (Joutel et al., 1996). Virtually all pathogenic mutations lead to an odd number of cysteine residues in one of the 34 epidermal growth factor (EGF) like repeats in the extracellular domain of NOTCH3 (N3ECD). The mutations result in degeneration of vascular smooth muscle cells (VSMC), in which *NOTCH3* is predominantly expressed in adult humans (Joutel et al., 2000). The main pathological findings are accumulation of N3ECD on degenerating VSMCs as well as fibrosis and thickening of arterial walls, stenosis of arterioles and lacunar infarcts (Miao et al., 2004, Ruchoux et al., 1995). In electron microscopy (EM) the pathognomonic feature of CADASIL is accumulation of granular osmiophilic material (GOM) in indentations of the VSMCs or in the extracellular space in close vicinity to VSMCs (Baudrimont et al., 1993, Ruchoux et al., 1995). The exact composition of GOM has not been elaborated, but an immunogold EM study suggested N3ECD to be a component of GOM (Ishiko et al., 2006).

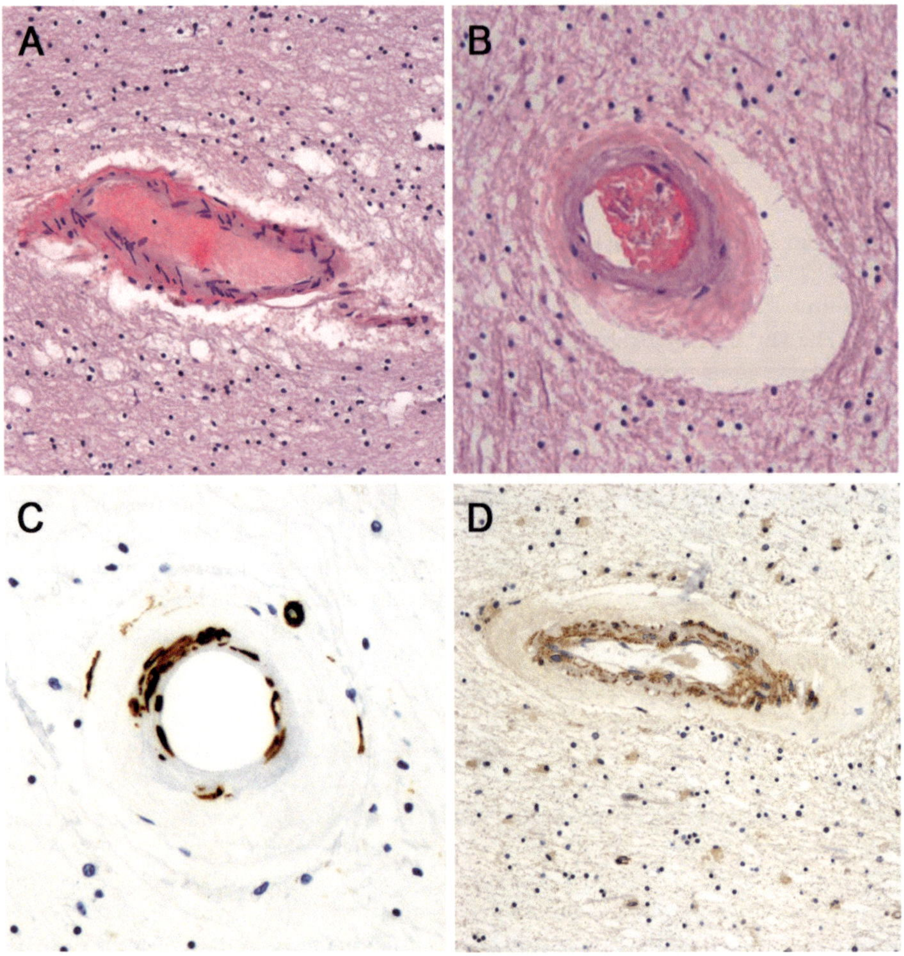

Fig. 1. Histopathological findings in CADASIL brain arteries. A) Small arteriole from the cerebral white matter of a control person. H&E staining. B) Corresponding arteriole from a CADASIL patient. Note the marked thickening of the wall. H&E staining. C) Degeneration of VSMCs is seen as decreased immunoreactivity for α-SMA. D) N3ECD has accumulated in the *tunica media* of an affected arteriole.

2.3 Vascular pathology

2.3.1 Brain arteries

Pathological changes are present in all small to medium-sized arteries of the body and in some veins and capillaries. In small arterioles in cerebral white matter (WM) histological stainings reveal markedly thickened walls with accumulation of N3ECD in the degenerating tunica media. This material is basophilic in H&E (Figure 1A and B) and red in PAS stainings. Decreased immunopositivity for α-smooth muscle actin (α-SMA) reveals degeneration of the VSMCs (Figure 1C). The accumulation of N3ECD can be verified by immunohistochemical staining (Figure 1D). Accumulation of extracellular matrix proteins, including various types of collagens and fibronectin and vimentin outside the degenerating VSMCs causes the thickening of the vessel walls (Figures 1A-D). On the basis of the stainings above CADASIL can be distinguished from the two other arteriopathies with thickened walls: In arteriolosclerosis (Binswanger disease) and cerebral amyloid angiopathy the walls are homogeneously stained, either like collagen or like amyloid. The brain arteries are usually not studied until post mortem, when the degeneration of VSMCs and the accumulation of GOM are already obvious at the LM level. Thus, EM examination is not needed and is usually not performed.

2.3.2 Dermal arterioles - appearance of GOM

Skin biopsies are most often performed and the specimens examined at earlier stages of CADASIL, often when the diagnosis is only suspected. In histological sections the skin usually looks relatively normal: the possible thickening of the walls of small arteries within the dermal connective tissue is difficult to discern. Thus, either EM or IHC examination is needed.

EM analysis of an arterial wall reveals enlarged subendothelial space and the degenerating VSMCs which appear irregularly shaped as they have lost their intercellular connections (Figure 2; Ruchoux and Maurage, 1997, Kalimo et al., 2008). As a striking and pathognomonic feature of CADASIL, GOM accumulates on VSMCs (Baudrimont et al., 1993, Ruchoux et al., 1995). Already before the gene defect was found, GOM was detected in skin biopsies from CADASIL patients (Ruchoux et al., 1994). So far GOM has not been described in any other disease entity: GOM is negative in both histological (e.g. Congo red and thioflavin) and immunohistochemical stainings for different amyloid angiopathies (Ragno et al., 1995, Ruchoux and Maurage, 1997). GOM accumulates in the arterial wall, in the *tunica media* and is usually detected in the close vicinity to VSMCs, often in small indentations of VSMC plasma membrane within the basal lamina (Figures 2 and 3A), which is usually irregularly thickened, or GOM lies free in the extracellular space (Figures 2 and 6C.). The indentations are often associated with caveolar structures (Figure 3A), but as caveolae are common structures of VSMCs, their pathogenetic significance is unclear. The size of GOM deposits is variable, ranging from 0.2 μm to 0.8 μm, and they are composed of 10-15 nm granules (Ruchoux and Maurage, 1997). GOM appears in EM as evenly electron dense or, as often, denser on the side which is towards the VSMC membrane (Figure 3A). The exact composition of GOM has not been fully clarified, but N3ECD is a component of GOM as demonstrated by immunoelectron microscopy (Ishiko et al., 2006). Moreover, with confocal microscopy, N3ECD immunoreactivity can be seen as dot-like accumulations on the arterial wall, in concordance with the appearance of GOM deposits in the EM (Figure 3B). The degeneration of VSMCs and the accumulation of GOM begin early and the morphological changes in arteries and the accumulation of GOM are already detectable before the age of 20 (Tikka et al., 2009)(Figure 3C).

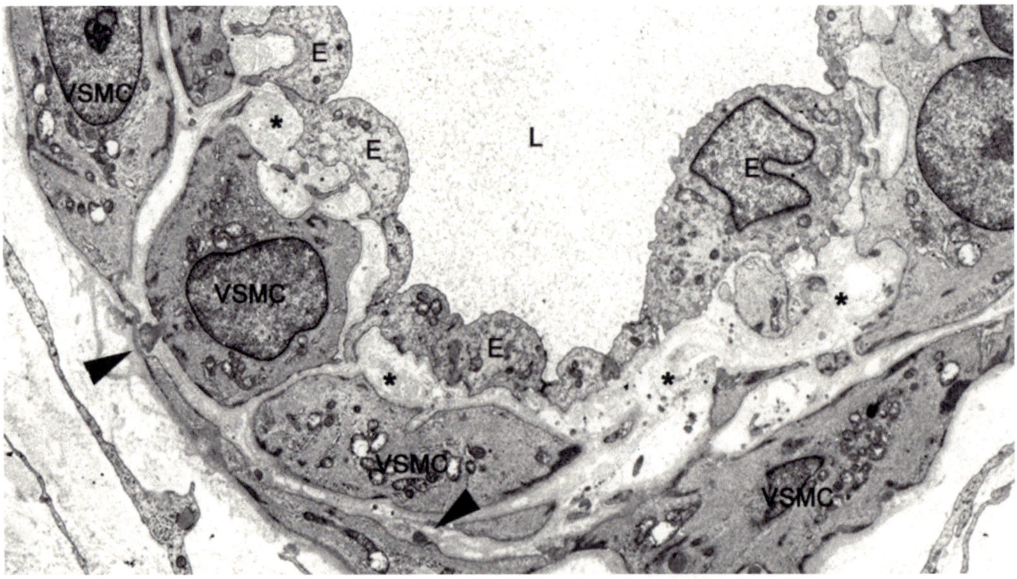

Fig. 2. EM micrograph of a dermal artery from a CADASIL patient. Characteristic vascular pathology is clearly detectable already in early age. Subendothelial space is widened (asterisks) and VSMCs are irregularly shaped and have lost their intercellular connections. Accumulation of GOM is seen in close vicinity of VSMCs. CADASIL patient with pArg133Cys mutation. L=arterial lumen, E=endothelial cell, VSMC=vascular smooth muscle cell. Two GOMs are pointed with arrowheads. Figure is reproduced with permission from *Future Neurology* (Kalimo et al., 2008)

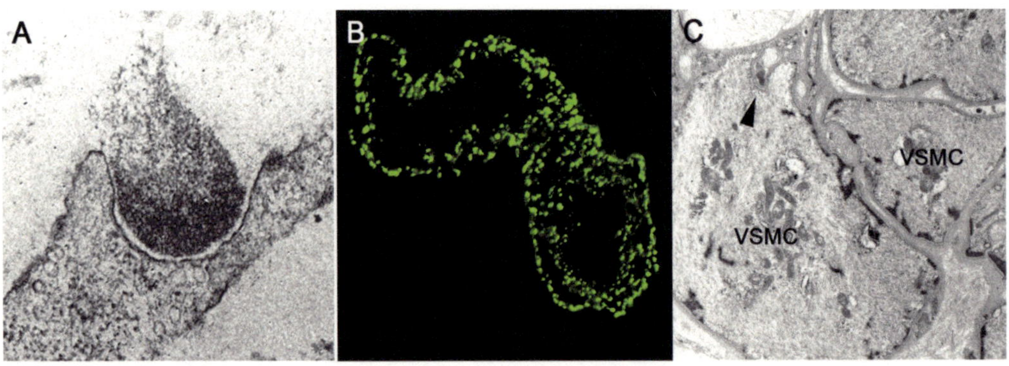

Fig. 3. Dermal artery of CADASIL patient. A) EM micrograph of CADASIL patient (p.Arg133C) showing characteristic GOM deposits in the intendation of VSMC with caveolar structures. B) Confocal microscopy reveals N3ECD immunoreactivity as dot-like accumulations in the arterial wall in concordance with GOM deposits. A 62 year-old patient carrying p.Tyr1069Cys mutation. C) Accumulation of GOM in an artery of 19 year-old CADASIL patient with mutation p.Arg133Cys. Figure B is reproduced with permission from *Future Neurology* (Kalimo et al., 2008)

3. Diagnosis of CADASIL

3.1 Clinical findings

CADASIL is suspected in patients with the typical clinical features, occasionally with positive family history. Patients are sometimes hypertensive, but it does not have any diagnostic significance. White matter alterations in brain T2-weighted MRI (O'Sullivan et al., 2001) are important clues. In T2w MRI an experienced radiologist can detect changes that are highly suggestive of CADASIL already in asymptomatic carriers of the gene defect (even before the age of 20). Hyperintensities on T2w and FLAIR MRI in temporopolar WM are nearly diagnostic of CADASIL (Figures 4A). In addition, cerebral periventricular WM and capsula externa hyperintensities are characteristic (Figure 4B; Chabriat et al., 1998). Laboratory examinations are usually non-rewarding or non-specific, i.e. the examinations may reveal risk factors of other cerebrovascular diseases.

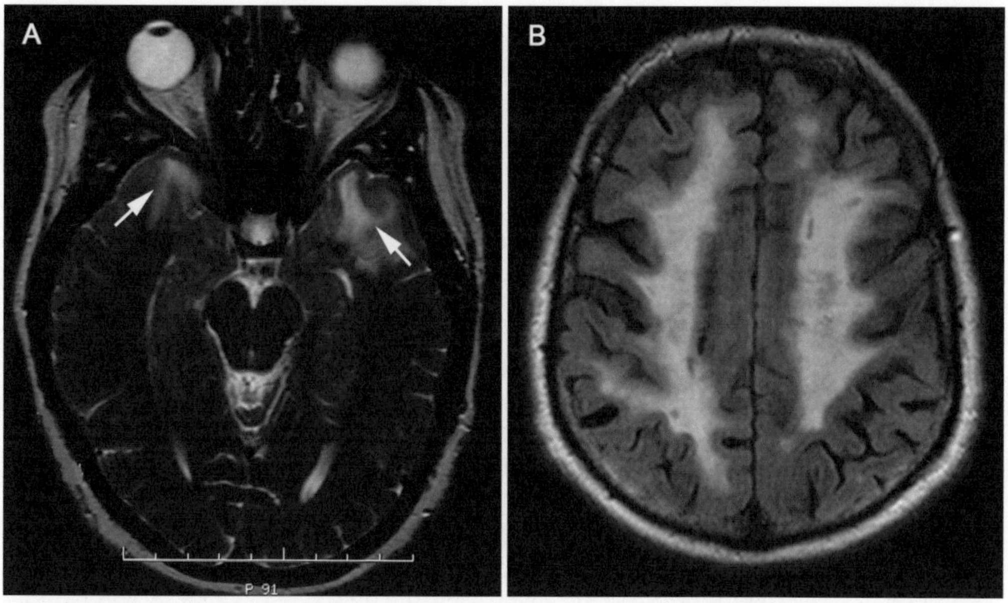

Fig. 4. MRI findings in CADASIL. Hyperintensities in anterior temporal lobes in T2-weighted MRI are characteristic early alterations in CADASIL. A 29-year-old female soon after her first transient ischemic attack. B) At an advanced stage of CADASIL FLAIR MRI shows extensive hyperintensities in the cerebral white matter (leukoaraiosis). Figure 4A is reproduced with permission of *Future Neurology* (Kalimo et al., 2008)

3.2 Genetic analysis

The definite verification of the diagnosis can be done by identifying a pathogenic mutation in the *NOTCH3* gene. However, over 200 different mutations in 20 different exons have been reported to cause CADASIL (Tikka et al., 2009, Junna et al. 2011 unpublished). Comprehensive analysis of all these exons is time consuming and costly. Thus, most diagnostic laboratories screen only the exons that according to the previous reports harbour majority of the mutations (Dotti et al., 2005, Escary et al., 2000, Joutel et al., 1997, Kalimo et al., 2002, Opherk et al., 2004). Of the all reported pathogenic *NOTCH3* mutations 62% locate in exons 3, 4, 5 and 8. Furthermore, to obtain 80 % coverage, additional investigation of exons 2, 6, 11 and 18 is required (Tikka et al., 2009). Mutation screening covering the whole region coding for EGF repeats (exons 2-24) is not realistic for all patients and for most laboratories.

3.3 Skin biopsy

Given the challenging factors complicating comprehensive genetic analyses it is fortunate that CADASIL is also possible to diagnose by skin biopsy using EM or IHC examination.

3.3.1 EM analysis

Although GOM has not been detected in any other disease and the specificity is considered to be 100% (Ebke et al., 1997, Mayer et al., 1999, Markus et al., 2002, Razvi et al., 2003) the reports on the sensitivity of detecting GOM in skin biopsy of patients with genetically verified CADASIL have been contradictory. Two earlier studies on a smaller number of patients suggested 100% sensitivity (Ebke et al., 1997, Mayer et al., 1999) in which Ebke et al. analysed one family with 8 patients (mutation not specified) and 5 controls suffering from sporadic leukoencephalopathies and Mayer et al. examined 14 patients (mutation not specified) from three unrelated families. Two more recent papers have reported a low sensitivity: Markus et al. (2002) reported GOM detected only in 8 patients out of 18, thus giving a sensitivity of only 44.4%. Razvi et al. (2003) suspected that the sensitivity might be even lower, although they did not give an exact number. In the latest EM study in a cohort of 131 CADASIL patients and 26 control subjects GOM was detected in all skin biopsies from mutation positive patients and in none of the control biopsies (Tikka et al., 2009). This study was a retrospective investigation of a combined patient material from Finland, Sweden and France comprising 131 patients, from whom both the genetic analysis and EM examination of skin biopsy were available. Skin biopsies from 26 mutation negative members in genetically proven CADASIL families served as controls.
This study showed that EM demonstration of GOM in skin biopsy is a highly reliable and practical method to screen for or even specifically diagnose CADASIL. Furthermore, the intensive search for mutations based on confidence in the diagnostic specificity of GOM resulted in discovery of four novel, previously unreported mutations, among them the first duplication of three codons (Tikka et al., 2009). Thus the detection of GOM in skin biopsies is a highly reliable diagnostic method: in this large cohort the congruence between *NOTCH3* mutations and presence of GOM was 100% (Tikka et al., 2009).

Technical requirements

When using EM analysis of skin biopsy as a diagnostic method in suspected CADASIL cases, special attention should be paid to the quality and analysis of the skin biopsy. The GOM is best detectable generally from medium sized or small arterioles (usually outer diameter 20-40 µm) in deep dermis or upper subcutis, but in a few cases GOM has been detected also in veins (Tikka et al. 2009, Fig. 6B) and capillaries (Lewandowska et al., 2010). The detection of fragmented lamina elastica interna as dark blue dots in toluidine blue semithin sections (Figure 5) is a good marker of representative arterioles. Technical factors in the processing of the samples may also influence the result. Since GOM is osmiophilic, the osmium tetroxide treatment should be adjusted such that GOM becomes sufficiently well contrasted. Furthermore, if GOM is not detected in the first vessel investigated, other vessels or even repeat biopsies should be examined. Besides, examination should be targeted rather to an artery/arteriole (with multiple layers of VSMCs and inner elastic lamina) than a vein or a capillary, since veins and capillaries are not always GOM positive (Figure 6). Of course, a prerequisite is that the investigator recognizes GOM correctly and distinguishes it from fallacious deposits like small clumps of cell debris or fragmented ECM proteins (Figure 7).

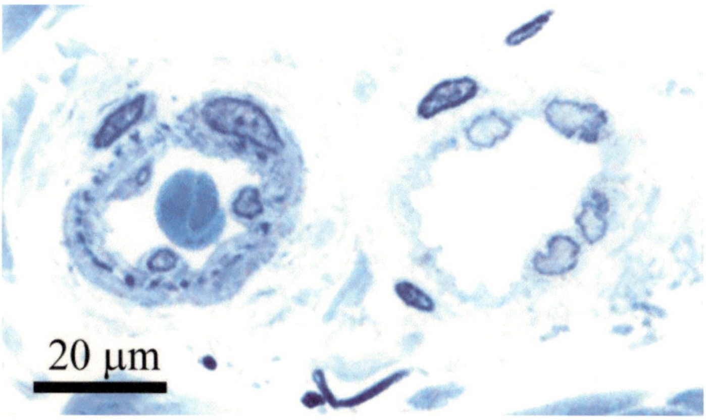

Fig. 5. Small arteriole and vein in skin biopsy. Note the thicker vessel wall and fragmented lamina elastica (dark blue dots beneath endothelial cell layer) in the arteriole. Toluide blue stained semithin epon section of a skin biopsy from CADASIL patient carrying p.Arg133Cys mutation. Figure is reproduced with permission of *Brain* (Tikka et al., 2009).

3.3.2 Immunohistochemistry

IHC showing accumulation of N3ECD in the tunica media of small arteries is another microscopic method to diagnose CADASIL, the availability of IHC being, of course, better than that of EM. Joutel et al. (2001) introduced IHC as a diagnostic tool in CADASIL. In that study they showed in a cohort of 39 patients (23 patients, 16 controls) that sensitivity of N3ECD staining was 96% and specificity 100%. Another study with a cohort of 41 *NOTCH3* mutation carriers, 21 controls and 10 hereditary cerebral hemorrhage with amyloidosis-Dutch (HCHWA-D) patients reported sensitivity of 85.4-90.2% and specificity of 95.2-100% (Lesnik Oberstein et al., 2003). Both studies reported false negatives which were associated with mutations in exon 11 (Joutel et al., 2001, Lesnik Oberstein et al., 2003). In addition, nonspecific staining is an inherent caveat of IHC producing false positives (Lesnik Oberstein et al., 2003). In the latest immunohistochemical study on 93 skin biopsies from subjects with suspected CADASIL the sensitivity and specificity of the skin biopsies were 97.7% and 56.5%, respectively though in familial cases the values improved to 100% and 81.5% (Ampuero et al., 2009). Specificity was limited in that study by incomplete sequencing of *NOTCH3* (sequenced exons: 2-6, 8, 11, 14, 18, 19, 22 and 23). Although IHC is relatively sensitive and highly specific, given the possibility of false negatives and positives, it should not be used as definitive tool for diagnostics but to help other methods of choice.

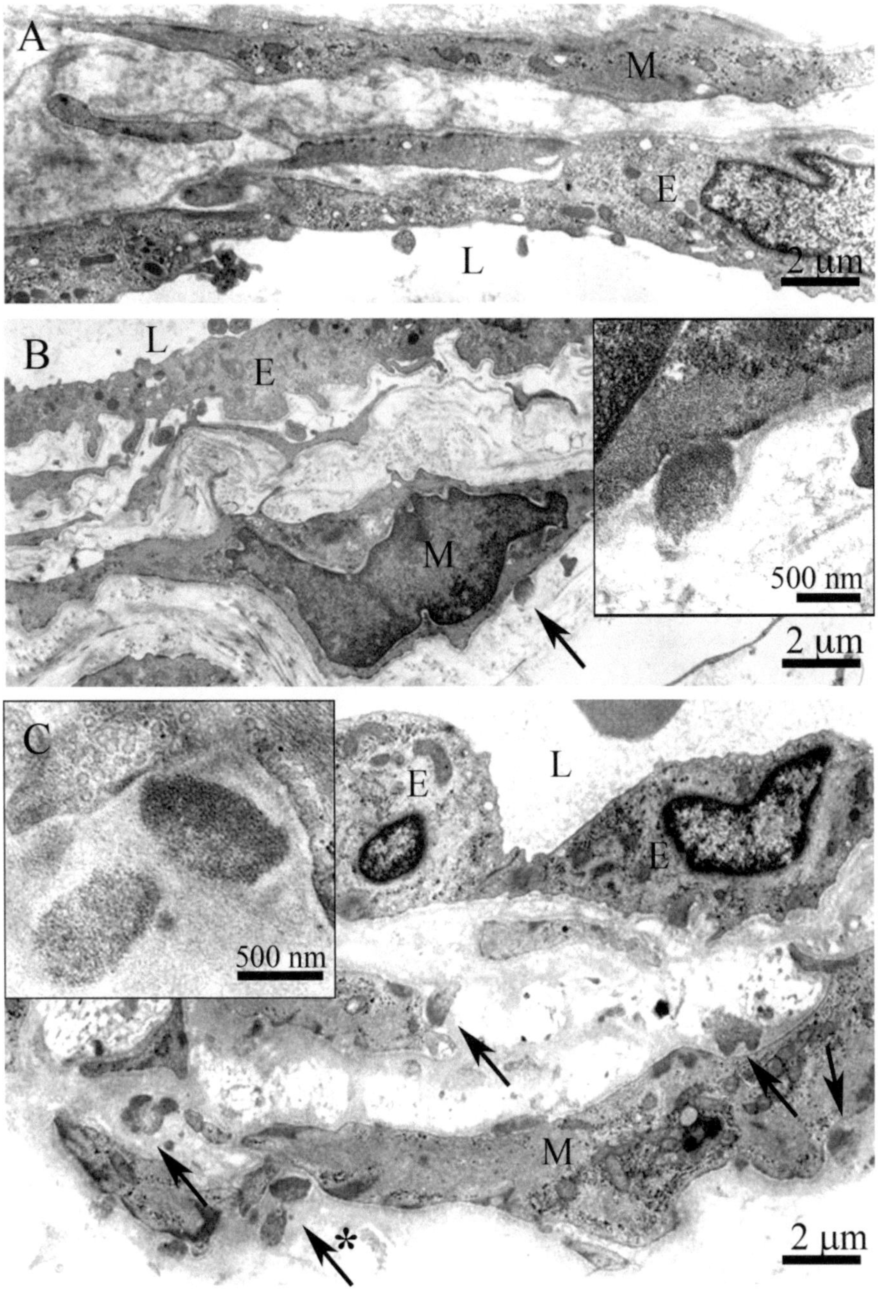

Fig. 6. GOM is usually detected in small arteries or arterioles and sometimes in veins and capillaries. A) The same vein as in figure 5 with no GOM. B) A vein from deep dermis showing one definite GOM (arrow) shown with higher magnification in the inset. C) The same arteriole as in figure 5 with several GOM deposits (five shown with arrows), one marked with asterisk is in the inset with higher magnification. L=lumen, E=endothelial cell, M=vascular smooth muscle cell. Figure is reproduced with permission of *Brain* (Tikka et al., 2009).

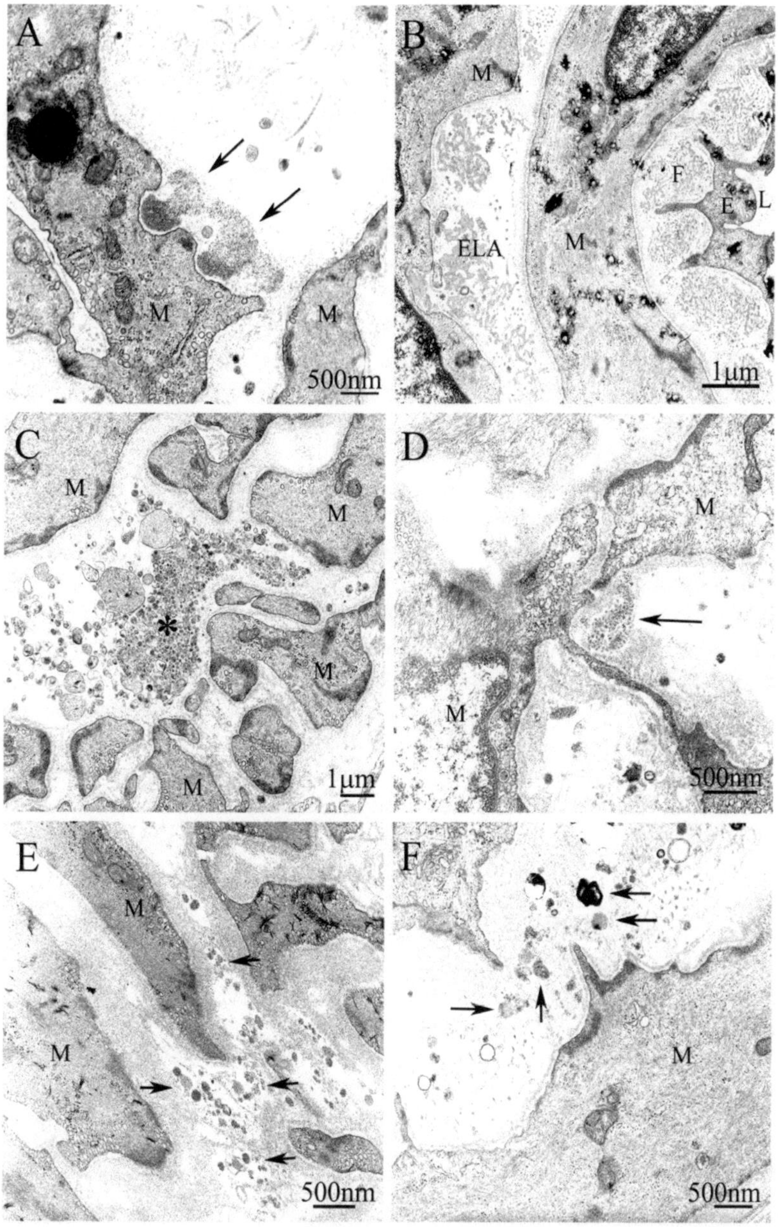

Fig. 7. Fallacious deposits which may lead the electron microscopist astray. A) A true GOM deposits with exceptional mushroom-like form (arrows) in CADASIL skin biopsy. Note the characteristic fine granular appearance of GOM. B) Fragments of elastica interna (ELA) and granular fibrillin network (F) in the widened subendothelial space in skin biopsy of a CADASIL suspect with no GOM and no *NOTCH3* mutation. C) Granular debris (asterisk) of unknown origin. D) Similar granular material as in C) (arrow) with misleading location in an indentation of VSMC. E and F) Small clumps of cell debris of different composition (arrows) possibly from degenerated cells. L=lumen, E=endothelial cell, M=vascular smooth muscle cell. Figure is reproduced with permission of *Brain* (Tikka et al., 2009).

3.4 Diagnostic workflow

What would be the most efficient strategy to confirm the clinical suspicion of CADASIL? Strategy strongly depends on the family history of patient and the mutational background in the population to which the suspected patient belongs. In families with a known mutation, the method of choice is, of course, to analyse directly that mutation. If the patient´s population harbours known founder or major mutations, the diagnostic workup is best to begin by first screening for those mutations. In populations with no known founder or other prevailing mutations, screening of the known mutational hot spot region of the *NOTCH3* gene should be the first genetic method to search for CADASIL. To obtain 80 % coverage of the reported CADASIL mutations investigation of exons 2-4, 5, 6, 8, 11 and 18 is required (Tikka et al., 2009 Supplement table 1). After these analyses EM or IHC analysis of a skin biopsy for detection of GOM or accumulation of N3ECD is highly recommended. Similar approach has been suggested by Peters et al. (2005). Mutation screening covering the whole region coding for EGF repeats (exons 2-24) is not realistic for all suspected patients and for most diagnostic laboratories.

N3ECD the immunostaining has been found reliable method in cases with at least a fair amount of accumulated N3ECD (Joutel et al., 2001). However, if only a small amount of the N3ECD has accumulated, e.g. at the early stage of the disease, ultrastructural resolution and characteristic appearance of GOM most likely make the EM analysis more reliable. We have detected GOM even in patients below the age of 20 years (Figure 3C). Besides, nonspecific staining producing false positives is an inherent caveat of immunohistochemistry (Lesnik Oberstein et al., 2003), which may cause problems also in CADASIL cases with only small amounts of N3ECD giving rise to false negatives. Moreover, EM examination provides also information about other pathological changes in the arterial wall, such as those due to hypertension, ageing and possibly even other hereditary arteriopathies (Brulin et al., 2002, Ruchoux et al., 2000, Ruchoux et al., 2002). The Swedish family with multi-infarct dementia was previously thought to be the first published pedigree with CADASIL (Sourander and Walinder, 1977). The absence of GOM in the arteries was an important piece of evidence in addition to the negative genetic analyses in the demonstration that this family suffers from another hereditary vascular dementia (Low et al., 2007). On the other hand, another cerebral small vessels disease caused by a novel type of pathogenic mutation (p.Leu1515Pro) in the exon 25 of *NOTCH3* outside the EGF like repeat rich domain, results in constitutively active NOTCH3 receptor (Fouillade et al., 2008). This leads to increased signaling in a ligand-independent fashion, possibly due to destabilization of the NOTCH3 heterodimer. Remarkably, in this single patient reported there is no deposition of N3ECD and GOM on VSMCs.

4. Conclusion

The strategy of the CADASIL workup should be based on logical evaluation of clinical findings, family history as well as on both genetic and morphological methods available. Demonstration of a known pathogenic mutation provides indisputable evidence for the disease and gives a practical tool to clarify genetic counselling in the family. In those cases, in which the mutation is not easy to identify or genetic analysis is not available, skin biopsy is easy to perform. IHC showing accumulation of N3ECD can also be used as a supportive method in diagnostic process although it should not be used as only method. Detection of GOM by EM should be preferable method when analysing skin biopsies given its high specificity and sensitivity. Neither is it time consuming nor excessively expensive. Importantly, it is invaluable in guiding, how far one should proceed with the genetic analyses.

5. Acknowledgment

For their skilful ultrastructural techniques we thank in Finland Ms. Virpi Myllys in Turku and Ms. Svetlana Zueva in Helsinki; in Sweden Ms. Madeleine Jarild in Uppsala and in France Ms. Sylvie Limol and Ms. Nathalie Goethink in Lille and Ms. Fabienne Arcanger in Tours.

6. References

Ampuero I, Alegre-Abarrategui J, Rodal I, Espana A, Ros R, Sendon JL, et al. On the diagnosis of CADASIL. J Alzheimers Dis 2009; 17: 787-94

Baudrimont M, Dubas F, Joutel A, Tournier-Lasserve E, Bousser MG. Autosomal dominant leukoencephalopathy and subcortical ischemic stroke. A clinicopathological study. Stroke 1993; 24: 122-5

Brulin P, Godfraind C, Leteurtre E, Ruchoux MM. Morphometric analysis of ultrastructural vascular changes in CADASIL: Analysis of 50 skin biopsy specimens and pathogenic implications. Acta Neuropathol 2002; 104: 241-8

Chabriat H, Levy C, Taillia H, Iba-Zizen MT, Vahedi K, Joutel A, et al. Patterns of MRI lesions in CADASIL. Neurology 1998; 51: 452-7

Dotti MT, Federico A, Mazzei R, Bianchi S, Scali O, Conforti FL, et al. The spectrum of Notch3 mutations in 28 italian CADASIL families. J Neurol Neurosurg Psychiatry 2005; 76: 736-8

Ebke M, Dichgans M, Bergmann M, Voelter HU, Rieger P, Gasser T, et al. CADASIL: Skin biopsy allows diagnosis in early stages. Acta Neurol Scand 1997; 95: 351-7

Escary JL, Cecillon M, Maciazek J, Lathrop M, Tournier-Lasserve E, Joutel A. Evaluation of DHPLC analysis in mutational scanning of Notch3, a gene with a high G-C content. Hum Mutat 2000; 16: 518-26

Fouillade C, Chabriat H, Riant F, Mine M, Arnoud M, Magy L, et al. Activating NOTCH3 mutation in a patient with small-vessel-disease of the brain. Hum Mutat 2008; 29: 452

Granild-Jensen J, Jensen UB, Schwartz M, Hansen US. Cerebral autosomal dominant arteriopathy with subcortical infarcts and leukoencephalopathy resulting in stroke in an 11-year-old male. Dev Med Child Neurol 2009; 51: 754-7

Ishiko A, Shimizu A, Nagata E, Takahashi K, Tabira T, Suzuki N. Notch3 ectodomain is a major component of granular osmiophilic material (GOM) in CADASIL. Acta Neuropathol (Berl) 2006; 112: 333-9

Joutel A, Favrole P, Labauge P, Chabriat H, Lescoat C, Andreux F, et al. Skin biopsy immunostaining with a Notch3 monoclonal antibody for CADASIL diagnosis. Lancet 2001; 358: 2049-51

Joutel A, Andreux F, Gaulis S, Domenga V, Cecillon M, Battail N, et al. The ectodomain of the Notch3 receptor accumulates within the cerebrovasculature of CADASIL patients. J Clin Invest 2000; 105: 597-605

Joutel A, Vahedi K, Corpechot C, Troesch A, Chabriat H, Vayssiere C, et al. Strong clustering and stereotyped nature of Notch3 mutations in CADASIL patients. Lancet 1997; 350: 1511-5

Joutel A, Corpechot C, Ducros A, Vahedi K, Chabriat H, Mouton P, et al. Notch3 mutations in CADASIL, a hereditary adult-onset condition causing stroke and dementia. Nature 1996; 383: 707-10

Kalimo H, Miao Q, Tikka S, Mykkanen K, Junna M, Roine S, et al. CADASIL: The most common hereditary subcortical vascular dementia. Future Neurology 2008; 3: 683

Kalimo H, Ruchoux MM, Viitanen M, Kalaria RN. CADASIL: A common form of hereditary arteriopathy causing brain infarcts and dementia. Brain Pathol 2002; 12: 371-84

Lesnik Oberstein SA, van Duinen SG, van den Boom R, Maat-Schieman ML, van Buchem MA, van Houwelingen HC, et al. Evaluation of diagnostic NOTCH3 immunostaining in CADASIL. Acta Neuropathol 2003; 106: 107-11

Lewandowska E, Szpak GM, Wierzba-Bobrowicz T, Modzelewska J, Stepien T, Pasennik E, et al. Capillary vessel wall in CADASIL angiopathy. Folia Neuropathol 2010; 48: 104-15

Low WC, Junna M, Borjesson-Hanson A, Morris CM, Moss TH, Stevens DL, et al. Hereditary multi-infarct dementia of the swedish type is a novel disorder different from NOTCH3 causing CADASIL. Brain 2007; 130: 357-67

Markus HS, Martin RJ, Simpson MA, Dong YB, Ali N, Crosby AH, et al. Diagnostic strategies in CADASIL. Neurology 2002; 59: 1134-8

Mayer M, Straube A, Bruening R, Uttner I, Pongratz D, Gasser T, et al. Muscle and skin biopsies are a sensitive diagnostic tool in the diagnosis of CADASIL. J Neurol 1999; 246: 526-32

Miao Q, Paloneva T, Tuominen S, Poyhonen M, Tuisku S, Viitanen M, et al. Fibrosis and stenosis of the long penetrating cerebral arteries: The cause of the white matter pathology in cerebral autosomal dominant arteriopathy with subcortical infarcts and leukoencephalopathy. Brain Pathol 2004; 14: 358-64

Opherk C, Peters N, Herzog J, Luedtke R, Dichgans M. Long-term prognosis and causes of death in CADASIL: A retrospective study in 411 patients. Brain 2004; 127: 2533-9

O'Sullivan M, Jarosz JM, Martin RJ, Deasy N, Powell JF, Markus HS. MRI hyperintensities of the temporal lobe and external capsule in patients with CADASIL. Neurology 2001; 56: 628-34

Peters N, Opherk C, Bergmann T, Castro M, Herzog J, Dichgans M. Spectrum of mutations in biopsy-proven CADASIL: Implications for diagnostic strategies. Arch Neurol 2005; 62: 1091-4

Ragno M, Tournier-Lasserve E, Fiori MG, Manca A, Patrosso MC, Ferlini A, et al. An italian kindred with cerebral autosomal dominant arteriopathy with subcortical infarcts and leukoencephalopathy (CADASIL). Ann Neurol 1995; 38: 231-6

Razvi SS, Davidson R, Bone I, Muir KW. Diagnostic strategies in CADASIL. Neurology 2003; 60: 2019,20; author reply 2020

Ruchoux MM, Brulin P, Brillault J, Dehouck MP, Cecchelli R, Bataillard M. Lessons from CADASIL. Ann N Y Acad Sci 2002; 977: 224-31

Ruchoux MM, Brulin P, Leteurtre E, Maurage CA. Skin biopsy value and leukoaraiosis. Ann N Y Acad Sci 2000; 903: 285-92

Ruchoux MM, Maurage CA. CADASIL: Cerebral autosomal dominant arteriopathy with subcortical infarcts and leukoencephalopathy. J Neuropathol Exp Neurol 1997; 56: 947-64

Ruchoux MM, Guerouaou D, Vandenhaute B, Pruvo JP, Vermersch P, Leys D. Systemic vascular smooth muscle cell impairment in cerebral autosomal dominant arteriopathy with subcortical infarcts and leukoencephalopathy. Acta Neuropathol (Berl) 1995; 89: 500-12

Ruchoux MM, Chabriat H, Bousser MG, Baudrimont M, Tournier-Lasserve E. Presence of ultrastructural arterial lesions in muscle and skin vessels of patients with CADASIL. Stroke 1994; 25: 2291-2

Sourander P, Walinder J. Hereditary multi-infarct dementia. morphological and clinical studies of a new disease. Acta Neuropathol 1977; 39: 247-54

Tikka S, Mykkanen K, Ruchoux MM, Bergholm R, Junna M, Poyhonen M, et al. Congruence between NOTCH3 mutations and GOM in 131 CADASIL patients. Brain 2009; 132: 933-9

Part 3

Research Applications of Human Skin Biopsy

10

The Clinicopathologic and Molecular Aspects of Non-Melanoma Skin Cancer

Anthony P. Tufaro[1,4], Nijaguna B. Prasad[2],
Anne C. Fischer[3] and Allan D. Hess[4]
[1]*Department of Plastic & Reconstructive Surgery, Johns Hopkins Medical Institutions, Baltimore, MD,*
[2]*Department of Surgery, Johns Hopkins Medical Institutions, Baltimore, MD,*
[3]*Department of Surgery and Cancer Immunobiology Institute, UT Southwestern Medical Center, Dallas TX*
[4]*Department of Oncology, Johns Hopkins Medical Institutions, Baltimore, MD, USA*

1. Introduction

Non-melanoma skin cancer (NMSC) is the most common form of malignancy. The annual incidence of NMSC had previously been estimated to be over one million cases per year in United States.(1) A recent study has shown that estimated burden of NMSC to have increased approximately to 3.5 million annual cases, affecting over 2 million people. (2,3)
Although the burden of NMSC measured in terms of mortality and morbidity is thought to be relatively modest, the direct costs of NMSC are substantial owing to its high incidence. In the US Medicare population, it is considered a major health care problem and among the five most costly cancers to treat based on the actual economics of this disease. (4,5) In fact the estimated treatment costs of NMSC exceeded $500 million/year a decade ago.(6) More common than all other cancers combined, NMSC has been associated metachronously with the development of other malignancies. (7,8)
In general, due to an underappreciation of its increasing prevalence and potential to be highly aggressive, NMSC has been relatively overlooked. While the molecular profiles of melanoma have been well characterized given its stature as the most lethal type of skin cancer, those for NMSC have lagged behind. In this chapter we discuss the numerous types of NMSC, their biologic variability and the various risk factors and etiologies. The etiologies for the subset of NMSC with the most mortality, cutaneous squamous cell carcinoma (cSCC) will be summarized. Despite the fact that the majority of these tumors present at early stages, cSCC accounts for the majority of NMSC deaths and 20% of all skin cancer- related deaths. (9,10) We will review the clinical approach and scientific methodologies that are used to analyze skin biopsies specifically evaluating differential gene transcription between patients who either have a definite propensity to develop cSCC or vary in their susceptibility to developing cSCC. In summary we will introduce where the field stands in the discovery of a molecular profile.

As the most frequent cancer in the US and worldwide, NMSC has been increasing in overall incidence since the 1960's at a rate of 3-8% per year.[11, 12] With over 3.5 million new diagnoses of NMSC per year in the United States, it is both the diversity of types, of which there are 82, and biologic variability in phenotype, that makes the analysis of NMSC even more challenging.[2]
Although the incidence of basal cell carcinoma (BCC) exceeds cSCC by a 5:1 ratio, cSCC is associated with the burden of mortality with a yearly disease-specific mortality rate of 1% per year as reported in the early 1990's.[13] Despite the fact that the majority of these tumors present at an early stage, cSCC accounts for the majority of NMSC deaths and 20% of all skin cancer- related deaths.[9,10] Recurrent NMSC carries a very poor prognosis with only a 50% cure rate.[14] In contrast malignant melanoma is the deadliest at 60% of skin cancer deaths, which explains the primary focus on melanoma, albeit it is the rarest skin cancer at 1% of skin malignancies.[15]
Most suspicious skin lesions are more often evaluated by a primary care physician than a dermatologist, but both face the need to identify if a lesion is malignant, premalignant or benign. To appreciate the breadth of the differential diagnosis, a study of 1215 biopsies from a primary care population were evaluated and 80% were benign lesions, 7% premalignant lesions, including actinic keratoses and lentigo maligna, with 13% being malignant. The malignancies included 73% BCC, 14% SCC, and 12% malignant melanoma.[16] There are multiple precursor skin lesions for NMSC and include Bowen's disease, SCC in situ (erythroplasia of Queyrat), and actinic keratoses.

2. Paradigm shift in staging guidelines

In light of the large number of low risk lesions with a cure rate of greater than 90% for the routine lesion, the significance of an increasing incidence of cSCC is not fully recognized, given the often quoted 5-year recurrence and metastatic rates of 8% and 5%, respectively.[10,17,18] With the diverse spectrum of lesions, clearly grouping the worst subset in with the high incidence of low grade lesions numerically minimizes the poor outcomes associated with the most aggressive lesions. In January 2010, the 7th Edition of the American Joint Committee on Cancer (AJCC) Staging Manual introduced a dramatic paradigm shift in the staging of cSCC to better incorporate known clinical predictors of poor outcome into the classification system and thus better group the diversity of lesions properly. It is this edition that has launched a better rationale to track lesions based on their aggressive characteristics and to more comprehensively stage lesions.
The recent changes to the AJCC Staging Manual focus on identifying clinical parameters that portend a worse prognosis to identify and stage appropriately that subset of cSCC that progresses to metastatic disease.[19] These factors include lesional size (> 2cm), and high risk features including a depth of invasion (>2mm, ≥Clark level IV), perineural invasion, tumor grade (poorly differentiated or un-differentiated), as well as high-risk anatomic sites (See Table 1). Tumor grade alone is significantly associated with mortality given a 5-year cure post therapy of 61.5% for poorly differentiated cSCC compared to 94.6% for well differentiated.[10] High risk histologic features were defined as showing poor differentiation, spindle cell characteristics, necrosis, high mitotic activity and deep invasion.[19] Both the depth of invasion and presence of perineural invasion significantly correlate with prognosis and >4mm thickness or depth of invasion of ≥Clark level IV are associated with a 2 fold increased rate of recurrence or 5-fold increase metastatic rate;

similarly, perineural invasion is associated with a 5-fold increase in both the recurrence rate and metastatic rate.(10,20) Although not identified in the 7th Edition of AJCC, other histologic features are important in prognosis and those include lymphovascular invasion and the presence of inflammatory features such as the presence of eosinophils and plasma cells.(21) cSCC in immunocompromised patients or those that arise in scars, sinus tracts or burns all demonstrate a more aggressive biologic phenotype with a greater metastatic rate of up to 40%.(10,22,24) So not only are subsets with a worse prognosis critical to correctly stage in order to appropriately recognize an unrecognized metastatic potential, but also recurrent disease or persistent disease both portent a worse survival of 78% 5-year survival.(20,25)

Histologic Differentiation
Poor differentiation
Spindle cell characteristics
Necrosis
High Mitotic Activity
Deep Invasion
Depth of Invasion
>2mm
Clark Level ^{3}IV
Perineural Invasion
High Risk Anatomic Sites
Nonglabrous Lip
Ear
Advanced T stage (T3 and T4)
Bony extension or involvement
Maxilla, mandible, orbit, temporal bone
Perineural invasion
Invasion of Skull base
Invasion of axial or appendicular skeleton

Table 1. High Risk Factors For NMSC Tumor Characteristics*

* 7th Edition of American Joint Commission on Cancer Staging Manual (19)

3. Overview of treatment

Standard surgical excision remains the mainstay of treatment of NMSC. The traditional surgical methods include excisional biopsy with appropriate margins or MOHS surgery for areas in which margins are limited by anatomy. These so called critical areas include the commissure of the lip, nasal ala or canthus of the eye as shown in Figure 1. Mohs surgery is a microscopically controlled procedure allowing for the narrowest surgical margin (1mm-1.5mm). Ideally, the Mohs resection should include 100% of the epidermal margin, but often 95% is conventional or at least 70% is accepted for frozen section analysis.[26] A conservative approach such as serial sectioning, proper staining technique, and a conservative Mohs margin (~at least 200 micrometer from the surgical margin) can assure the lowest recurrence rate. The use of frozen sections for margin control increases the cure rate of conventional surgical excision to be comparable with Mohs excisions.

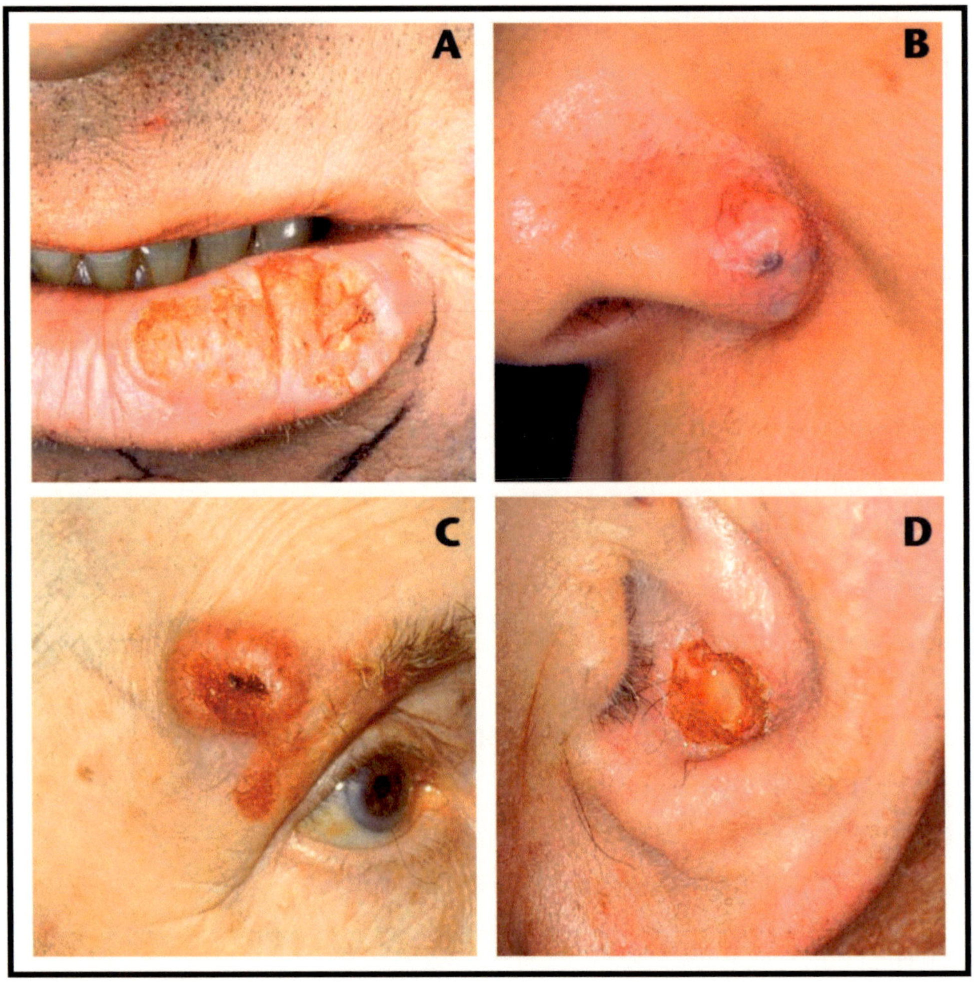

Fig. 1. Clinical presentations of Non-melanoma Skin cancer cutaneous squamous. Cell carcinoma (A and D) Basal Cell Carcinoma (B and C). Courtesy from Skin Cancer Guide CA.

Larger lesions should be biopsied with an incisional technique. A scalpel or a 2 or 3 mm. dermatologic punch can be used. The biopsy should avoid any area that appears to contain necrotic tissue. It is often best to biopsy at the apparent margin of the malignant lesion with normal skin. The biopsy should be "full thickness", including epidermis, dermis and subcutaneous tissue. This will allow adequate evaluation of the depth of invasion and allow for surgical planning. Small lesions can be excised with a 0.5 to 1 cm. margin. Larger lesions will require a 1cm. or wider margin

Traditional histology of skin tissue uses vertical sectioning with the subcutaneous tissue at the bottom and the epidermis at the top. In contrast, Mohs surgery uses tangential or horizontal sectioning. Thus the samples from biopsies are typically formalin-fixed paraffin-embedded tissue blocks or frozen tissue specimens from Mohs surgery. These tissue specimens are first analysed for histologic review or evaluated by Mohs mapping. The mapping combined with the unique "smashing the pie pan" method of processing such that the corollary of the blood covered surgical margin is an aluminum pie pan. The top of the pie is the crust covered surface of the skin and the goal is to flatten this specimen into one flat sheet, mark it, stain it, and examine it under the microscope.(27)

Notably there are many nonsurgical modalities, including cryosurgery, electrodessication and curettage, radiotherapy and intralesional therapies. However, all these later approaches lose the benefit of pathologic analysis. Thus it is easy to understand why capturing the actual incidence of NMSC has been difficult. In the era of personalized medicine, molecular markers have been used in many tumors to prognosticate and risk stratify patients. Given the relative lack of recognition of the growing incidence of cSCC and the inability to track the worst subset of cSCC given the abundance of low risk lesions and the practice of not banking or staging lesions, these molecular studies have been relatively limited compared to the field of melanoma.

4. Risk factors

Multiple etiologies exist for cSCC, including environmental, genetic, altered immunity and virally mediated. The high incidence of cSCC and BCC is primarily attributed to sun exposure and the mutagenic effects of ultraviolet (UV) light worsened by geographic latitude.(11,28) Cutaneous SCC and BCC are more common in fair skinned patients and anatomic sites exposed to the sun, such as head, neck and extremities: head and neck is the most common site. Other known risk factors are male sex, advanced age, immunosuppression (induced or acquired), human papilloma viruses (HPV), chronic inflammation and genetic diseases manifested in the skin.(28-30) Genetically inherited skin conditions that have a known propensity of risk for developing cSCC are albinism, xeroderma pigmentosum, and epidermodysplasia verruciformis.(9,31-32) The strongest risk factors for NMSC mirror the etiologies and include Caucasian race, older age 55-75 years of age, male sex, a prior diagnosis of NMSC confers a 10-fold risk for recurrence, and immunosuppression, as well as genetic, chemical and environmental factors (See Table 2). Likewise sites of chronic inflammation, such as scars, sinus tracts, and burns, can also demonstrate more aggressive clinical behavior and a greater propensity to metastasize with an overall metastatic rate of 40%.(10,22)

Significant Risk Factors
Caucasian
Immunosuppression
Previous NMSC or precursor lesion
Age 55-75
Male sex
Genetic Risk Factors
Blue eyes
Fair skin
Celtic ancestry
Genetic Syndromes
Xeroderma Pigmentosum
Albinism
Epidermodysplasia verruciformis
Basal cell nevus syndrome
Chemical Exposure
Coal Tar
Tobacco
Environmental Exposure
Ionizing radiation
Primary Inflammatory skin disorder
Chronic wounds, burns, scars

Table 2. Potential Risk Factors for NMSC

5. Immunologic altered host state

Several studies have demonstrated an association between an enhanced risk of NMSC and immunosuppression in patients with inflammatory bowel disease (IBD), rheumatoid arthritis (RA) and solid-organ transplants.(33- 35) Malignant lesions develop within 10 years after organ transplantation. The prevalence of NMSC in renal transplant recipients (RTR) is 5% and from 10% to 27% at 2 and 10 years, respectively, but increases up to 40% to 60% at 20 years.(36) In the long-term follow-up, this represents an increase of 12 to 90 times the NMSC-risk in the general population.(35) Similarly, in heart transplant recipients, the cumulative risk rose from 4.3% at 1 year up to 43.8% at 7 years after transplantation.(37,38)

More importantly, the incidence and risk of malignancy particularly cSCC is significantly elevated in post-transplant patients compared to other patient populations. Immunosuppression is associated with a disproportionate increase in the incidence of cSCC of up to 64-250 times greater than that in the general population compared to the 10-fold increased risk in BCC. This disproportionate increase causes a reversal of the expected 5:1ratio of BCC: cSCC in immunocompetent individuals to a range between 1:1.8 and 1:15 in those that are immunosuppressed.(39,40)

Furthermore, immunosuppression significantly impacts the biology and aggressiveness of cSCC. In solid organ transplant patients, cSCC tumors tend to be numerous, exhibit a strong propensity to recur and metastasize at a high rate regardless of lesional size.(41) Skin malignancies in transplant recipients has some features that differ from those in the general population; (i) multiple sites are involved, (ii) the cancers occur in younger age-group (30 years vs. 60 years), (iii) the cancers are more aggressive and recur more frequently, and (iv) the squamous cell type is more common than basal cell.(42)

6. Viral pathogenesis

The increased incidence of cSCC in immunocompromised patients compared to BCC suggests a mechanism of viral pathogenesis. Evidence of HPV has been reported in cSCC in organ transplant patients with up to 80% of lesions containing HPV DNA as well as the presence of a higher viral load of HPV DNA.(43,44) However the variable quantity of HPV in immunocompetent individuals can range between 27-70% depending on detection techniques.(32,44) Thus the type of HPV, β-papillomavirus species 2, may be more often associated with cSCC as opposed to the total amount of HPV DNA present.[32]

Three theories have been suggested for the mechanism of HPV carcinogenesis: 1) UV radiation induced immunosuppression to explain an enhanced interaction between HPV and UV radiation, 2) E6/E7 oncoprotein-related changes in p53 and Rb tumor suppressor gene, and 3) integration of HPV DNA disrupting genomic stability.(32,45,46). Viral expression of E6 and E7 oncoproteins can inactivate p53 and Rb tumor suppressor genes, leading to an uncontrolled system of cell proliferation and apoptosis.(47)

Association of viral pathogens such as human papillomavirus (HPV) with head and neck squamous cell cancer (HNSCC), especially oropharyngeal cancer has been recognized over the past two decades. HPV16 is the most common genotype in these tumours, whereas HPV6 and HPV11 can also be found in a minority of these cancers, implying that these low-risk HPV types are not entirely benign in HNSCC. HPV DNA is closely associated with poorly differentiated cancers, positive lymph nodes and late-stage disease, which portend a worse diagnosis. HPV status is also associated with p16 expression and HPV+ tumours are less likely to harbour p53 mutations.(48) A subset of HNSCC patients who had HPV 16 infection confers a better prognosis. On the other hand, β papillomaviruses (β- HPVs) also play a role in the tumorigenesis of cSCC as shown by both European and US studies.(49) However, no high-risk types have been identified although there is an association of β species 1 in SCC. Other viruses, such as polyomavirus (MCPyV) have been shown to be causative agent in Merkel cell carcinoma.(50)

7. Allelic imbalance and loss of heterozygosity

The genetic progression model for head and neck squamous cell carcinoma (HNSCC) demonstrates that loss of heterozygosity (LOH) is common during the progression from

premalignant lesion to malignant tumors.[51] Tumor suppressor genes (TSGs) are usually found in the area of loss rendering the cells more susceptible to tumorigenesis.[52]
Several regions of chromosomal loss are identified in HNSCC. One of the most common regions, 9p21, has been reported in both HNSCC and cSCC.[53,54] This region contains several TSGs, including p16INK4A (CDKN2A), p15INK4B and MTAP. Allelic imbalances are also found in other regions of cSCC, including LOH on 3p, 2q, 8p, and 13 and allelic gain on 3q and 8q.[55] Such studies indicate that allelic imbalance and LOH are recognized and relevant events in cSCC and can be used for early diagnosis and tumor surveillance.

8. Epigenetics

Epigenetics is the inheritance of genetic information that is altered in gene expression without changes in the DNA sequence. Epigenetic alterations include DNA methylation and histone modifications, which consist of methylation, acetylation, phosphorylation, ubiquitination, and sumoylation. Changes in genomic DNA methylation associated with cancer include global DNA hypomethylation and gene-specific hyper- or hypomethylation. All of these modifications of gene expression have been associated with the development of various tumor types, including HNSCC and cSCC.[56,57] A higher frequency of FOXE1 promoter hypermethylation has been documented in SCCs (55%) which was seen in association with a complete absence of or downregulated gene expression, indicating that FOXE1 is a crucial player in development of cutaneous SCC.[56]
Promoter DNA methylation gene panels have been described for screening of primary HNSCC, for determination of tumor recurrence, and assessment of margin status during surgery.[58,59] However, a determination of methylation gene panels relevant in cSCC is yet to be established. A combination of different genes from different pathways may allow for a better determination of the aggressiveness of cSCC to determine prognosis.

9. RNA and MiRNA

Messenger RNA (mRNA) and microRNA (MiRNA) profiles have been described in both HNSCC and cSCC.[60] MiRNAs play a role in regulation of mRNA. Several mRNA biomarkers for cSCC were identified, including CCR10, CCL27, MUC4, p16, MMP2 and MMP9.[61] A recent study has demonstrated that a distinct microRNA profile is modulated by UV radiation.[62]

10. Mitochondrial mutation

Mitochondrial mutation in HNSCC has been well reported; however, only a few studies show the association of mitochondrial DNA mutation and cSCC.[63] Several regions of mitochondrial DNA were reported, including displacement-loop (D-loop) and other regions.[64,65] Therefore, mitochondrial mutations may correlate in the future with the phenotypic behavior of cSCC.

11. Conclusions

The molecular mechanisms that underlie the development of cutaneous skin cancers are poorly understood. Even the spectrum of biologic behavior has been slow to be characterized given the previously very generic clinical criteria used to distinguish low risk lesions from more aggressive lesions. Recent changes in the classification of the staging paradigm have better captured this more aggressive subset to allow for a more precision in identifying the worst subset. Thus molecular analysis can potentially profile that subset with biomarkers chosen to best correlate with the biologic phenotype.

12. References

[1] Jemal A, Siegel R, Ward E, Murray T, Xu J, Thun MJ. Cancer Statistics, 2007. CA Cancer J Clin 2007;57:43-66

[2] Rogers HW, Weinstock MA, Harris AR, Hinckley MR, Feldman SR, Fleischer AB, Coldiron BM Incidence estimate of nonmelanoma skin cancer in the United States, 2006. Arch Dermatol, 2010; 146:283-287

[3] Long MD, Kappelman MD, Pipkin CA Nonmelanoma skin cancer in inflammatory bowel disease: A review. Inflamm Bowel Dis 2011; 17(6): 1423-1427.

[4] Housman TS, Feldman SR, Williford PM, Fleischer AB, Jr., Goldman ND, Acostamadiedo JM, Chen GJ Skin cancer is among the most costly of all cancers to treat for the Medicare population. J Am Acad Dermatol 2003;48:425-429

[5] Housman TS, Williford PM, Feldman SR, Teuschler HV, Fleischer AB, Jr., Goldman ND, Balkrishnan R, Chen GJ Nonmelanoma skin cancer: an episode of care management approach. Dermatol Surg 2003; 29:700-711.

[6] Gloster HM, Jr., Brodland DG. The epidemiology of skin cancer. Dermatol Surg 1996; 22:217-226.

[7] Friedman GD, Tekawa IS 2000 Association of basal cell skin cancers with other cancers (United States). Cancer Causes Control 2000; 11:891-897

[8] Efird JT, Friedman GD, Habel L, Tekawa IS, Nelson LM Risk of subsequent cancer following invasive or in situ squamous cell skin cancer. Ann Epidemiol 2002; 12:469-475

[9] Alam M, Ratner D. Cutaneous squamous cell carcinoma. N Engl J Med. 2001:344:975-83.

[10] Rowe DE, Carroll RJ, Day CL Jr. Prognostic factors for local recurrence, metastasis, and survival rates in squamous cell carcinoma of the skin, ear, and lip. Implications for treatment modality selection. J Am Acad Dermatol. 1992;26:976-90.

[11] Ramos J, Villa J, Ruiz A, Armstrong R, Matta J. UV dose determines key characteristics of nonmelanoma skin cancer. Cancer Epidemiol Biomarkers Prev 2004;13:2006-11.

[12] Diepgen TL, Mahler V. The epidemiology of skin cancer. Br J Dermatol 2002;146 (Suppl):1-6.

[13] M.A.Weinstock, "Epidemiologic investigation of nonmelanoma skin cancer mortality: the Rhode Island Follow Back Study," Journal of Investigative Dermatology, 1994; 102:6 (6S-9S)

[14] Garner KL, Rodney WM. Basal and squamous cell carcinoma. Primary Care 2000;27:447-458

[15] Skin Tumours. In: Sauer GC, Hall JC, eds. A Manual of Skin Diseases. Philadelphia, Pa: Lippincott- Raven, 1196:342.

[16] Jones TP, Boiko PE, Piepkorn MW. Skin Biopsy indications in primary care practice: a population-based study. JABFP 1996;9-397-404.

[17] Czarnecki D, Staples M, Mar A, Giles G. and Meehan C. Metastases from squamous cell carcinoma of the skin in southern Australia. Dermatology 1994;189(1):52-54.

[18] Jackson A. Prevention, early detection and team management of skin cancer in primary care: contribution to the health of the nation objectives. British Journal of General Practice 1995:45(391):97-101.

[19] Edge SE, Byrd DR, Compton CC et al. AJCC Cancer Staging Manual, Springer, New York, NY, USA, 7th Edition, 2009.

[20] Buethe D, Warner C. Miedler J, and Cockerell CJ. Focus Issue on Squamous Cell Carcinoma: Practical Concerns Regarding the 7th Edition AJCC Staging Guidelines. Journal of Skin Cancer 2011: Article ID 156391:9

[21] Quadvlieg PJF, Creytens DHKV, Epping GG et al. Histopathological characteristics of metastasizing squamous cell carcinoma of the skin and lips. Histopathology 2006:49(3):256-264.

[22] Cherpelis B.S., Marcusen C. and Lang P.G. Prognostic factors for metastasis in squamous cell carcinoma of the skin. Dermatologic Surgery 2002;28(3):268-273.

[23] Novick M, Gard DA., Hardy SB, and Spira M. Burn scar carcinoma: a review and analysis of 46 cases. Journal of Trauma 1977:17(10):809-817.

[24] Andruchow JL, Veness MJ, Morgan GJ et al. Implications for clinical staging of metastatic cutaneous squamous carcinoma of the head and neck based on a multicenter study of treatment outcomes. Cancer 2006:106(5):1078-1083.

[26] Gross, Kenneth Gary; Steinman, Howard K.; Rapini, Ronald P. 1999. Mohs Surgery: Fundamentals and Techniques. Saint Louis: Mosby. p.62.

[27] Maloney, Mary E. 1999. Surgical dermatopathology. Malden, Mass: Blackwell Science. pp. 1111–7.

[28] Preston DS, Stern RS. Nonmelanoma cancers of the skin. N Engl J Med. 1992; 327:1649-62.

[29] Ulrich C, Schmook T, Sachse MM, et al. Comparative epidemiology and pathogenic factors for nonmelanoma skin cancer in organ transplant patients. Dermatol Surg. 2004;30:622-7.

[30] Chapter 29: Cutaneous squamous cell carcinoma and other cutaneous carcinomas. In: Edge ES, Byrd DR, Compton CC, Fritz AG, Greene FL, Trotti A, et al, editors. AJCC cancer staging manual. 7th ed. New York: Springer; 2010.

[31] Barksdale Sk, O'Connor N, Barnhill R. Prognostic factors for cutaneous squamous cell and basal cell carcinoma. Determinants of risk of recurrence, metastasis, and development of subsequent skin cancers. Surg Oncol Clin N Am. 1997;6:625-638.

[32] Dubina M and Goldenberg G. Viral- Associated Nonmelanoma Skin Cancers: A Review. Am J Dermatopathol 2009:31(6):561-573.

[33] Long MD, Herfarth HH, Pipkin CA, Porter CQ, Sandler RS, Kappelman MD Increased risk for non-melanoma skin cancer in patients with inflammatory bowel disease. Clin Gastroenterol Hepatol 2009;8:268-274

[34] Chakravarty EF, Michaud K, Wolfe F Skin cancer, rheumatoid arthritis, and tumor necrosis factor inhibitors. J Rheumatol 2005; 32:2130-2135

[35] Gutierrez-Dalmau A, Campistol JM Immunosuppressive therapy and malignancy in organ transplant recipients: a systematic review. Drugs 2007; 67:1167-1198

[36] Ulrich C, Kanitakis J, Stockfleth E, Euvrard S Skin cancer in organ transplant recipients--where do we stand today? Am J Transplant 2008;8:2192-2198

[37] Espana A, Martinez-Gonzalez MA, Garcia-Granero M, Sanchez-Carpintero I, Rabago G, Herreros J A prospective study of incident nonmelanoma skin cancer in heart transplant recipients. J Invest Dermatol 2000;115:1158-1160
[38] Espana A, Redondo P, Fernandez AL, Zabala M, Herreros J, Llorens R, Quintanilla E Skin cancer in heart transplant recipients. J Am Acad Dermatol 1995;32:458-465
[39] Jensen P, Hansen S, Moller B, et al. Skin cancer in kidney and heart transplant recipients and different longterm immunosuppressive therapy regimens. J Am Acad Dermatol 1999;40 (1):177-186
[40] Penn I. Malignancy. Surg Clin North Am 1994;74:1247-57.
[41] Moloney FJ, Comber H, O'Lorcain P, et al. A population-based study of skin cancer incidence and prevalence in renal transplant recipients. Br J Dermatol 2006;154:498-504.
[42] Sheil AG, Disney AP, Mathew TH, Amiss N, Excell L Cancer development in cadaveric donor renal allograft recipients treated with azathioprine (AZA) or cyclosporine (CyA) or AZA/CyA. Transplant Proc 1991;23:1111-1112
[43] De Villiers EM, Lavergne D, McLaren K, et al. Prevailing papillomavirus types in non-melanoma carcinomas of the skin in renal allograft recipients. Int J Cancer. 1997;73:356-361.
[44] Harwood CA, Surentheran T, Mc Gregor JM, et al. Human papilloma-virus infection and non-melanoma skin cancer in immunosuppressed and immunocompetent individuals. J Med Virol. 2000;61:289-297.
[45] Asgari MM, Kiviat NB, Critchlow CW et al. Detection of human papillomavirus DNA in cutaneous squamous cell carcinoma among immunocompetent individuals. J Invest Dermatol. 2008:128:1409-1417.
[46] Forslund O, Ly H, Reid C, et al. A broad spectrum of human papillomavirus types is present in the skin of Australian patients with non-melanoma skin cancers and solar keratosis. Br J Dermatol. 2003;149:64-73.
[47] Zur Hausen H. Papillomaviruses and cancer:from basic studies to clinical application. Nat Rev Cancer 2002;2:342-350
[48] Syrjanen S. The role of human papillomavirus infection in head and neck cancers. Ann Oncol 2010; S7:vii243-vii245
[49] Patel AS, Karagas MR, Perry AE, Nelson HH. Exposure profiles and human papillomavirus infection in skin cancer: an analysis of 25 genus beta-types in a population-based study. J Invest Dermatol. 2008;128(12):2888-93.
[50] Feng H, Shuda M, Chang Y, Moore PS. Clonal integration of a polyomavirus in human Merkel cell carcinoma. Science 2008;319(5866):1096-100.
[51] Reed AL, Califano J, Cairns P, Westra WH, et al. High Frequency of p16 (CDKN2/MTS-1/INK4A) inactivation in head and neck squamous cell carcinoma. Cancer Research 1996;56(16):3630-3.
[52] Van Doorn R, Gruis NA, Willemze R, Van der Velden PA, Tensen CP. Aberrant DNA methylation in cutaneous malignancies. Semin Oncol 2005;32(5):479-87.
[53] Van der Riet P, Nawroz H, Hruban RH, Corio R, Tokino K, Koch W, Sidransky D. Frequent loss of chromosome 9p21-22 early in head and neck cancer progression. Cancer Research. 1994;54(5):1156-8.

[54] Gray SE, Kay E, Leader M, Mabruk M. Analysis of p16 expression and allelic imbalance/loss of heteroxygosity of 9p21 in cutaneous squamous cell carcinomas. J Cell Mol Med 2006;10(3):778-88.

[55] Purdie KJ, Lambert SR, The MT, Chaplin T, Molloy G, et al. Allelic imbalances and microdeletions affecting the PTPRD gene in cutaneous squamous cell carcinomas detected using single nucleotide polymorphism microarray analysis. Genes Chromosomes Cancer. 2007:46(7):661-9.

[56] Venza I, Visalli M, Tripodo B, De Grazia G, et al. FOXE1 is a target for aberrant methylation in cutaneous squamous cell carcinoma. Br. J Dermatol 2010:162(5):1093-7.

[57] Laing ME, Cummins R, O'Grady A, O'Kelly P et al. Aberrant DNA methylation associated with MTHFR C677T genetic polymorphism in cutaneous squamous cell carcinoma in renal transplant patients. Br. J. Dermatol. 2010;163(2):345-52.

[58] Costello JF, Fruhwald MC, Smiraglia DJ, Rush LJ. Aberrant CpG-island methylation has non-random and tumour type specific patterns. Nat Genet. 2000;24(2):101-2.

[59] Esteller M, Corn PG, Baylin SB, Herman JG. A gene hypermethylation profile of human cancer. Cancer Res. 2001;61(8):3225-9.

[60] Yu J, Ryan DG, Getsios S, Oliveira-Fernandes M, Fatima A, Lavker RM. MicroRNA-184 antagonizes microRNA-205 to maintain SHIP2 levels in epithelia. Proc Natl Acad Sci 2008;105(49):193000-5.

[61] Dang C, Gottschling M, Manning K, O'Currain E, Schneider S et al. Identification of dysregulated genes in cutaneous squamous cell carcinoma. Oncol Rep. 2006; 16(3):513-9.

[62] Dziunycz P, Iotzova-Weiss G, Eloranta JJ, Lauchli S, et al. Squamous cell carcinoma of the skin shows a distinct microRNA profile modulated by UV radiation. J Invest Dermatol 2010:130(11):2686-9.

[63] Durham SE, Krishnana KJ, Betts J, Birch- Machin MA. Mitochondrial DNA damage in non-melanoma skin cancer. Br J Cancer 2003;88(1):90-5.

[64] Prior SL, Griffiths AP, Lewis PD. A study of mitochondrial DNA D-loop mutations and p53 status in nonmelanoma skin cancer. Br J. Dermatol 2009;161(5):1067-71.

[65] Harbottle A, Birch-Machin MA. Real-time PCR analysis of a 3895 bp mitochondrial DNA deletion in nonmelanoma skin cancer and its use as a quantitative marker for sunlight exposure in human skin. Br J Cancer. 2006;94(12):1887-93.

11

Stress Hormone and Skin Disease

Jung Eun Kim and Hyun Jeong Park
Department of Dermatology, College of Medicine, The Catholic University of Korea, Korea

1. Introduction

Stress activates several neural pathways. The main stress response systems are the locus coeruleus, sympathetic-adrenal medullary system, and the hypothalamic - pituitary - adrenal (HPA) axis (Zhang et al., 2005). Stressors stimulate the paraventricular nuclei of the hypothalamus, where corticotropin-releasing hormone (CRH) and arginine vasopressin (AVP) are synthesized. CRH is a central component of the HPA axis and regulates the expression of pro-opiomelanocortin (POMC) and POMC-derived peptides (adrenocorticotropin (ACTH), α-melanocyte-stimulating hormone (α-MSH) and β-endorphin) from the anterior pituitary gland (Chrousos, 1998). CRH stimulates AVP secretion and AVP has synergistic effect with CRH, particularly under chronic stress. Pituitary ACTH stimulates adrenal cortisol and glucocorticoid production. Stress influences cellular and humoral immune responses by releasing glucocorticoid, catecholamine, and CRH and POMC peptide secretion as well as by altering cytokine profiles (Elenkov & Chrousos, 1999).

The skin is directly exposed to various environmental stresses. Skin should be able to defense immediately against these stressors and reestablish tissue homeostasis. Recent studies have identified the existence of a peripheral stress response system equivalent to the central HPA axis in the skin. CRH, urocortin, POMC-derived peptides, and their receptors are expressed in normal skin. Response to local CRH stimulation in melanoncytes and fibroblasts confirmed the presence of a fully functional local HPA axis (Slominski et al., 2007). Stress hormone of the HPA axis produced locally under stress enables the skin to regulate the local homeostasis.

CRH, the main coordinator of the stress response can be secreted by various skin cells including epidermal and hair follicle keratinocytes, sebocytes and mast cells (Kono et al., 2001). The peptide acts through CRH receptor (CRH-R), which belong to the calcitonin/vasoactive intestinal peptide (VIP)/growth hormone-releasing hormone subfamily of G protein-coupled receptors. These include CRH-R1 and CRH-R2, both being subdivided into CRH-R1α/1β and CRH-R2α/2β. CRH-R1 is the major receptor in the epidermis and dermis. CRH-R2 is the predominant type of receptor in adnexal structures (Chalmers et al., 1996; Pisarchik & Slominski, 2004; Slominski et al., 2001).

CRH has a pleiotropic effect in the skin depending on the cell type and experimental growth conditions. CRH stimulates diverse signaling pathways via CRH-R1 activation, which modulates proliferation, differentiation, apoptosis and pro- or anti-inflammatory activities of skin cells (Elenkov & Chrousos, 1999; O'Kane et al., 2006).

CRH activates various cells to release the pro-inflammatory cytokines. For example, CRH stimulates interleukin (IL)-6 release by keratinocytes (Zbytek et al., 2002) and IL-1β release by monocytes (Paez Pereda et al., 1995). Skin mast cells function as "sensors" of environmental and emotional stress (Theoharides et al., 2010). There have been a few evidences that CRH-induced activation of mast cells may explain the phenomenon of stress-related exacerbation of cutaneous inflammatory diseases. Mast cells express CRH-R1 (Cao et al., 2005). CRH and urocortin activates skin mast cells and increases vascular permeability in humans, through activation of CRH-R1 (Theoharides et al., 1998). Stress-induced mast cell degranulation is mediated by CRH, neurotensin, and substance P (SP) in the rat skin (Singh et al., 1999). CRH and urocortin stimulated selective release of vascular endothelial growth factor (VEGF) and IL-6, respectively from mast cells through CRH-R1 activation without degranulation (Theoharides et al., 2010; Zhou et al., 2010). Moreover, human mast cells can produce CRH and urocortin (Kempuraj et al., 2004).

On the while, CRH has anti-inflammatory activity. In rat injury models, CRH attenuated vascular leakage and reduced edema through pituitary ACTH and CRH-R2 (Wei & Gao, 1991). The peptide diminishes NF-kB activation in epidermal melanocytes (Zbytek et al., 2006) and inhibits IL-18 expression through the mitogen-activated protein kinase (MAPK) signaling pathway in human HaCaT keratinocytes (Park et al., 2005). IL-18 is a key mediator of peripheral inflammation and host defense responses. On the while, ACTH stimulates human keratinocytes to secrete IL-18 through melanocortin receptor 1(MC1R), melanocortin receptor 2 (MC2R), p38 and ERK MAPK pathways. Since CRH inhibits IL-18 expression in HaCaT cells, IL-18 may play an important role on the negative feedback loop of CRH regulation (Park et al., 2007). This provides insights on the pathophysiology of stress-related skin diseases.

Stress or an abnormal response to stressors has been found to modify the course of skin disorders. A few studies revealed dysregulated central and peripheral HPA expression in some stress-exacerbating skin diseases. This review focuses on what is known about the distribution and function of stress hormone in the representative stress-exacerbating skin diseases such as atopic dermatitis (AD), psoriasis, and alopecia areata (AA). By summarizing the literature, this comprehensive review may help clinicians understand "stress hormone and skin disease" better.

2. Psoriasis

Psoriasis is a polygenic disease that is characterized by keratinocyte hyperproliferation, abnormal differentiation and chronic inflammation. Many psoriatic patients believe that there is a causal relationship between stressors and their disease outcome. Earlier retrospective studies have suggested that exacerbation of psoriasis occur a few weeks to months after a stressful event (Gupta et al., 1988). Recently, Verhoeven et al. have found a positive significant correlation between preceding daily stressors and Psoriasis Area and Severity Index and itch 4 weeks later through a prospective study (Verhoeven et al., 2011). It has been suggested that exacerbations of psoriasis after stress might be related to alteration of the HPA axis and the release of neuropeptides.

Earlier studies have found a blunted HPA axis function in psoriatic patients during exposure to the acute stressor (Arnetz et al., 1985; Richards et al., 2005). The hyporesponsiveness of HPA axis might result in exaggerated inflammatory responses due to the diminished suppressive effect of the low level of cortisol. This may explain why psoriatic patients are more vulnerable to the influence of stressors on their symptoms. Recent study revealed that peak levels of daily stressors were related to an increase in disease severity a month later, and the highest levels of daily stressors were also significantly associated with a lower cortisol level. Furthermore, patients with persistently high levels of stressors had lower mean cortisol levels (Evers et al., 2010).

However, two studies by Karanikas et al. and Buske-Kirschbaum et al. detected no alteration of the HPA axis function in psoriasis and suggested that the systemic HPA axis response could be normal in a T helper type 1 (Th1)-dominant inflammatory condition (Karanikas et al., 2009; Buske-Kirschbaum et al., 2006).

After psychosocial stress, psoriasis patients showed increased number of activated T cell with a shift towards a Th1-derived cytokine profile and increased number of cutaneous lymphocyte-associated antigens-positive T cells and natural killer cells in the circulation, which was pathologically relevant in aggravation of psoriatic plaques (Buske-Kirschbaum et al., 2007; Schmid-Ott et al., 2009).

β-endorphin is one of the POMC-related peptides. The peptide is produced by the HPA axis but can be secreted by immune cells. Psoriatic patients with actively spreading plaque lesions showed increased levels of β-endorphin in sera. β-endorphin may be produced by inflammatory cells in psoriatic lesions rather than activation of HPA axis by chronic stress (Glinski et al., 1994). The presence of high levels of β-endorphin in psoriatic lesions might induce SP-mediated neurogenic inflammation and have an antinociceptive effect on peripheral sensory nerve function (Glinski et al., 1994). This may be responsible for the absence of itching in psoriatic lesions in the majority of psoriasis patients.

There have been some conflicting results of peripheral HPA axis expression in psoriatic lesions. Prior studies reported that CRH/CRH-R expression was increased in the affected epidermis (Kono et al., 2001; O'Kane et al., 2006). We previously reported increased expression of CRH in various clinical subtypes of psoriasis (Kim et al., 2007). CRH treatment on HaCat cell lines induced proliferation/differentiation (Zbytek & Slominski, 2005; Slominski et al., 2006). Aberrant CRH/CRH-R1 expression in active psoriatic lesions might result in disharmony in proliferation/differentiation.

Many researchers focus on the proinflammatory role of CRH. CRH may activate mast cells via a CRH-R-dependent mechanism, leading to the release of histamine with increased vascular permeability (Theoharides et al., 1998). The proinflammatory cytokine IL-1, 6, and tumor necrosis factor (TNF)-α secreted by mast cells are upregulated in psoriatic skin. They are recognized as potent stimulators of CRH and POMC production in human skin (Tsigos & Chrousos, 2002).

In contrast, Tagen et al. and Zhou et al. found increased serum CRH and decreased lesional skin CRH/CRH-R1 gene expression and suggested that downregulated CRH/CRH-R1 expression in psoriatic lesion may be the result of negative feedback of systemic CRH elevation (Tagen et al., 2007; Zhou et al., 2009). CRH could downregulate pro-inflammatory cytokine IL-18 as we previously reported (Park et al., 2005). In this view, CRH might have protective function from developing the psoriatic lesions.

Altered CRH/CRH-R expression was observed not only in the psoriatic skin but also in the psoriatic arthritis. Upregulation of CRH-R1α mRNA and peptide in the endothelial cells and mast cells of inflamed synovium was observed in patients with psoriatic arthritis. CRH potentially play a role through angiogenesis or inflammatory effects in psoriatic arthritis (McEvoy et al., 2001).

SP, one of the stress neuropeptides, is suggested to have a role of neurogenic inflammation in the pathogenesis of psoriasis. Expression of SP and its receptor correlated with the severity of depression and was associated with low level of cortisol, which indicates chronic stress (Remröd C et al., 2007; Amatya et al., 2011). SP also play a critical role in stress-induced mast cell degranulation in mice (Kawana et al., 2006).

In conclusion, exposure to real life- and experimental stressors showed altered HPA axis in psoriatic patients. Dysregulated HPA activity might result in changes of immune responses and peripheral CRH levels. CRH-induced mast cell activation plays an important role in stress-induced psoriasis exacerbation. Inflammatory mediators released from psoriatic lesions not only interact with peripheral HPA axis, but also may influence central HPA axis. The stress-dependent mechanism of CRH and POMC-related peptides with the symptom of psoriasis should be studied further.

3. Atopic dermatitis

AD is a chronic, inflammatory, allergic skin disease, provoked by the imbalance of Th1/ T helper type 2 (Th2) immune responses. Epidemiological and experimental studies suggest that psychological stress triggers the symptom of AD. This phenomenon has been explained by the finding that activation of the HPA axis by stress aggravates the symptoms, mainly by inducing a shift toward Th2 cell phenotype.

After stress, blunted HPA axis responsiveness and increased reactivity of the sympathetic adrenomedullary system in atopic patients was demonstrated (Buske-Kirschbaum et al., 2010). Interestingly, neonates with a parental atopic history and elevated cord IgE were found to show significantly increased responsiveness of the HPA axis to the heel prick stress, which may be due to maternal stress hormonal effect or which may increase the vulnerability to develop AD in later life (Buske-Kirschbaum et al., 2004). Adolescents with AD had an attenuated cortisol response to laboratory stress (Wamboldt et al., 2003). However, Afsar et al. identified that children with AD do not have different basal cortisol levels nor more anxiety compared with normal children (Afsar et al., 2010).

Dendritic cells (DCs) promote allergic immune responses by inducing Th2 cell differentiation. Recently, Lee et al. detected CRH-R1α, 1β, 2α mRNA and CRH-R1, CRH-R2 protein in mononuclear cell-derived dendritic cells in AD patients. IL-18 is a potent inducer of Th1 responses. CRH significantly decreased the expression of IL-18 in DCs of AD patients. Stress-induced CRH may enhance Th2 immune responses by acting directly on DCs via CRH-R and aggravate the clinical manifestations in AD (Lee et al., 2009).

Increased levels of β-endorphin in the sera had been considered as a biological marker for severe AD (Lee et al., 2006; Glinski et al., 1994, 1995). The increased neuropeptide has been suggested to be produced from lesional inflammatory cells rather than activation of central HPA axis by chronic stress. Stress-related pruritus may be associated with a systemic pruritic effect of β-endorphin (Glinski et al., 1995).

Altered POMC-related gene expression also influences the development of postinflammatory hyperpigmentation. Increased plasma α-MSH levels and MC1R and MC3R expression in the skin and intestine, respectively was associated with pigmentation of AD in an NC/Nga mouse model. The changes were completely blocked by pretreating with MC1R antagonist or MC3R antagonist (Hiramoto et al., 2010).

There have been several attempts to reveal how various stressors could affect central and peripheral HPA axis in AD animal models.

Amano et al. demonstrated that psychological stress by itself could develop AD-like skin lesions along with concomitant increase of serum immunoglobulin E in NC/Nga mice. The lesions were not induced by treatment with CRH antagonist (Amano et al., 2008).

Orita et al. demonstrated that AD-like lesions in NC/Nga mice was exacerbated by strong exercise but ameliorated by mild exercise. Plasma a-MSH, transforming growth factor- β (TGF- β) and lesional SP expression correlated with exacerbation of the symptom. Plasma levels of β-endorphin increased by the mild exercise. Exercise-induced stress differently affects the symptom of AD and stimulates POMC-related hormone depending on the strength of exercise (Orita et al., 2011). β-endorphin has been known to strengthen natural immunity and proper exercise might be helpful to control the symptom of AD by stimulating the HPA axis and inducing balanced Th1/Th2 immunity.

AD is also exacerbated by stress through mast cell activation (Katsarou-Katsari et al., 1999) Mast cells in the presence of stem cell factor (SCF) and IL-4, produce mostly Th2 predominant cytokines (Bischoff et al., 2001) and release neuropeptide such as SP and nerve growth factor (NGF) (Theoharides et al., 2010; Xiang & Nilsson, 2000).

Computer-induced stress or video games-induced stress enhanced allergen specific immune responses with elevated levels of plasma SP, VIP and NGF, with concomitant increase of Th2 cytokines, in patients with AD (Kimata, 2003).

There have been little studies about local stress hormone expression in AD lesions. Recently, Oh et al. reported that CRH and SP expression was not different between AD lesions and normal, whereas NGF and neuropeptide Y (NPY) expression was significantly higher in the epidermis of affected skin of four AD patients, although the result was not quantitated (Oh et al., 2010). Increased expression of NGF in AD lesions was supported by Dou et al. (Dou et al., 2006). NGF and NPY have been known to be related with anxiety. Anxiety score positively correlated with pruritus in AD patients (Oh et al., 2010). Stress aggravates pruritus by lowering the itching threshold (Gieler et al., 2003; Paus et al., 2006). For the mechanism, increased contacts of nerve and mast cells have been suggested. The neuropeptides NGF and NPY might have a role to activate intraepidermal mast cells in AD lesion and contributes to stress-induced pruritus (Oh et al., 2010).

Blunted HPA axis responses to stressors are shown in AD patients. In general, stress negatively impact the severity of AD by down-regulating cellular immunity and enhancing humoral immunity. CRH, and POMC-related peptide hormones, as well as neuropeptide SP, NGF, and NPY modulate immunological and inflammatory response under stress.

4. Alopecia areata

The hair follicle (HF) is a unique mini organ that has immune-privilege (IP) during the anagen phase. Several factors are involved in the maintenance of HF-IP. Those include absence of MHC class I molecules expression, and upregulation of immunosuppressant such as Insulin-like growth factor-1, TGF- β1, ACTH, α-MSH and cortisol (Ito, 2010). The hair follicles have their own local equivalent of the HPA axis, termed the brain-hair follicle axis (BHA) (Arck et al., 2003). There have been few evidences that BHA hormones modulate the hair cycle (Maurer et al., 1997; Slominski et al., 1998).

4.1 Normal hair follicle HPA axis

In normal human hair follicle, CRH/CRH-R2 is expressed in the outer root sheath (ORS) and hair bulb (Arck et al., 2003). CRH-R2 plays an important role in modulating hair cycle and is detectable in the cells-derived from HF keratinocytes and dermal papilla fibroblasts. In murine HF, the highest intensity of CRH occur during anagen IV/VI, and the lowest levels are found during catagen and telogen (Roloff et al., 1998)

CRH induce POMC mRNA and peptide in human HFs in vitro. Moreover, CRH stimulates cortisol secretion by organ-cultured human HFs that also possess feedback systems (Ito et al., 2005)

ACTH is solely expressed in ORS of anagen HFs and its concentration significantly increases during anagen and stimulates intrafollicular cortisol production (Ito et al., 2005). α-MSH is detected in ORS and hair matrix during anagen (Paus et al., 1999). The POMC peptide and cortisol production contribute to the anagen-dependent immune-suppression.

4.1.1 Stress hormone and hair follicle mast cells

Perifollicular mast cells play an important role in human hair cycling. Degranulation of mast cells abruptly increase just before the onset of catagen. Inhibition of mast cell degranulation can delay catagen development in the murine hair cycle (Ito et al., 2010). It was recently reported that CRH induces differentiation of human HF precursors into mast cells (Ito et al., 2010). CRH-induced mast cell degranulation is mediated by SCF stimulation in human HFs (Kumamoto et al., 2003).

4.1.2 Stress and substance P

Neuropeptides, SP, are expressed in the hair follicles and also affect the hair growth cycle (Maurer et al., 1997; Zhou et al., 2006). SP facilitates catagen development by promotion of mast cell degranulation and also induces a loss of IP markers in HFs (Arck et al., 2001; Peters et al., 2007).

4.2 Alopecia areata and hair follicle HPA axis

AA is a hair cycling disorder, which is characterized by early catagen development. The condition is initiated by the collapse of the anagen-specific IP. Anagen HFs are attacked by inflammatory cells and move prematurely into catagen.

Many patients often experience development or recurrence of AA after trauma or stressful events. It was hypothesized that the chronic inflammatory state of AA might modify the HPA axis and subsequent stress responses or abnormal expression of HPA axis-related hormone itself might implicate the development of AA (Ito et al., 2010).

4.2.1 Central HPA axis in Alopecia areata

AA mice have a significantly blunted systemic HPA response to acute physiological stress and a defective adaptation to repeated psychological stress. Increased expression of hypothalamic AVP following stress exposure increased pituitary POMC under both basal and stress conditions. AVP has been known to potentiate the effects of CRH under chronic stressed conditions. An increased AVP appears to be critical for maintaining pituitary responsiveness to repeated stress (Zhang et al., 2009).

4.2.2 Peripheral HPA axis in Alopecia areata

In our previous study, the epidermis and pilosebaceous units of AA lesion showed intense expression of CRH, ACTH and α-MSH peptides (Kim et al., 2006). Enhanced CRH/CRH-R2 expression in human AA lesion was obtained by others (Katsarou-Katsari et al., 2001) but CRH was not detected in some studies (Zhang et al., 2009).

Upreguated CRH/CRH-R2 and ACTH peptide and insufficient glucocorticoid and higher glucocorticoid receptor levels in affected skin of human AA have been reported. Recently, Guo et al. revealed increased MC2R mRNA and decreased MC2R protein expression in AA lesions. They hypothesized that these reciprocal changes indicated a defect of post-transcriptional control of MC2R gene expression. Stressors activate CRH/CRH-R system, then increase ACTH, which upregulates MC2R mRNA expression. However, due to decreased MC2R protein, ACTH cannot produce sufficient amount of cortisol (Guo et al., 2010, 2011).

Hyper-active BHA axis was observed in not only in the HFs but also in the lymph nodes of AA mice. Increased POMC mRNA levels with decreased Nr3c1 levels in HFs and lymph nodes were detected. Nr3c1 is a mineralocorticoid receptor and is activated by cortisol. Thus, the findings suggest that there may be a negative feedback mechanism in BHA axis of AA mice (Zhang et al., 2009). Stress hormone release from the skin may modulate AA-associated inflammation. Plasma ACTH levels and lesional ACTH receptor expression were positively correlated to TNF-α expression in AA mouse skin (Zhang et al., 2009).

4.2.3 Stress-induced perifollicular neurogenic inflammation

Early catagen development is characteristic of AA. SP and its receptor, NGF, and mast cells play key roles in stress-induced perifollicular neurogenic inflammation. SP plays an important role in catagen development. It causes MHC-class I based IP to collapse (Peters et al., 2007). The number of SP-immunoreactive nerve fibers increase during early stage of AA, and decrease during advanced stage. SP and SP-degrading enzymes are highly expressed in the skin of AA-affected humans (Toyoda et al., 2001) and in the C3H/HeJ mouse model (Siebenhaar et al., 2007). AA onset may require stress-induced SP expression in the skin (Peters et al., 2006, 2007). Exposure to stress increase expression of SP (Arck et al., 2001, 2003). Sound stress upregulated SP protein expression and activated mast cells with premature catagen development in CBA/J mice, and neurokinin1 receptor antagonist normalized most stress-induced alterations (Maurer et al., 1997)

AA patients have highly active central and peripheral HPA tone. HPA activity has positive correlation with Th1 cytokine activity in AA mice. There may be interactions between systemic HPA hormones, expression levels of cutaneous HPA hormone receptors, and proinflammatory cytokine production in AA skin.

5. Skin tumors

We previously investigated CRH and POMC-related hormone expression in benign and malignant skin tumors. CRH, ACTH and α-MSH expression of skin cancer was increased compared with normal and precancerous skin lesions, consistent with prior results (Kim et al., 2006; Slominski et al., 2004). Immunoreactivity of CRH expression increased in line with malignant tendency (Kim et al., 2006).

CRH is known to have endothelial cell chemotaxis and angiogenesis through CRH-R (Arbiser et al., 1999). CRH can enhance cell migration ability by ERK1/2 pathway in murine melanoma cell line (Yang et al., 2007). Yang et al. reported that CRH-POMC axis can also control metalloproteinase expression (Yang et al., 2002). CRH can stimulate tumor growth in vivo (Arbiser et al., 1999).

CRH may play a role in tumorigenesis in certain types of skin cancer by promoting angiogenesis and migration. Psychosocial stress might be related to the development and progression of tumors. However, whether the elevated expression of CRH-POMC is a cause or a result in carcinogenesis needs further studies.

6. Acne and seborrhea

CRH/CRH-R2 system is normaly expressed in human sebaceous gland (Kono et al., 2001) and regulate sebaceous lipid synthesis (Zouboulis et al., 2002).

Acne is an inflammatory disorder of the pilosebaceous unit. Increased CRH and CRH-binding protein immunoreactivity was observed in the sebaceous gland cells of acne lesions (Ganceviciene et al., 2009). *Propionibacterium acnes* increased the CRH expression in the epidermis (Isard et al., 2009). CRH-activating pathways which affect keratinocyte differentiation, lipogenic activity and inflammatory processes lead to the development of formation of the microcomedo and inflammatory acne lesions (Ganceviciene et al., 2009). This might be the reason why stress exacerbates the symptom of acne and seborrhea.

7. Urticaria and contact dermatitis

Stress-induced CRH expression increases the disease severity of type IV delayed hypersensitivity and chronic contact dermatitis through CRH-R1-expressing mast cell activation (Dhabhar & McEwen, 1999; Kaneko et al., 2003). Enhanced vascular permeability and vasodilation by CRH is expected to involve the pathomechanism of aggravation of urticaria or contact dermatitis after stress (Theoharides et al., 1998; Crompton et al., 2003). Furthermore, urticarial lesions from patients with chronic urticaria have shown increased expression of CRH-R1 and histidine decarboxylase, which is a mast cell-related gene and regulates the production of histamine (Papadopoulou et al., 2005). CRH/CRH-R and mast cells seems to participate in the pathogenesis of chronic urticaria under the stress.

8. Conclusion

Skin has its own equivalent of the central HPA axis and responses to various stressors. HFs also possess unique form of the HPA axis dependent on hair cycle. Aberrant CRH-POMC expression was observed in stress-exacerbating inflammatory skin disorders and malignant skin tumors. Stress hormone showed unique expression patterns in each disease, and some inconsistent expression results have been reported in an identical disease.

Skin HPA axis modulates inflammatory mediators in response to various stressors. Peripheral HPA axis in the skin may interact with central HPA axis with a feedback loop of inflammatory responses.

We summarized the role of HPA-related hormone in stress-related skin diseases. Impact of stress and stress hormone on the disease development, course, response to treatment, and stress management should be studied further.

9. Acknowledgment

This work was supported by the National Research Foundation of Korea (NRF) grant funded by the Korea government (MEST) (2011-0001390) and Basic research program through the NRF funded by the Ministry of Education, Science and Technology (2010-0002431). We thank Dr. Eujin Cho for English editing.

10. References

Afsar, FS., Isleten, F., & Sonmez, N. Children with atopic dermatitis do not have more anxiety or different cortisol levels compared with normal children. *Journal of cutaneous medicine and surgery*, Vol.14, No.1, (January-February 2010), pp.13-18, ISSN: 1203-4754

Amano, H., Negishi, I., Akiyama, H., & Ishikawa, O. Psychological stress can trigger atopic dermatitis in NC/Nga mice: an inhibitory effect of corticotropin-releasing factor. *Neuropsychopharmacology*, Vol.33, No.3, (February 2008), pp.566-573, ISSN: 1740-634X

Amatya, B., El-Nour, H., Holst, M., Theodorsson, E., & Nordlind, K. Expression of tachykinins and their receptors in plaque psoriasis with pruritus. *The British Journal of Dermatology*, (February 2011), Epub ahead of print, ISSN: 0007-0963

Arbiser, JL., Karalis, K., Viswanathan, A., Koike, C., Anand-Apte, B., Flynn, E., Zetter, B., & Majzoub, JA. Corticotropin-releasing hormone stimulates angiogenesis and epithelial tumor growth in the skin. *Journal of Investigative Dermatology*, Vol.113, No.5, (November 1999), pp. 838-842, ISSN: 0022-202X

Arck, PC., Handjiski, B., Hagen, E., Joachim, R., Klapp, BF., & Paus, R. Indications for a 'brain-hair follicle axis (BHA)': inhibition of keratinocyte proliferation and up-regulation of keratinocyte apoptosis in telogen hair follicles by stress and substance P. *The FASEB journal : official publication of the Federation of American Societies for Experimental Biology*, Vol.15, No.13, (November 2001), pp. 2536–2538, ISSN: 0892-6638

Arck, PC., Handjiski, B., Peters, EM., Peter, AS., Hagen, E., Fischer, A., Klapp, BF., & Paus, R. Stress inhibits hair growth in mice by induction of premature catagen development and deleterious perifollicular inflammatory events via neuropeptide substance P-dependent pathways. *The American journal of pathology*, Vol.162, No.3, (March 2003), pp.803-814, ISSN: 0002-9440

Arnetz, BB., Fjellner, B., Eneroth, P., & Kallner, A. Stress and psoriasis: psychoendocrine and metabolic reactions in psoriatic patients during standardized stressor exposure. *Psychosomatic medicine*, Vol.47, No.6, (November-December 1985), pp.528-541, ISSN: 0033-3174

Bischoff, SC., Sellge, G., Manns, MP., & Lorentz, A. Interleukin-4 induces a switch of human intestinal mast cells from proinflammatory cells to Th2-type cells. *International archives of allergy and immunology*, Vol.124, No.1-3, (January-March 2001), pp.151-154, ISSN: 1018-2438

Buske-Kirschbaum, A., Geiben, A., Höllig, H., Morschhäuser, E., & Hellhammer, D. Altered responsiveness of the hypothalamus-pituitary-adrenal axis and the sympathetic adrenomedullary system to stress in patients with atopic dermatitis. *The Journal of clinical endocrinology and metabolism*, Vol.87, No.9, (September 2002), pp.4245-4251, ISSN: 0021-972X

Buske-Kirschbaum, A., Fischbach, S., Rauh, W., Hanker, J., & Hellhammer, D. Increased responsiveness of the hypothalamus-pituitary-adrenal (HPA) axis to stress in newborns with atopic disposition. *Psychoneuroendocrinology*, Vol.29, No.6, (July 2004), pp.705-711, ISSN: 0306-4530

Buske-Kirschbaum, A., Ebrecht, M., Kern, S., & Hellhammer, DH. Endocrine stress responses in TH1-mediated chronic inflammatory skin disease (psoriasis vulgaris)--do they parallel stress-induced endocrine changes in TH2-mediated inflammatory dermatoses (atopic dermatitis)? *Psychoneuroendocrinology*, Vol.31, No.4, (May 2006), pp.439-446, ISSN: 0306-4530

Buske-Kirschbaum, A., Kern, S., Ebrecht, M., & Hellhammer, DH. Altered distribution of leukocyte subsets and cytokine production in response to acute psychosocial stress in patients with psoriasis vulgaris. *Brain, behavior, and immunity*, Vol.21, No.1, (January 2007), pp.92-99, ISSN: 0889-1591

Buske-Kirschbaum, A., Ebrecht M., & Hellhammer, DH. Blunted HPA axis responsiveness to stress in atopic patients is associated with the acuity and severeness of allergic inflammation. *Brain, behavior, and immunity*, Vol.24, No.8, (November 2010), pp.1347-1353, ISSN: 0889-1591

Cao, J., Papadopoulou, N., Kempuraj, D., Boucher, WS., Sugimoto, K., Cetrulo, CL., & Theoharides, TC. Human mast cells express corticotropin-releasing hormone (CRH) receptors and CRH leads to selective secretion of vascular endothelial growth factor. *Journal of Immunology*, Vol.15, No.174, (June 2005), pp. 7665-7675, ISSN: 0022-1767

Chalmers, DT., Lovenberg, TW., Grigoriadis, DE., Behan, DP., & De Souza, EB. Corticotropin-releasing factor receptors: from molecular biology to drug design. *Trends in pharmacological sciences*, Vol.17, No.4, (April 1996), pp.166-172, ISSN: 0167-7691

Chrousos, GP. Stressors, stress, and neuroendocrine integration of the adaptive response. *Annals of the New York Academy of Sciences*, Vol.30, No.851, (June 1998), pp. 311-335, ISSN: 0077-8923

Crompton, R., Clifton, VL., Bisits, AT., Read, MA., Smith, R., & Wright, IM. Corticotropin-releasing hormone causes vasodilation in human skin via mast cell-dependent pathways. *The Journal of clinical endocrinology and metabolism*, Vol.88, No.11, (November 2003), pp. 5427-5432, ISSN: 0021-972X

Dhabhar, FS., & McEwen, BS. Enhancing versus suppressive effects of stress hormones on skin immune function. *Proceedings of the National Academy of Sciences of the United States of America*, Vol. 2, No.96, (February 1999), pp. 1059–1064, ISSN: 0027-8424

Dou, YC., Hagströmer, L., Emtestam, L., & Johansson, O. Increased nerve growth factor and its receptors in atopic dermatitis: an immunohistochemical study. *Archives of dermatological research*, Vol.298, No.1, (June 2006), pp. 31-37, ISSN: 0340-3696

Elenkov, IJ., & Chrousos, GP. Stress hormones, Th1/Th2 patterns, pro/anti-inflammatory cytokines and susceptibility to disease. *Trends in endocrinology and metabolism : TEM.*, Vol.10, No.9, (November 1999), pp.359–368, ISSN: 1043-2760

Evers, AW., Verhoeven, EW., Kraaimaat, FW., de Jong, EM., de Brouwer, SJ., Schalkwijk, J., Sweep, FC., & van de Kerkhof, PC. How stress gets under the skin: cortisol and stress reactivity in psoriasis. *The British Journal of Dermatology*, Vol.163, No.5, (November 2010), pp. 986-991, ISSN: 0007-0963

Ganceviciene, R., Graziene, V., Fimmel, S., & Zouboulis, CC. Involvement of the corticotropin-releasing hormone system in the pathogenesis of acne vulgaris. *The Britsh Journal of Dermatology*, Vol.160, No.2, (February, 2009), pp.345-352, ISSN: 0007-0963

Ganceviciene, R., Böhm, M., Fimmel, S., & Zouboulis, CC. The role of neuropeptides in the multifactorial pathogenesis of acne vulgaris. *Dermatoendocrinology*, Vol.1, No.3, (May 2009), pp. 170-176, ISSN: 1938-1980

Gieler, U., Kupfer, J., Niemeier, V., & Brosig, B. Psyche and skin: what's new? *Journal of the European Academy of Dermatology and Venereology : JEADV.*, Vol.17, No.2, (March 2003), pp.128-130, ISSN: 0926-9959

Glinski ,W., Brodecka, H., Glinska-Ferenz, M., & Kowalski, D. Increased concentration of beta-endorphin in sera of patients with psoriasis and other inflammatory dermatoses. *The British Journal of Dermatology*, Vol.131, No.2, (August 1994), pp.260-264, ISSN: 0007-0963

Glinski, W., Brodecka, H., Glinska-Ferenz, M., & Kowalski, D. Neuropeptides in psoriasis: possible role of beta-endorphin in the pathomechanism of the disease. *International Journal of Dermatology*, Vol.33, No.5, (May 1994), pp.356-360, ISSN: 0011-9059

Glinski, W., Brodecka, H., Glinska-Ferenz, M., & Kowalski, D. Increased concentration of beta-endorphin in the sera of patients with severe atopic dermatitis. *Acta dermato-venereologica*, Vol.75, No.1, (January 1995), pp.9-11, ISSN: 0001-5555

Guo, HW., Deng, J., Yang, XC., Zhong, BY., Shen, Z., Yang, SY., Liu, BH., & Hao, F. Melanocortin receptor type 2 (MC2R, ACTH receptor) expression in patients with alopecia areata. *Experimental Dermatology*, Vol.19, No.11, (November 2010), pp.1020-1022, ISSN: 0906-6705

Guo, HW., Deng, J., Yang, XC., Yang, SY., Liu, BH., & Hao, F. An implication for post-transcriptional control: reciprocal changes of melanocortin receptor type 2 mRNA and protein expression in alopecia areata. *Medical Hypotheses*, Vol.76, No.1, (January 2011), pp. 122-124, ISSN: 0306-9877

Gupta, MA., Gupta, AK., Kirkby, S., Weiner, HK., Mace, TM., Schork, NJ., Johnson, EH., Ellis, CN., & Voorhees, JJ. Pruritus in psoriasis. A prospective study of some psychiatric and dermatologic correlates. *Archives of dermatology*, Vol.124, No.7, (July 1988), pp.1052-1057, ISSN: 0003-987X

Hiramoto, K., Kobayashi, H., Ishii, M., Sato, E., & Inoue, M. Increased alpha-melanocyte-stimulating hormone (alpha-MSH) levels and melanocortin receptors expression associated with pigmentation in an NC/Nga mouse model of atopic dermatitis. *Experimental Dermatology*, Vol.19, No.2, (February 2010), pp. 132-136, ISSN: 0906-6705

Isard, O., Knol, AC., Castex-Rizzi, N., Khammari, A., Charveron, M., & Dréno, B. Cutaneous induction of corticotropin releasing hormone by *Propionibacterium acnes* extracts. *Dermatoendocrinology*, Vol.1, No.2, (March 2009), pp.96-99, ISSN: 1938-1980

Ito, N., Ito, T., Kromminga, A., Bettermann, A., Takigawa, M., Kees, F., Straub, RH., & Paus, R. Human hair follicles display a functional equivalent of the hypothalamic-pituitary-adrenal axis and synthesize cortisol. *The FASEB journal : official publication of the Federation of American Societies for Experimental Biology*, Vol.19, No.10, (August 2005), pp.1332-1334, ISSN: 0892-6638

Ito, N., Sugawara, K., Bodó, E., Takigawa, M., van Beek, N., Ito, T., & Paus, R. Corticotropin-releasing hormone stimulates the in situ generation of mast cells from precursors in the human hair follicle mesenchyme. *Journal of Investigative Dermatology*, Vol.130, No.4, (April 2010), pp. 995-1004, ISSN: 0022-202X

Ito, T. Hair follicle is a target of stress hormone and autoimmune reactions. *Journal of Dermatological Science*, Vol.60, No.2, (November 2010), pp. 67-73, ISSN: 0923-1811

Kaneko, K., Kawana, S., Arai, K., & Shibasaki, T. Corticotropin-releasing factor receptor type 1 is involved in the stress-induced exacerbation of chronic contact dermatitis in rats. *Experimental Dermatology*, Vol.12, No.1, (February 2003), pp. 47–52, ISSN: 0906-6705

Karanikas, E., Harsoulis, F., Giouzepas, I., & Griveas, I. Stimulation of the hypothalamic-pituitary-adrenal axis with corticotropin releasing hormone in patients with psoriasis. *Hormones (Athens, Greece)*, Vol.6, No.4, (October-December 2007), pp.314-320, ISSN: 1109-3099

Karanikas, E., Harsoulis, F., Giouzepas, I., Griveas, I., & Chrisomallis, F. Neuroendocrine stimulatory tests of hypothalamus-pituitary-adrenal axis in psoriasis and correlative implications with psychopathological and immune parameters. *The Journal of dermatology*, Vol.36, No.1, (January 2009), pp.35-44, ISSN: 0385-2407

Katsarou-Katsari, A., Filippou, A., & Theoharides, TC. Effect of stress and other psychological factors on the pathophysiology and treatment of dermatoses. *International journal of immunopathology and pharmacology*, Vol.12, No.1, (January-April 1999), pp.7-11, ISSN: 0394-6320

Katsarou-Katsari, A., Singh, LK., & Theoharides, TC. Alopecia areata and affected skin CRH receptor upregulation induced by acute emotional stress. *Dermatology*, Vol.203, No.2, (2001), pp.157-161, ISSN: 1018-8665

Kawana, S., Liang, Z., Nagano, M., & Suzuki, H. Role of substance P in stress-derived degranulation of dermal mast cells in mice. *Journal of dermatological science*, Vol.42, No.1, (January 2006), pp. 47-54, ISSN: 0923-1811

Kempuraj, D., Papadopoulou, NG., Lytinas, M., Huang, M., Kandere-Grzybowska, K., Madhappan, B., Boucher, W., Christodoulou, S., Athanassiou, A., & Theoharides ,TC. Corticotropin-releasing hormone and its structurally related urocortin are synthesized and secreted by human mast cells. *Endocrinology*, Vol. 145, No.1,(January 2004), pp. 43-48, ISSN: 0013-7227

Kim, JE., Cho, DH., Kim, HS., Kim, HJ., Lee, JY., Cho, BK., & Park, HJ. Expression of the corticotropin-releasing hormone-proopiomelanocortin axis in the various clinical types of psoriasis. *Experimental Dermatology*, Vol.16, No.2, (February 2007), pp.104-109, ISSN: 0906-6705

Kim, HS., Cho, DH., Kim, HJ., Lee, JY., Cho, BK., & Park, HJ. Immunoreactivity of corticotropin-releasing hormone, adrenocorticotropic hormone and alpha-melanocyte-stimulating hormone in alopecia areata. *Experimental Dermatology*, Vol.15, No.7, (July 2006), pp. 515-522, ISSN: 0906-6705

Kim, MH., Cho, D., Kim, HJ., Chong, SJ., Lee, KH., Yu, DS., Park, CJ., Lee, JY., Cho, BK., & Park, HJ. Investigation of the corticotropin-releasing hormone-proopiomelanocortin axis in various skin tumours. *The British Journal of Dermatology*, Vol.155, No.5, (November 2006), pp. 910-915, ISSN: 0007-0963

Kimata, H. Enhancement of allergic skin wheal responses and in vitro allergen-specific IgE production by computer-induced stress in patients with atopic dermatitis. *Brain, behavior, and immunity*, Vol.17, No.2, (April 2003), pp.134-138, ISSN: 0889-1591

Kimata, H. Enhancement of allergic skin wheal responses in patients with atopic eczema/dermatitis syndrome by playing video games or by a frequently ringing mobile phone. *European journal of clinical investigation*, Vol.33, No.6, (June 2003), pp. 513-517, ISSN: 0014-2972

Kono, M., Nagata, H., Umemura, S., Kawana, S., & Osamura, RY. In situ expression of corticotropin-releasing hormone (CRH) and proopiomelanocortin (POMC) genes in human skin. *The FASEB journal : official publication of the Federation of American Societies for Experimental Biology*, Vol.15, No.12, (October 2001), pp. 2297–2299, ISSN: 0892-6638

Kumamoto, T., Shalhevet, D., Matsue, H., Mummert, ME., Ward, BR., Jester, JV., & Takashima, A. Hair follicles serve as local reservoirs of skin mast cell precursors. *Blood*, Vol. 1, No.102, (September 2003), pp.1654-1660, ISSN: 0006-4971

Orita, K., Hiramoto, K., Inoue, R., Sato, EF., Kobayashi, H., Ishii, M., & Inoue, M. Strong exercise stress exacerbates dermatitis in atopic model mice, NC/Nga mice, while proper exercise reduces it. *Experimental Dermatology*, Vol.19, No.12, (December 2010), pp.1067-1072, ISSN: 0906-6705

Lee, CH., Chuang, HY., Shih, CC., Jong, SB., Chang, CH., & Yu, HS. Transepidermal water loss, serum IgE and beta-endorphin as important and independent biological markers for development of itch intensity in atopic dermatitis. *The British Journal of Dermatology*, Vol.154, No.6, (June 2006), pp.1100-1107, ISSN: 0007-0963

Lee, HJ., Kwon, YS., Park, CO., Oh, SH., Lee, JH., Wu, WH., Chang, NS., Lee, MG., & Lee, KH. Corticotropin-releasing factor decreases IL-18 in the monocyte-derived dendritic cell. *Experimental Dermatology*, Vol.18, No.3, (March 2009), pp. 199-204, ISSN: 0906-6705

Maurer, M., Fischer, E., Handjiski, B., von Stebut, E., Algermissen, B., Bavandi, A., & Paus, R. Activated skin mast cells are involved in murine hair follicle regression (catagen). *Laboratory investigation; a journal of technical methods and pathology*, Vol.77, No.4, (October 1997), pp. 319-332, ISSN: 0023-6837

McEvoy, AN., Bresnihan, B., FitzGerald, O., & Murphy, EP. Corticotropin-releasing hormone signaling in synovial tissue from patients with early inflammatory arthritis is mediated by the type 1 alpha corticotropin-releasing hormone receptor. *Arthritis and rheumatism*, Vol.44, No.8, (August 2001), pp. 1761-1767, ISSN: 0004-3591

Oh, SH., Bae, BG., Park, CO., Noh, JY., Park, IH., Wu, WH., & Lee, KH. Association of stress with symptoms of atopic dermatitis. *Acta dermato-venereologica*, Vol.90, No.6, (November 2010), pp.582-588, ISSN: 0001-5555

O'Kane, M., Murphy, EP., & Kirby, B. The role of corticotropin-releasing hormone in immune-mediated cutaneous inflammatory disease. *Experimental Dermatology*, Vol.15, No.3, (March 2006), pp.143-153, ISSN: 0906-6705

Papadopoulou, N., Kalogeromitros, D., Staurianeas, NG., Tiblalexi, D., & Theoharides, TC. Corticotropin-releasing hormone receptor-1 and histidine decarboxylase expression in chronic urticaria. *Journal of Investigative Dermatology*, Vol.125, No.5, (November 2005), pp. 952-955, ISSN: 0022-202X

Park, HJ., Kim, HJ., Lee, JH., Lee, JY., Cho, BK., Kang, JS., Kang, H., Yang, Y., & Cho, DH. Corticotropin-releasing hormone (CRH) downregulates interleukin-18 expression in human HaCaT keratinocytes by activation of p38 mitogen-activated protein kinase (MAPK) pathway. *Journal of Investigative Dermatology*, Vol.124, No.4, (April 2005), pp.751-755, ISSN: 0022-202X

Park, HJ., Kim, HJ., Lee, JY., Cho, BK., Gallo, RL., & Cho, DH. Adrenocorticotropin hormone stimulates interleukin-18 expression in human HaCaT keratinocytes. *Journal of Investigative Dermatology*, Vol.127, No.5, (May 2007), pp.1210-1216, ISSN: 0022-202X

Paez Pereda, M., Sauer, J., Perez Castro, C., Finkielman, S., Stalla, GK., Holsboer, F., & Arzt, E. Corticotropin-releasing hormone differentially modulates the interleukin-1 system according to the level of monocyte activation by endotoxin. *Endocrinology*, Vol.136, No.12, (December 1995), pp.5504-5510, ISSN: 0013-7227

Paus, R., Botchkarev, VA., Botchkareva, NV., Mecklenburg, L., Luger, T., & Slominski, A. The skin POMC system (SPS). Leads and lessons from the hair follicle. *Annals of the New York Academy of Sciences*, Vol.20, No.885, (October 1999), pp.350-363, ISSN: 0077-8923

Paus, R., Schmelz, M., Biro, T., & Steinhoff, M. Frontiers in pruritus research: scratching the brain for more effective itch therapy. *The Journal of clinical investigation*, Vol.116, No.5, (May 2006), pp. 1174 - 1186, ISSN: 0021-9738

Peters, EM., Arck, PC., & Paus, R. Hair growth inhibition by psychoemotional stress: a mouse model for neural mechanisms in hair growth control. *Experimental Dermatology*, Vo.15, No.1, (January 2006), pp.1–13, ISSN: 0906-6705

Peters, EM., Liotiri, S., Bodo, E., Hagen, E., Biro, T., Arck, PC., & Paus, R. Probing the effects of stress mediators on the human hair follicle: substance P holds central position.

The American journal of pathology, Vol.171, No.6, (December 2007), pp.1872–1886, ISSN: 0002-9440

Pisarchik, A., & Slominski, A. Molecular and functional characterization of novel CRFR1 isoforms from the skin. *European journal of biochemistry / FEBS,* Vol.271, No.13, (July 2004), pp.2821-2830, ISSN: 0014-2956

Remröd, C., Lonne-Rahm, S., & Nordlind, K. Study of substance P and its receptor neurokinin-1 in psoriasis and their relation to chronic stress and pruritus. *Archives of dermatological research,* Vol.299, No.2, (May 2007), pp.85-91, ISSN: 0340-3696

Richards, HL., Ray, DW., Kirby, B., Mason, D., Plant, D., Main, CJ., Fortune, DG., & Griffiths, CE. Response of the hypothalamic-pituitary-adrenal axis to psychological stress in patients with psoriasis. *The British journal of dermatology,* Vol.153, No.6, (December 2005), pp.1114-1120, ISSN: 0007-0963

Roloff, B., Fechner, K., Slominski, A., Furkert, J., Botchkarev, VA., Bulfone-Paus, S., Zipper, J., Krause, E., & Paus, R. Hair cycle-dependent expression of corticotropin-releasing factor (CRF) and CRF receptors in murine skin. *The FASEB journal : official publication of the Federation of American Societies for Experimental Biology,* Vol.12, No.3, (March 1998), pp. 287-297, ISSN: 0892-6638

Rupprecht, M., Hornstein, OP., Schlüter, D., Schäfers, HJ., Koch, HU., Beck, G., & Rupprecht, R. Cortisol, corticotropin, and beta-endorphin responses to corticotropin-releasing hormone in patients with atopic eczema. *Psychoneuroendocrinology,* Vol.20, No.5, (1995), pp. 543-551, ISSN: 0306-4530

Siebenhaar, F., Sharov, AA., Peters, EM., Sharova, TY., Syska, W., Mardaryev, AN., Freyschmidt-Paul, P., Sundberg, JP., Maurer, M., & Botchkarev, VA. Substance P as an immunomodulatory neuropeptide in a mouse model for autoimmune hair loss (alopecia areata). *Journal of Investigative Dermatology,* Vol.127, No.6, (June 2007), pp.1489–1497, ISSN: 0022-202X

Singh, LK., Pang, X., Alexacos, N., Letourneau, R., & Theoharides, TC. Acute immobilization stress triggers skin mast cell degranulation via corticotropin releasing hormone, neurotensin, and substance P: A link to neurogenic skin disorders. *Brain, behavior, and immunity,* Vol.13, No.3, (September 1999), pp. 225-239, ISSN: 0889-1591

Singh, LK., Boucher, W., Pang, X., Letourneau, R., Seretakis, D., Green, M., & Theoharides, TC. Potent mast cell degranulation and vascular permeability triggered by urocortin through activation of corticotropin-releasing hormone receptors. *The Journal of pharmacology and experimental therapeutics,* Vol.288, No.3, (March 1999), pp.1349-1356, ISSN: 1521-0103

Schmid-Ott, G., Jaeger, B., Boehm, T., Langer, K., Stephan, M., Raap, U., & Werfel, T. Immunological effects of stress in psoriasis. *The British Journal of Dermatology,* Vol.160, No.4, (April 2009), pp.782-785, ISSN: 0007-0963

Slominski, A., Botchkareva, NV., Botchkarev, VA., Chakraborty, A., Luger, T., Uenalan, M. & Paus, R. Hair cycle-dependent production of ACTH in mouse skin. *Biochimica et biophysica acta,* Vo.19, No.1448, (November 1998), pp.147–152, ISSN: 0006-3002

Slominski, A., Wortsman, J., Luger, T., Paus, R., & Solomon, S. Corticotropin releasing hormone and proopiomelanocortin involvement in the cutaneous response to stress. *Physiological reviews,* Vol.80, No.3, (July 2000), pp.979-1020, ISSN: 0031-9333

Slominski, A., Wortsman, J., Pisarchik, A., Zbytek, B., Linton, EA., Mazurkiewicz, JE., & Wei, ET. Cutaneous expression of corticotropin-releasing hormone (CRH), urocortin, and CRH receptors. *The FASEB journal : official publication of the Federation of American Societies for Experimental Biology,*Vol.15, No.10, (August 2001), pp.1678-1693, ISSN: 0892-6638

Slominski, A., Pisarchik, A., Tobin, DJ., Mazurkiewicz, JE., & Wortsman, J. Differential expression of a cutaneous corticotropin-releasing hormone system. *Endocrinology*, Vol.145, No.2, (February 2004), pp.941–950, ISSN: 0013-7227

Slominski, A., Zbytek, B., Pisarchik, A., Slominski, RM., Zmijewski, MA., & Wortsman, J. CRH functions as a growth factor/cytokine in the skin. *Journal of cellular physiology*, Vol.206, No.3, (March 2006), pp.780-791, ISSN: 0021-9541

Slominski, A., Wortsman, J., Tuckey, RC., & Paus, R. Differential expression of HPA axis homolog in the skin. *Molecular and cellular endocrinology*, Vol.265-266, (February 2007), pp. 143-149, ISSN: 0303-7207

Tagen, M., Stiles, L., Kalogeromitros, D., Gregoriou, S., Kempuraj, D., Makris, M., Donelan, J., Vasiadi, M., Staurianeas, NG., & Theoharides,TC. Skin corticotropin-releasing hormone receptor expression in psoriasis. *Journal of Investigative Dermatology*, Vol.127, No.7, (July 2007), pp. 1789-1791, ISSN: 0022-202X

Theoharides, TC., Singh, LK., Boucher, W., Pang, X., Letourneau, R., Webster, E., & Chrousos, G. Corticotropin-releasing hormone induces skin mast cell degranulation and increased vascular permeability, a possible explanation for its proinflammatory effects. *Endocrinology*, Vol.139, No.1, (January 1998), pp. 403-413, ISSN: 0013-7227

Theoharides, TC., Alysandratos, KD., Angelidou, A., Delivanis, DA., Sismanopoulos, N., Zhang, B., Asadi, S., Vasiadi, M., Weng, Z., Miniati, A., & Kalogeromitros, D. Mast cells and inflammation. *Biochimica et biophysica acta*, (December 2010), Epub ahead of print, ISSN:0006-3002

Toyoda, M., Makino, T., Kagoura, M., & Morohashi, M. Expression of neuropeptide-degrading enzymes in alopecia areata: an immunohistochemical study. *The British Journal of Dermatology*, Vol.144, No.1, (January 2001) pp.46–54, ISSN: 0007-0963

Tsigos, C., & Chrousos, GP. Hypothalamic-pituitary-adrenal axis, neuroendocrine factors and stress. *Journal of psychosomatic research*, Vol.53, No.4, (October 2002), pp. 865-871, ISSN: 0022-3999

Verhoeven, EW., Kraaimaat, FW., Jong, EM., Schalkwijk, J., van de Kerkhof, PC., & Evers, AW. Effect of daily stressors on psoriasis: a prospective study. *Journal of Investigative Dermatology*, Vol.129, No.8, (August 2009), pp. 2075-2077, ISSN: 0022-202X

Wamboldt, MZ., Laudenslager, M., Wamboldt, FS., Kelsay, K., & Hewitt, J. Adolescents with atopic disorders have an attenuated cortisol response to laboratory stress. *The Journal of allergy and clinical immunology*, Vol.111, No.3, (March 2003), pp. 509-514, ISSN: 0091-6749

Wei, ET., & Gao, GC. Corticotropin-releasing factor: an inhibitor of vascular leakage in rat skeletal muscle and brain cortex after injury. *Regulatory peptides*, Vol.25, No.33, (April 1991), pp. 93-104, ISSN: 0167-0115

Xiang, Z., & Nilsson, G. IgE receptor-mediated release of nerve growth factor by mast cells. *Clinical and experimental allergy : journal of the British Society for Allergy and Clinical Immunology*, Vol.30, No.10, (October 2000), pp. 1379-1386, ISSN: 0954-7894

Yang, EV., Bane, CM., MacCallum, RC., Kiecolt-Glaser, JK., Malarkey, WB., & Glaser, R. Stress-related modulation of matrix metalloproteinase expression. *Journal of neuroimmunology*, Vol.133, No.1-2, (December 2002), pp. 144-150, ISSN: 0165-5728

Yang, Y., Park, H., Yang, Y., Kim, TS., Bang, SI., & Cho, D. Enhancement of cell migration by corticotropin-releasing hormone through ERK1/2 pathway in murine melanoma cell line, B16F10. *Experimental Dermatology*, Vol.16, No.1, (January 2007), pp.22-27, ISSN: 0906-6705

Zbytek, B., Mysliwski, A., Slominski, A., Wortsman, J., Wei, ET., & Mysliwska, J. Corticotropin-releasing hormone affects cytokine production in human HaCaT keratinocytes. *Life sciences*, Vol.18, No.70, (January 2002), pp.1013-1021, ISSN: 0024-3205

Zbytek, B., Pikula, M., Slominski, RM., Mysliwski, A., Wei, E., Wortsman, J., & Slominski, AT. Corticotropin-releasing hormone triggers differentiation in HaCaT keratinocytes. *The British Journal of Dermatology*, Vol.152, No.3, (March 2005), pp. 474-480, ISSN: 0007-0963

Zbytek, B., & Slominski, AT. Corticotropin-releasing hormone induces keratinocyte differentiation in the adult human epidermis. *Journal of cellular physiology*, Vol.203, No.1, (April 2005), pp.118-126, ISSN: 0021-9541

Zbytek, B., Pfeffer, LM., & Slominski, AT. CRH inhibits NF-kappa B signaling in human melanocytes. *Peptides*, Vol.27, No.12, (December 2006), pp. 3276-3283, ISSN: 0196-9781

Zhang, X., Sliwowska, JH., & Weinberg, J. Prenatal alcohol exposure and fetal programming: effects on neuroendocrine and immune function. *Experimental biology and medicine (Maywood, N.J.)*, Vol.230, No.6, (June 2005), pp. 376-388, ISSN: 1535-3699

Zhang, X., Yu, M., Yu, W., Weinberg, J., Shapiro, J., & McElwee, KJ. Development of alopecia areata is associated with higher central and peripheral hypothalamic-pituitary-adrenal tone in the skin graft induced C3H/HeJ mouse model. *Journal of Investigative Dermatology*, Vol.129, No.6, (June 2009), pp.1527-1538, ISSN: 0022-202X

Zhou, Z., Kawana, S., Aoki, E., Katayama, M., Nagano, M., & Suzuki, H. Dynamic changes in nerve growth factor and substance P in the murine hair cycle induced by depilation. *The Journal of dermatology*, Vol.33, No.12, (December 2006), pp.833–841, ISSN: 0385-2407

Zhou, C., Yu, X., Cai, D., Liu, C., & Li, C. Role of corticotropin-releasing hormone and receptor in the pathogenesis of psoriasis. *Medical Hypotheses*, Vol.73, No.4, (October 2009), pp.513-515, ISSN: 0306-9877

Zhou, CL., Yu, XJ., Chen, LM., Jiang, H., & Li, CY. Corticotropin-releasing hormone attenuates vascular endothelial growth factor release from human HaCaT keratinocytes. *Regulatory peptides*, Vol.25, No.160, (February 2010), pp.115-120, ISSN: 0167-0115

Zouboulis, CC., Seltmann, H., Hiroi, N., Chen, W., Young, M., Oeff, M., Scherbaum, WA., Orfanos, CE., McCann, SM., & Bornstein, SR. Corticotropin-releasing hormone: an autocrine hormone that promotes lipogenesis in human sebocytes. *Proceedings of the National Academy of Sciences of the United States of America*, Vol.14, No.99, (May 2002), pp. 7148-7153, ISSN: 0027-8424

12

Use of Reconstructed Skin Specimens to Analyze *Stratum corneum* Remodeling and Epidermal Modifications

Paolo U. Giacomoni, Kelly Dong, Donald Collins,
Nadine Pernodet and Daniel Yarosh
Clinique Laboratories, Melville, NY
Estee Lauder Research Park, Melville, NY
USA

1. Introduction

The epidermis is the epithelial tissue lining the dermis. It is constituted of differentiating keratinocytes distributed in successive layers according to their degree of differentiation. It contains cycling cells with neurological, immune and sensorial functions, such as Langerhans cells, melanocytes, Swan cells, Merkel cells. The upper layers of the epidermis are constituted by fully differentiated corneocytes which constitute the *stratum corneum* or horny layer.

The *stratum corneum* constitutes the interface between the body and the outside world. It modulates the exchanges of oxygen and water vapor with the environment. It harbors enzymes which contribute to its healthy maintenance. Some enzymes help the steady state renewal of the surface by cutting the inter-corneocyte bonds and allowing outer-layer corneocytes to be shed. Others catalyze the synthesis of factors of moisturization, such as urea. Other enzymes such as RNase fight viral infections while the colonization of the skin by film forming microorganisms is averted by proteases like trypsin and chymotrypsin. Defensins, specific peptides in the *stratum corneum* originating from sebaceous gland, exert an efficient anti-bacterial action.

The *stratum corneum* reflects and refracts visible light and is thus partially responsible for the image of the individual in the eyes of the observer. When the *stratum corneum* is not in its optimal state, it is felt as conferring dryness, roughness, lack of flexibility, or general discomfort to the skin. Learning about the structure of the *stratum corneum*, and about ways to modify it to achieve a smooth, supple, flexible, extensible, translucent, shiny surface is one of the objects of surface biochemistry and of cosmetically-oriented scientific research.

Reconstructed skin specimens can be prepared by mixing fibroblasts in a collagen suspension, allowing it to gellify and seeding keratinocytes on the top of it. Air exposed keratinocytes do differentiate and the cells can be kept alive for several days by feeding growth medium underneath the specimen (Prunieras *et al*, 1983).

It is possible to explore the structure of the *stratum corneum* of reconstructed skin and to investigate the chemical or physical-chemical parameters which contribute to its structure. The absence of sebaceous glands, sweat glands, blood vessels or nervous endings makes it

simpler to study the effect of particular chemicals on the structure of the horny layer because of the absence of components difficult to control such as sebum lipids or sweat salts. Reconstructed skin specimens can also be used to assess the synthesis of molecules relevant to the structure and to the physiology of keratinocytes in the latest stages of differentiation. For instance, filaggrin (**fil**ament **aggr**egating prote**in**) is derived from the maturation of Pro-filaggrin which is a major component of keratohyalin granules (Sandiland *et al*, 2009, Chen *et al*, 2008). During differentiation, Pro-filaggrin is dephosphorylated and cleaved by serine proteases to form monomeric filaggrin which then binds to and condenses keratin filaments to trigger squame biogenesis. Within the squames, filaggrin is citrullinated by peptidyl-arginine de-aminases. This promotes its unfolding (from keratin) and further degradation by Caspase 14 to generate hygroscopic amino acids in the biogenesis of the so called Natural Moisturizing Factors, to which urea is eventually added, as the final catabolite of arginine *via* the action of arginase. Reconstructed skin specimens can be treated with biochemical moieties to explore their effect on filaggrin maturation and degradation.
Reconstructed skin specimens can also be prepared to contain melanocytes mixed with keratinocytes (Klausner *et al*, 1995). These specimens (MelanoDerm) allow one to explore the effect of specific treatments on the synthesis, the turnover and the overall accumulation of melanin. Melanocytes in the basal layer spontaneously produce melanin, allowing the specimens to progressively darken.

2. Materials and methods

2.1 Analysis of the stratum corneum

Specimens of reconstructed skin were purchased from MatTek Corporation (Ashland, MA) and were as described (Hayden *et al*, 2003). Upon reception, the specimens were dipped in growth medium EFT-400-ASY as provided by MatTek Corp, and incubated overnight at 37° C in a CO_2 oven. After incubation, the growth medium was removed and the test material, dissolved in water or ethanol, was added (40 µl per specimen) and allowed four hours at room temperature. After this incubation, as much as possible of the 40 µl were removed with a micro-pipette and the specimen fixed with 2.5% glutaraldehyde in water, for 44 hours, then stored in 70% ethanol and processed for histology analysis as described (Sheehan & Hrapchak, 1987, or in the Manual of Histologic Staining Methods of the Armed Forces Institute of Pathology -Third Edition). Upon punching a "biopsy" in the specimen of treated or untreated reconstructed skin, fixed with 2.5% glutaraldehyde, MatTek rafts were removed from ring and placed in a tissue cassette. Samples were processed through Ethanol, xylene, and paraffin for 11 hours on a TissueTek VIP tissue processor. Samples were bisected and embedded in Blue Ribbon Embedding Media (cat# 3801360) from Surgipath (Richmond, IL). Sections were cut at 5 microns on a RM2135 microtome from Leica Microsystems (Bannockburn, IL) and placed on Surgipath Apex glass slides (cat# 3800082). Slides were heated overnight at 70 degrees C. Slides were stained with Hematoxylin and Eosin-Phloxine (cat #s S2697 & S176) from Poly-Scientific (Bay Shore, NY) and coverslipped with resinous mounting media. Microscopy analysis allows one to assess the percent of "damaged" surface which is visible in one microscope field. Figure 1 displays typical histology images. In our experimental conditions (magnification x10), every section was comprised in four fields and eight sections per biopsy were examined. The percent damage in every field (determined as described in the legend of figure 1) were added to yield a number, the parameter of damage or d-value, which is equal to or larger than zero and smaller than or equal to 3,200 ($0 \leq d \leq 3{,}200$).

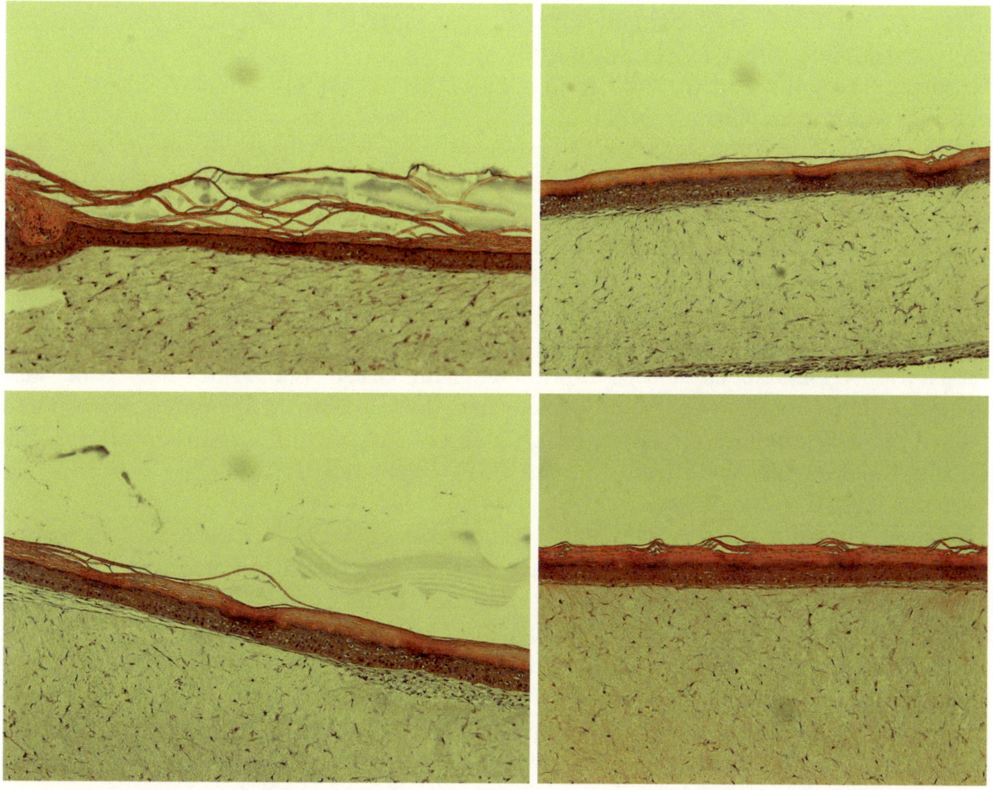

Fig. 1. Calculating d-value from histology images. The percent of surface damage in a field can be determined while observing the sections under the microscope. The top-left image has 100% surface damage, the top-right image has ~57% surface damage, the bottom-left image has ~52% damage, and the bottom-right image has 42% damage. The sum of the percent damage per field, summed over the 32 fields of eight sections, yields the damage parameter or d-value.

2.2 Surface remodeling

2.2.1 Chemicals used for surface remodeling experiments

Acrylates: Daitosol 5000 AD, Daitosol 5000 SJ, Daitosol 4000 SJT and Daitosol 5000 STY (Acrylates/Ethylhexyl Acrylate copolymers and Acrylates co-polymers) were from Kobo (South Plainfield, NJ). Galactorabinan was from Elemente (Jericho, NY). Styleze was from International Specialty Products (Wayne, NJ) and Simulgel was from Seppic (Paris, France).

Alkylated silicones. SF1632 and SF 16 42 were from Kobo (South Plainfield, NJ).

Ceramides. ω-3 ceramides from linen, ω-6 ceramides from wheat, primrose, cotton and safflower, as well as ω-9 ceramides were from Solabia (Pantin, France) and Lipowheat (total ceramides from wheat) were from Hitex-Lavipharm (Pentaparc, France).

Polysaccharides and muchopolysaccharides. Hyaluronic acid was from CPN (Dolni Dobrouc, Czech Republic). Unitamuron (poly-saccharide), and Unichondrin (mucho-poly-saccharide) were from Induchem (Volketswil, Switzerland). Fucogel, Glycofilm, Glycolift, Fucocert were from Solabia (Pantin, France), Fucoidan YSK was from Yaizu Suisankagaku Industries (Shizuoka, Japan) Crystalhyal, Stimulhyal and Soligel were from Soliance

(Allendale, NJ), Clearogel (scleroglucan) was from MMP (Plainfield, New Jersey). Maltrin (maltodextrin) was from GPC (Muscatine, Iowa).

Hydrolyzed proteins. Sericin, Silk Peptides, Silk Powder and Silk Amino Acids were from Sandream Enterprises (Chatam, NJ).

Proteins and Protein/polysaccharide mixtures Uniprosyn (oat proteins) was from Induchem (Volketswil, Switzerland). Reductine and Tensine were from Silab (Brive, France). Argatensyl was from Cognis (Pulnoy, France). Vegetensor was from Alban Muller (Vincennes, France). Functional keratin was from Keratech (Christchurch, NZ).

Hydrogenated poly-isobutenes. Perleam and Perleam 4 were from Rossow USA (Highland, NJ)

Lecithins and Hydrogenated Lecithins. Cerasome and Lipoid SLM were from Lipoid GmbH (Ludwigshafen, Germany). Liposomes with Green Tea, White Tea, Aloe Vera, Guarana, White Hibiscus were from Cosmetochem (Steinhausen, Switzerland), Merospheres were from AGI-dermatics (Freeport, NY). LipidureA, Lipidure B, Lipidure PMP,Lipidure NR and Lipidure NA were from Rossow USA (Highlands, NJ). Edemin was from Res Pharma (Trezzo d' Adda, Italy).

Exfoliators. Salicylic acid encapsulated in liposomes under the trade names Catezomes (~20% salicylic acid) or Salisomes (~10% Salicylic acid) was from BASF (Florham Park, NJ)

Lipids and Lipido-peptides Pellicer was fromAsahi Kasei Corp (Tokyo, Japan). N-Acetyl-L-Hydroxyproline was from Kyowa Hakko Bio Co.-Presperse (Somerset, NJ). Vitaskin E was from Solabia (Pantin, France). Buckwheat (capric/caprylic acid triglyceride) was from Barnet (Englewood Cliffs, NJ), Linoleamide was from Solabia (Pantin, France). Skinmimics was from Evonik (Essen, Germany). Lutein was from Kemin, Zenigloss was from Ultra (Red bank, NJ). Phytantriol (tetra-methyl-hexadecane) was from DSM (Kaiseraugst, Switzerland). Koboguard 5400 SQ (hydrogenated polycyclopentadiene) was from Kobo (South Plainfield, NJ).

Saccharides. Pulpactyl, Cohesium and Recoverine were from Silab (Brive, France)

Surfactants and Emulsifiers. Arlacel 165 (glyceryl stearate) was from Uniqema (New Castle, De). Olivoil glutamate was from Kalichem (Botticino Sera, Italy). Net-Won (tetra-alkyl-ammonium hectoride, polyglyceryl isostearate, polyglyceryl-6-polyricinoleate) was from Barnet (Edgewood Cliffs, NJ). Neogloss (isodecyl neopentanoate) and Crystalcast (ß-sitosterol, cetyl alcohol, stearyl alcohol, sucrose stearate/distearate) were from MMP (Plainfield, NJ). Dermofat (octadecanoic acid) was from Alzo International (Sayreville, NJ).

Gums. Easyliance (Acacia Senegal Gum and Hydrolyzed Rhizobian Gum) was from Soliance (Allendale, NJ)

Succinamides. Chitosan succinamide was from MMP (South Plainfield, NJ)

Poly-imides. Aquaflex was from International Specialty Products (Wayne, NJ)

Silanol-polysaccharides and PEG-silicones. Zenester was from Ultra (Red Bank, NJ). Epidermosil was from Exsymol (Montecarlo, Monaco).

Polyurethanes. Baycusan 1000, Baycusan 1003 and Baycusan 1004 were from Bayer (Leverkusen, Germany).

Plant aqueous extracts Dansonyl, Dulcemin and Vegeseryl were from Cognis (Pulnoy, France), Caviar Lime, Pepperberry, Tasmanian pepper, Riberry, Kakadu, Illiwara and Bush Plum were from Southern Cross Botanical (Knockrow, NSW, Australia). Dragon was from IBR (Rehovot, Israel).Hydra Kanzu and Ejitsu Rose were from Barnet (Englewood Cliffs, NJ)

2.2.2 Procedure to test

The test materials were applied on the top of MatTek specimens at concentrations ranging between 1 and 3 % in water (w/v). In some instances concentrations were kept lower (0.1%) to avoid excessive viscosity or gels. In some instances (e.g. with poly-acrylates) dose-response curves were generated, with concentrations ranging from 3% to 15%. Plant-derived ceramides were not soluble in water or in ethanol, so the tested material was the supernatant of a dispersion of those materials at 1% in ethanol.

2.3 Analysis of filaggrin catabolism and metabolism

Altermonas macleodi exopolysacharrides were from Unipex Innovations (Quebec, Canada) and Aquaflex (water extract of *Citrullus vulgaris*) was from Barnet (Englewood, NJ). They were dissolved at 1% or 3% in growth medium and were applied on the top of the MatTek specimens in a 100 µl volume

Upon incubation at 37 C for 2-24 hours, the specimens were fixed with 10% Formalin for 24 hours at room temperature and sections were prepared for immunohistochemistry analysis. Sections were treated with citrate buffer and heated to achieve antigen retrieval and incubated with commercially available anti-filaggrin antibody from Abcam (Cambridge, UK) followed by incubation with the secondary antibody, Vulcan Red alkphos chromagen and finally counterstained with Hematoxylin/Eosine.

2.4 Analysis of melanocyte-containing reconstructed skin

2.4.1 Tissue culture

Melanocyte-containing epidermis on dermis equivalent MelanoDerm) was as described (Klausner *et al*, 1995, Klausner, 1997). MelanoDerm B inserts (Lot #10790, Kit E & Lot #11625, Kit B) from MatTek (Ashland, MA) were stored at 4°C upon receipt. The inserts were incubated in 1 mL of maintenance media (Cat#EPI-100-NMM-113, Lot# 012309TTF & Lot# 040909TTE, MatTek) for 1 h at 37°C in a 5% CO_2 humidified incubator. Then the inserts were placed on top of culture stands (Cat# MEL-STND, MatTek) in 5 mL maintenance media in 6 well plates. The inserts were kept in the incubator when not receiving treatments or being photographed. Maintenance media were changed every other day.

2.4.2 Chemicals and treatments

Cyclohexadecanol was purchased from Barnet (Englewood, NJ). Kojic acid was from Sigma (Saint Louis, MO). The inserts were treated with non-ionic, oil in water emulsions containing 1% Cyclohexadecanol or 0.5% Cyclohexadecanol or 2% Kojic Acid daily (except for weekends) for 21 days. 2.3 µl of each emulsion were pipetted so that the amount of lotion left on the insert was 2 µl after application with the tip of a sterile glass rod. Prior to application, the inserts were washed by vigorously pipetting Phosphate Buffered Saline (PBS) (Cat#DPBS-100, Lot# 043007tvka, MatTek) on the surface, with two changes of PBS.

2.4.3 Microscopy

Each day the inserts were observed under 300x magnification with a Nikon Diaphot (Ontario, NY) microscope. Pictures were taken daily after washing and prior to treatment. Each insert was placed in a sterile 24-well plate, a small amount of PBS was pipetted below the insert, and then the plate was placed on to the microscope stage. The intensity of the melanin in the melanocytes was analyzed with the D.E. Light program. Macroscopic photographs were also taken with an Olympus SZH10 stereo microscope at 0.7X magnification.

2.4.5 Histology

After 14 days the inserts were rinsed in PBS and then fixed by incubating overnight in 10% formalin (Cat# HT501128) from Sigma (Saint Louis, MO) at 4°C. Then the inserts were placed in small containers filled with PBS and sent to Paragon Bioservices Inc (Baltimore, MD. for sectioning and staining with the Fontana-Masson stain. Pictures were taken at 400X with an Olympus BX60 microscope. The area of the section occupied by melanin was determined with the D.E. Light program.

2.4.6 Viability

The alamar blue viability test was performed as described (Ahmed *et al*, 1994; Hamid *et al*, 2004). A 10% alamar blue solution was made by combining 12 mL alamar blue (Cat#DAL1100, Lot# 149661SA) from Invitrogen) (Carlsbad, CA) with 108 mL maintenance media. The maintenance media was removed from each well and replaced with 5 mL of 10% alamar blue in each well. The inserts were incubated in 10% alamar blue for 2 h and then removed. The fluorescence of the medium in each well was measured on the Spectra Max Gemini XPS fluorescent plate reader (Molecular Devices, Sunnyvale, CA) at 530 nm excitation and 590 nm emission.

The viability test was done every week.

2.4.7 Melanin quantitative assay

After treatment with test materials and incubation for several days (up to three weeks) the specimens were removed from the plastic insert and placed in 250 µl Solvable (Cat#6NE9100, lot#140-090101) from Perkin Elmer (Waltham, MA) in a 1.7 mL microfuge tube. Tissues were incubated overnight at 60°C. Samples were vortexed and then centrifuged at 13,000 rpm for 5 minutes. 200 µl of the samples were pipetted into a 96-well plate read at 490 nm on the spectrophotometer and measured against melanin standards.

For spectro-photometrical measurements of melanin, tissues were removed from the plastic insert and placed in 250 µl Solvable in a 1.7 mL microfuge tube, incubated overnight at 60°C, vortexed and then centrifuged at 13,000 rpm for 5 minutes. 200 µl of the supernatant of every sample were transferred into the wells of a 96-well plate and read at 490 nm on the spectrophotometer Spectramax 190 (Molecular Devices, Sunnyvale, CA) and measured against melanin standards.

3. Results

3.1 Structure of the *stratum corneum*

The d-values of the *stratum corneum* of 58 untreated specimens displayed a unimodal distribution centered around a d-value = 500 with a 90 % confidence interval situated between 200 and 1,500 (Figure 2). Treating the specimens with water or ethanol did not result in striking differences as far as the d-values are concerned (data not shown). The distribution histogram for all the treated specimens (n=140) is reported in Figure 3. This histogram represents a multi-modal distribution centered at 0-100, 500 and 1100. This result seems to indicate that certain treatments might indeed reduce the d-value of the untreated specimens, whereas other treatments might damage the surface or leave it as in the control. In order to point out treatments which efficiently reduce the d-values of the surface, the distribution histograms of the d-values after treatment with substances belonging to the same chemical family, have been plotted (Figures 4 - 8). Treating the specimens with specific chemical families such as some polysaccharides, hydrogenated lecithins, plant-derived ceramides and proteins associated to polysaccharides resulted in a reduction of the d-values to values comprised between 0 and 200, as displayed in Figures 4-7. Two alkylated silicones gave d-values d=0. (data not shown). The addition of salicylic acid-containing liposomes (an exfoliator) also dramatically reduces the d-value (data not shown). On the other hand, acrylates or polyacrylates (Figure 8), hydrolyzed proteins, mono- or oligosaccharides, hydrogenated poly-isobutenes, styrene-acrylate co-polymers (data not shown) do not reduce the d-value, and sometimes they increase it. In some instances, detergents and silicones provide d-values close to zero, but detergents also dramatically reduce the thickness of the *stratum corneum* and the treatment with some silicones seems to provoke pyknotic nuclei and periplasmic edema in a majority of keratinocytes below the horny layers (data not shown).

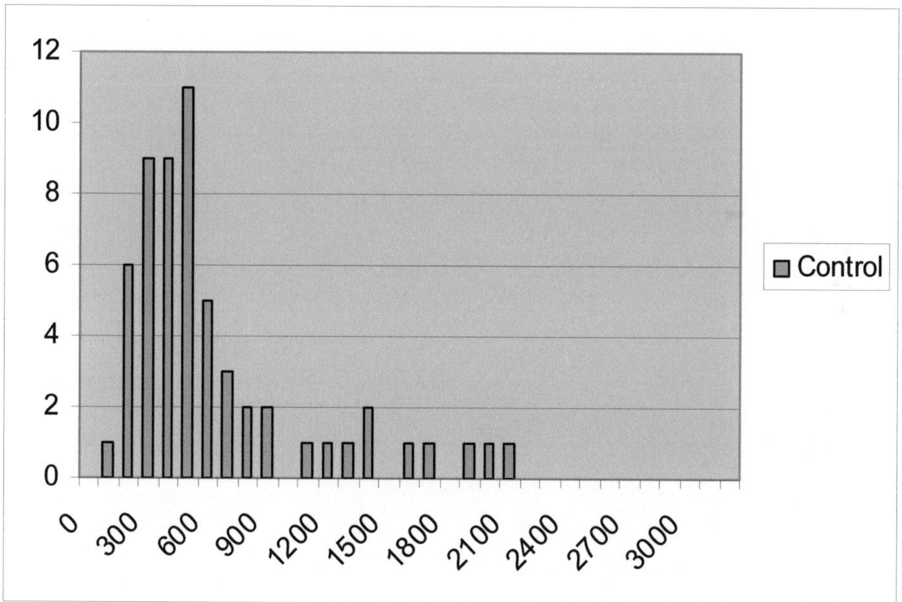

The plot represents a uni-modal distribution centered at d=500

Fig. 2. Histogram of distribution of d-values for 58 untreated controls.

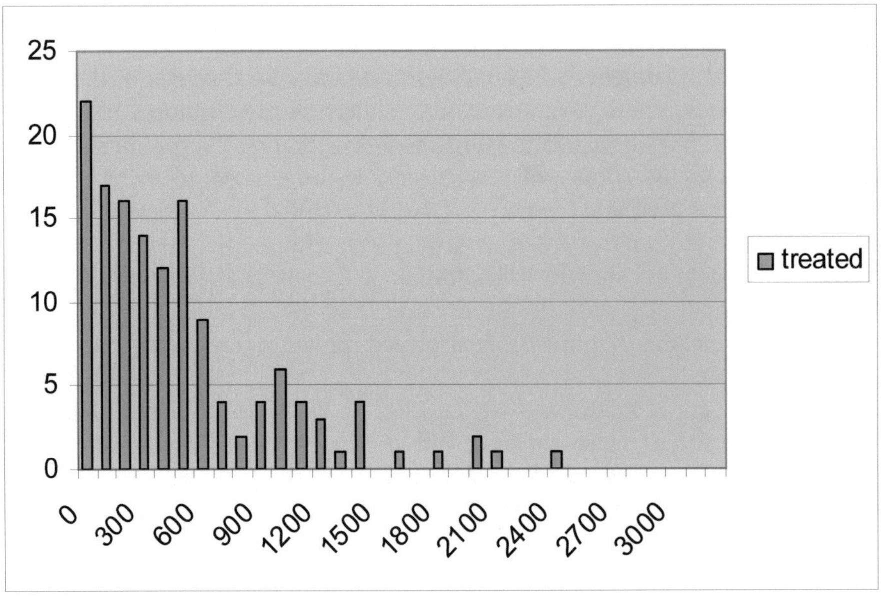

The plot represents a multi-modal distribution centered at 0-100, 500 and 1100.

Fig. 3. Histogram of distribution of d-values for 140 differently treated samples.

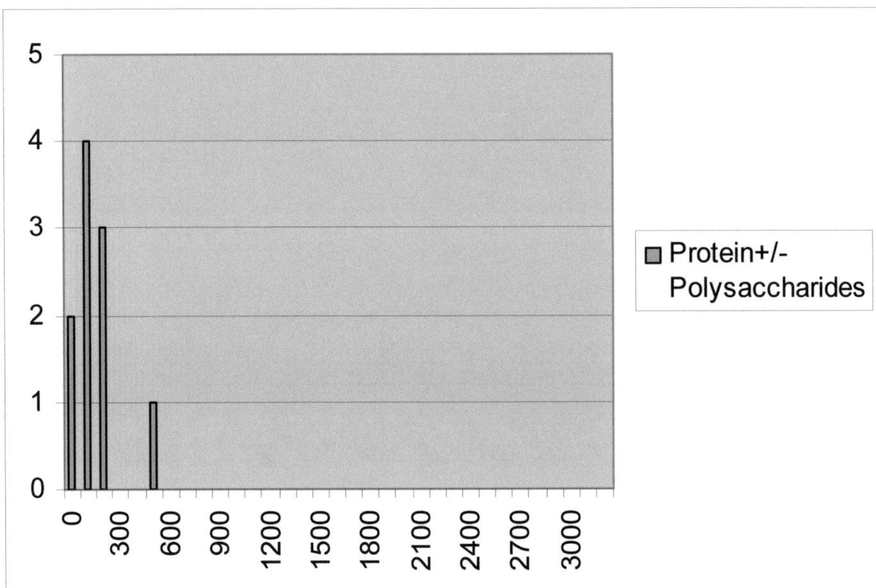

Fig. 4. Histogram of distribution of d-values for specimens treated with ten protein-polysaccharide mixtures.

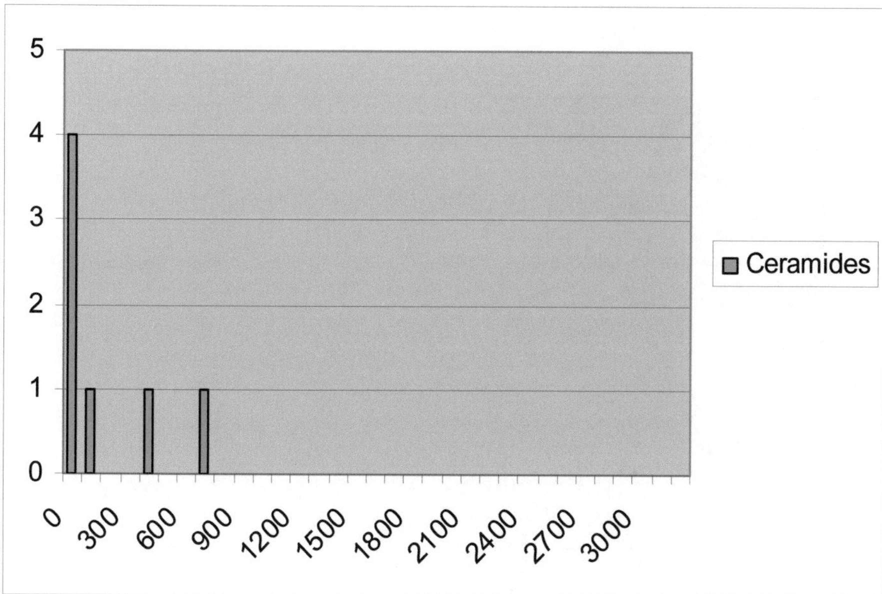

Fig. 5. Histogram of distribution of d-values for specimens treated with seven plant-derived ceramides

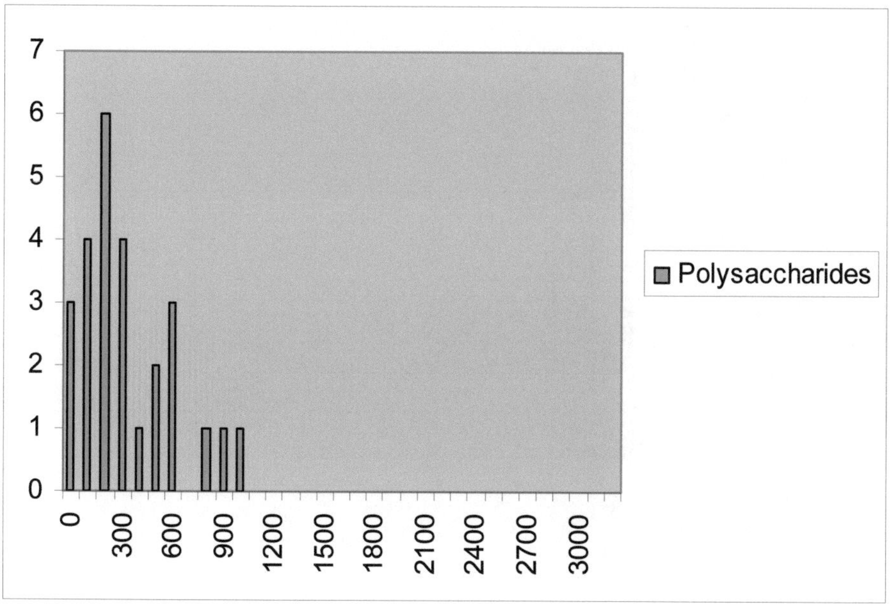

Fig. 6. Histogram of distribution of d-values for specimens treated with 26 polysaccharides

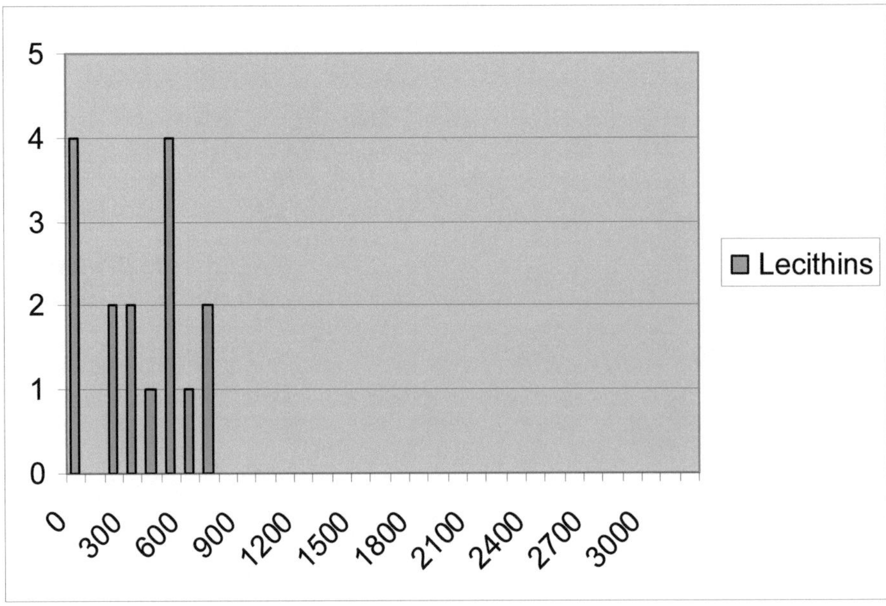

The three hydrogenated lecithins used in this study gave d-values d= 0 or 83 or 252.

Fig. 7. Histogram of distribution of d-values for specimens treated with 16 lecithins.

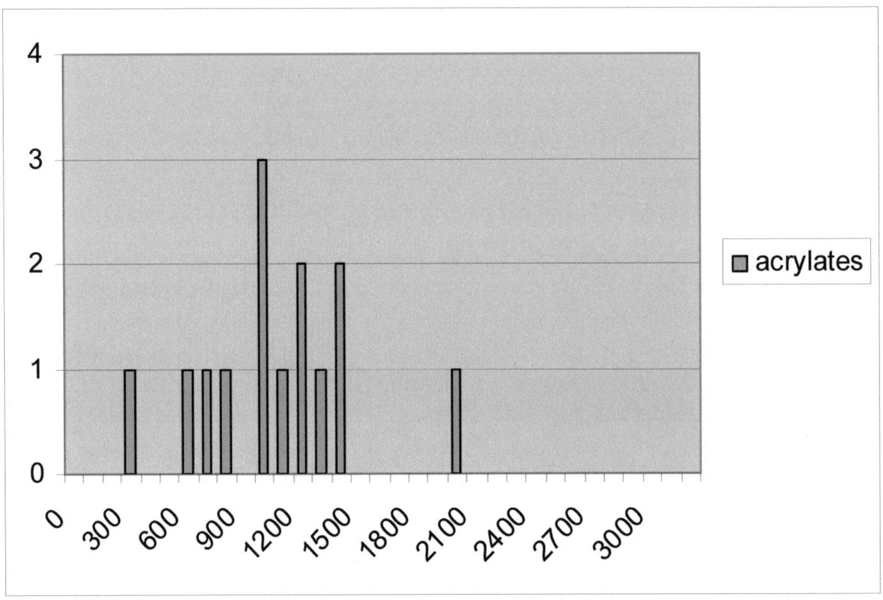

Fig. 8. Histogram of distribution of d-values for 14 specimens treated with acrylates or polyacrylates.

3.2 Analysis of filaggrin

Filaggrin (filament aggregating protein) matures from pro-filaggrin which is a major component of the keratohyalin granule. During the maturation process, pro-filaggrin is dephosphorylated and cleaved by serine proteases to form monomeric filaggrin which binds to and condenses keratin filaments to trigger squame biogenesis (Figure 9a). We have observed that 2 and 24 hours after topical treatment with bacterial exo-polysaccharides, the *stratum corneum* staining associated with filaggrin was dramatically increased (Figure 9b). Similar results were obtained with water extracts from *Citrullus vulgaris* (Figure 9c). These results indicate that the *stratum corneum* can be stained with anti-filaggrin antibodies as early as two hours after treatment, and that this effect lasts for at least twenty four hours. The kinetics aspects of these results are in keeping with the suggestion that bacterial exo-polysaccharide stimulates more the maturation of pro-filaggrin than the induction of the expression of the gene of pro-filaggrin.

Media 2 hour

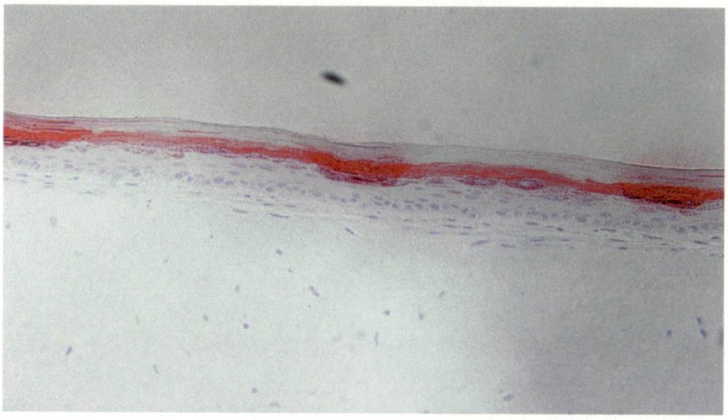

Media 24 hour

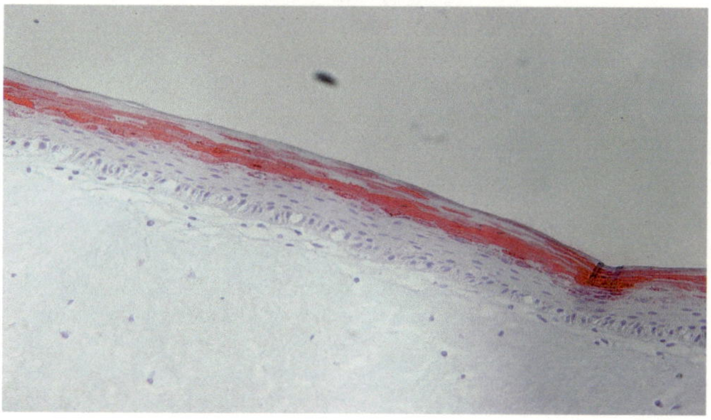

Fig. 9a. Filaggrin in the *stratum corneum* of MatTek specimens after 2 (top panel) or 24 hours (bottom panel). Media-treated control

Exo H 1% 2 hour

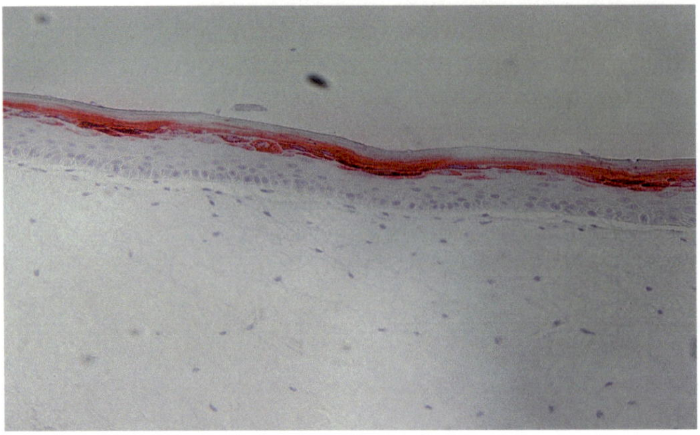

Exo H 1% 24 hour

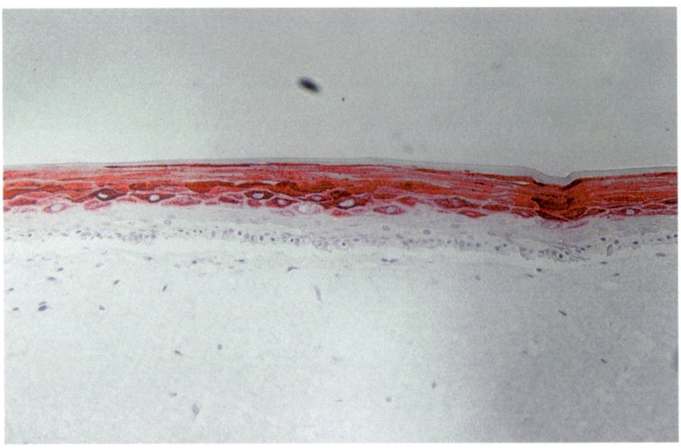

Fig. 9b. Filaggrin in the *stratum corneum* of MatTek specimens after 2 (top panel) or 24 hours (bottom panel). Samples treated with Bacterial Exopolysaccharide H (Exo H). Histology sections from ExoH-treated MatTek specimens, after 2 (top panel) and 24 (bottom panel) hours incubation.

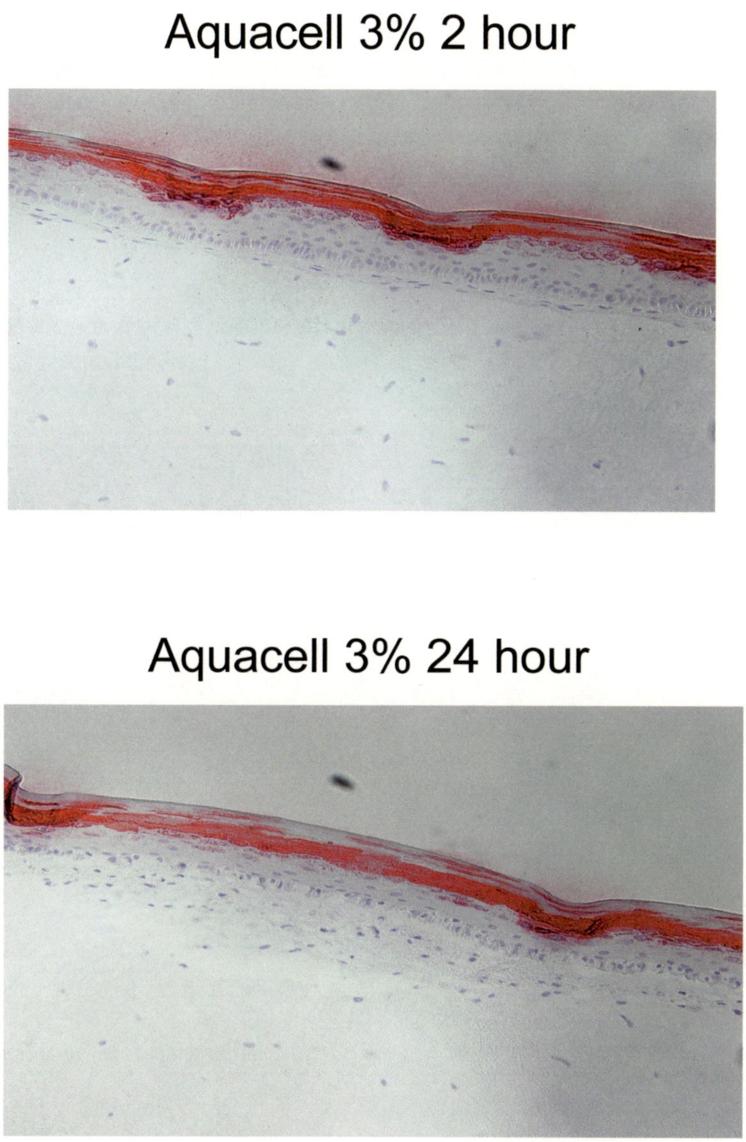

Fig. 9c. Filaggrin in the *stratum corneum* of MatTek specimens after 2 or 24 hours. Histology sections from Aquacell-treated MatTek specimens, after 2 (top panel) and 24 (bottom panel) hours incubation.

3.3 Analysis of pigmentation in melanoderm specimens

3.3.1 Viability

Cyclohexadecanol and kojic acid did not affect the viability at 7, 14, or 21 days (data not shown).

3.3.2 Histology sections

Figure 10 shows histology sections of MelanoDerm B specimens treated with 2% kojic acid or with 0.5% and 1% Cyclohexadecanol

After two weeks of daily treatment with 2% kojic acid or 0.5% or 1% cyclohexadecanol, the surface occupied by melanin in Melanoderm sections stained with Fontana-Masson staining decreased by 20%, 31% and 45% respectively. When melanin is assessed spectrophotometrically, the reduction induced by 0.5% or by 1% cyclohexadecanol is 27% and 29% respectively.

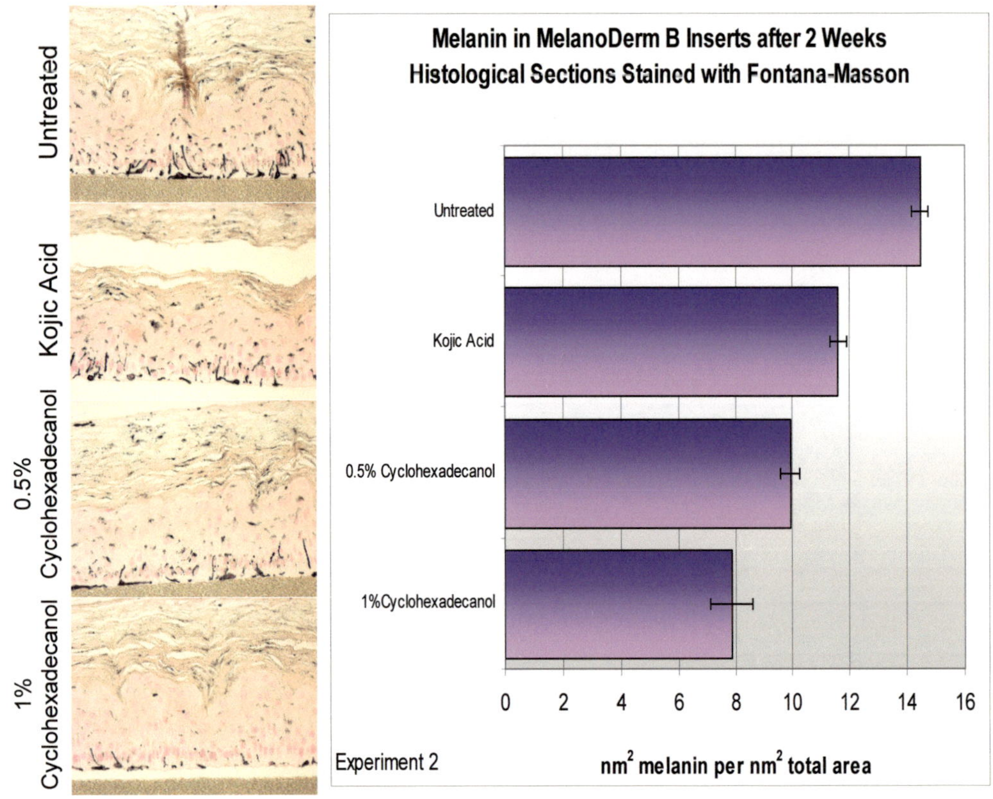

Fig. 10. Determination of melanin in Fontana-Masson stained sections of biopsies from differently treated MelanoDerm specimens

4. Discussion

Models of reconstructed skin have been prepared, which allow one to analyze large number of biopsies without infringing the ethical code which limits the experimentations on human volunteers. Cosmetics address healthy skin and reconstructed skin is suitable for cosmetic studies. The outer layer of the surface of the skin, the *stratum corneum*, plays an important role in skin smoothness, moisturization and color, it is therefore important to have a reproducible methodology at hand, to study the effects of xenobiotics on its structure and properties. Reconstructed skin is appropriate to undergo biopsy treatment and allows one to screen xenobiotics for their cosmetic properties. The structure of the horny layer is smoother after treatment with substances belonging to defined chemical classes, whereas other chemicals do not reduce the roughness of the surface, and sometimes they increase it. These results are helpful in guiding the formulation chemist in selecting ingredients for cosmetic products aimed at the smoothening of the skin.

Biopsies from specimens treated with bacterial exopolysaccharides or water extracts from *Citrullus vulgaris* increase the *stratum corneum* immuno-staining associated with filaggrin within hours after application, in keeping with an action on the maturation process more than with the induction of gene expression. This method is helpful for the formulation chemist in selecting ingredients for cosmetic products aimed at improving the overall moisturization of the epidermis.

Biopsies punched in melanocytes-containing specimens after two weeks of daily treatment with kojic acid or 0.5% or 1% cyclohexadecanol indicate that the surface occupied by melanin in histology sections stained with Fontana-Masson staining decreased by 20%, 31% and 45% respectively. These results indicate that MelanoDerm is appropriate to experiments aiming at selecting ingredients for topical application to reduce the visibility of surface discoloration

5. References

Ahmed, S.A., Gogal, R.M., & Walsh, J.I. (1994) A new rapid and simple non-radioactive assay to monitor and determine the proliferation of lymphocytes: an alternative to [^{3}H]-Thymidine incorporation assay. J. Immunol. Methods 170, 211-224

Chen, H., Ho,J.C.C., Sandilands, A., Chan, Y.C., Giam, Y.C., Evans, A.T., Lane, E.B., and McLean, W.H.I. (2008) Unique and Recurrent Mutations in the Filaggrin Gene in Singaporean Chinese Patients with Ichthyosis Vulgaris. J. Invest Dermatol 128, 1669–1675

Klausner, M. (1997).. "Latest *In Vitro* Testing Methods for Skin Care, Cosmetics, and Household Products," Presented at International Business Conference, Washington, D.C.,

Klausner, M., Kubilus, J., Neal, P.J. Initial characterization of an epidermal model containing functional melanocytes J. Invest. Dermatology, 104(4), 616, Abstr. # 370 (1995).

Manual of Histologic Staining Methods of the Armed Forces Institute of Pathology (Third Edition). American Registry of Pathology (Luna, Lee G., HT(ASCP) (editor)), McGraw Hill Publishers, New York 1960

Hayden, P.J., Kubilus, J., Burnham, B., Jackson, G.R. and Klausner, M. Epiderm full thickness (EPIDERM-FT™), a dermal – based dermal-epidermal skin model with a fully developed basement membrane The Toxicologist, 72, S1, 158 (2003).

Pruniéras M, Régnier M, Woodley D. (1983) Methods for cultivation of keratinocytes with an air-liquid interface. J Invest Dermatol. 81 : 28s-33s.

Sheehan, B.B. and Hrapchak, D.C.; (1987) Theory and Practice of Histotechnology; p138, CV Mosby

Sandilands, A., Sutherland, C, Irvine, A.D. and McLean, W.H.I. (2009) Filaggrin in the frontline: role in skin barrier function and disease Journal of Cell Science 122, 1285-1294

13

Keratinocyte Culture Techniques in Medical and Scientific Applications

Stefanie Kuhn, Christine Radtke,
Christina Allmeling, Peter M. Vogt and Kerstin Reimers
Department of Plastic, Hand and Reconstructive Surgery, Medical School Hannover, Germany

1. Introduction

Human skin is a complex organ essentially organized in a thin non-vascular epidermis, a thick collagenous dermis, and subcutaneous fat tissue called hypodermis. The epidermis is subdivided into five layers termed: stratum corneum, stratum lucidum, stratum granulosum, stratum spinosum, and stratum germinativum. Furthermore, skin appendages, like hair follicles and glands, are derived from the epidermis but project deep into the dermis (Priya et al, 2008). They fulfil specialized functions for body homeostasis and temperature control.

Cellular differentiation and growth follow precise temporal and spatial patterns. In the epidermis constant replacement of cells lost by desquamation in the outer layers by cells of the basal layers takes place (Atiyeh & Costagliola, 2007). The basal layers of the epidermis retain two cell populations with different proliferation capacity: stem cells with high potential for self-renewal have low level proliferation rates but retain their ability to generate daughter cells throughout life; other cells display high frequencies of cell divisions but finally are destined for terminal differentiation. These cells are called transit-amplifying (TA) cells. Epidermal stem cells have been found in the bulge region of hair follicles and in the epidermal bottom of the deep rete ridges (Lorenz et al, 2009). After wounding, keratinocyte stem cells contribute to wound closure by giving rise to daughter cells which migrate to the site of defect (Ito et al, 2005).

Human keratinocyte stem cells and TA cells can be differentiated by their panel of cell surface marker gene expression; while stem cell markers CD29 and CD49f are highly expressed in both cell types, the transferring receptor CD71 is expressed in higher amounts in the rapidly proliferating TA cells (Lorenz et al, 2009). Moreover, keratinocyte stem cells have the ability to grow clonogenically with the number of colony-forming units, obtained per mm^2 skin biopsies, varying between 94 and 3190. The growth potential of clonogenic keratinocytes can be differentiated by the morphological appearance of the colonies: colonies with significant growth potential (holoclones and meroclones) contain mostly small cells and have a regular round appearance, paraclones, however, contain large, terminally differentiated cells and appear rather irregular (Ronfard et al, 2000). Due to the restricted growth potential of terminally differentiated cells colony-forming units increase when kept under ideal culture conditions. Conditions supporting keratinocyte differentiation, however, decrease growth potential of the culture.

2.1 Cultured epithelial autografts

In the treatment of burn surgery, considerable technical progress in intensive care management, ventilation, resuscitation and nutrition, directed in specialized burn centres, greatly improved the survival rates of severely burned patients. Early tangential excision and quick skin grafting to limit inflammation and restore skin barrier function are applied at large wounds changing the repair process basically from wound healing to graft-take (Ehrlich, 2004). Beside the clear advantages of an early restoration of the outer barrier of the body thus preventing infection, fluid loss and catabolism, the practice of grafting minimizes granulation tissue to the thin space between skin graft and wound bed leading to scar reduction (Ehrlich, 2004). In the same time autologous material used for split thickness skin autografts is limited by massive tissue destruction and/or unsuited donor sites (e.g. hands and face). In order to replace autografts a number of approaches have been developed, essentially they are either based on the use of acellular matrices, transfer of cultured cells or a combination of both.

Since the 80ties of the last century the use of autologous keratinocytes has been reported by different burn centres and established as an alternative for severely burned patients with little donor skin (De Corte et al, 2011). Keratinocyte transplantation after burns and in chronic wound treatment is potentially useful in clinical practice to improve functional outcome in burn patients. After the establishment of keratinocyte growth on a mitotically inactivated and lethally irradiated feeder layer of murine embryonic fibroblasts (Rheinwald & Green, 1975) first clinical application of graftable epithelia (cultured epithelial autografts, CEA) for treatment of burns was reported by O'Connor et al. in 1981 (Atiyeh & Costagliola, 2007). However, general use of CEA in burn treatment is hampered by the extensive infrastructure needed for production of CEA as well as high costs. Technical problems include CEA susceptibility to infection due to a high vulnerability of cultured epithelial sheets to bacterial proteases and toxins. Take rates are variable and depend to a large extent on skilled preparation of the wound bed (Atiyeh & Costagliola, 2007). Histological analyses of the grafts indicate delay in rete ridge formation and basement membrane maturation leading to prolonged skin fragility after wound healing (Rennekampff et al, 1996, Hernon et al, 2006). Critical disadvantages like the loss of clonogenic cells by enzymatic separation of the epithelial sheets from the feeder layers and alteration of integrin expression patterns by high cellular density in the sheets still are in need of technical refinements (Ronfard et al, 2000, Poumay & Pittelkow, 1995). As an alternative to enzymatic treatment, for example use of Ca^{2+}-chelating agents or temperature-responsive culture dishes have been proposed (Ebara et al, 2003, Inoue et al, 2006). Nevertheless, due to the capability of epidermal cells to extensive expansion, CEA is an important means for treatment of large skin defects without the possibility of conventional skin transfer. As an example a 3 cm^2 biopsy is sufficient to cover the body surface of an adult after a 5,000-10,000 fold expansion in a culture period of 3-4 weeks (Williamson et al, 1995).

The growth potential of epidermal cells led to the innovative approach to graft keratinocyte single cell suspensions in non-solid delivery devices e.g. fibrin sealants or lactate solutions (Cervelli et al, 2010, Horch et al, 1998) or microcarriers (Seland et al, 2011). Aerosol spraying techniques have been developed when 2005 the first commercial system Recell® was introduced into clinical practice (Gravante et al, 2007).

Full-thickness skin wounds treated with split thickness autografts, transplanted keratinocytes or CEA with little or no dermal parts tend to poor stability, excessive contracture and scarring. Therefore, many different dermal substitutes are already available commercially, e.g. acellular human or animal dermis like human Alloderm® (Lifecell Corporation, Branchburg, NJ) and porcine Strattice™ (Lifecell Corporation, Branchburg, NJ). Other substitutes are biological derivates, mostly collagen I, like Integra™ (Integra Life Science, Plainsboro, NJ) and Matriderm® (Dr. Suwelack Skin & Health Care, Billerbeck, Germany), or substitutes combining synthetic material with biological material like polyglactin Dermagraft® (Advanced BioHealing, LaJolla, CA) (van der Veen et al, 2010) or Biobrane® (Bertek Pharmaceuticals, Morgantown, WV). Biological constructs might be seeded with autologous or allogenic cells, e.g. Epicel® (Genzyme Tissue Repair) or Apligraf® (Organogenesis, Canton, MA). Interestingly, in contrast to allogenic keratinocytes which provoke strong rejection after restoration of immunocompetence, allogenic fibroblasts are tolerated by the host enabling preparation of fibroblast seeded dermal substitutes prior to use (Coulomb et al, 1998). Nevertheless, autologous cells are favoured by recent reports in terms of functional and aesthetic outcome (Atiyeh & Costagliola, 2007).

Recent progress in innovative approaches, e.g. tissue engineering of living skin equivalents as well as cell transplantation and gene therapies, led to an urgent demand of obtaining pure cell cultures in sufficient amounts and quality. A major obstacle to achieve this aim is the standardization of keratinocyte preparation and the maintenance of pure proliferative cultures. Another potential problem for clinical application of cultured human keratinocytes is the use of serum because of safety issues. Other companies offer recombinant growth factors and enzymes for animal-free production of cell therapeutics like trypsin-like mann, E. (1995). Cultured epithelial autograft: five years of clinical2.**2 Pharmaceutical**

2.2 Pharmaceutical equivalents

Living skin equivalents are not only needed in clinical applications but also in the vast field of experimental research, including the pharmacological and cosmetic industry as in vivo animal experiments should be replaced by in vitro experiments if appropriate. Therefore, alternatives urgently need to be developed. Keratinocytes have been cultured in vitro in a two-dimensional (2D) fashion for a long time, using feeder layers of fibroblasts. Now, the culture of keratinocytes is possible using a special keratinocyte medium without serum which is important for the future use of the cells in animal or human applications (see above). Nevertheless, an organotypic - that is three-dimensional (3D) - culture of skin cells is an important issue as it mimics the natural skin and presents better interaction of the different skin cells.

Skin equivalents have been produced and improved already for a long time, including primary cells or cell lines (Schoop et al, 1999, Marionnet et al, 2006). Now, numerous 3D different skin equivalents exist - either commercially available or in-house equivalents (see below). They may comprise different kinds of cells, materials and structures. Some only include the epidermis while others represent a complete skin containing also a dermis. Also, some use de-epidermized dermis with others being made of fibroblasts integrated into a collagen gel with keratinocytes seeded on top. Constantly, new 3D skin equivalents are being generated and tested for many different purposes.

2.2.1 Use of skin equivalents as alternatives to animal testing

Evaluation of cosmetic ingredients is mainly done by irritancy, toxicity and corrosive testing. Up to now the rabbit Draize test has been used for this purpose, consisting of determination of oedema / erythema after topical application of the test substance. But apart from the animals suffering pain, the prediction of the irritancy potential is not always correct (Macfarlane et al, 2009). As the 3D skin equivalents are physiologically similar to natural skin they present an alternative to animal testing (Mertsching et al, 2008). As such, they can be used for the testing of drugs, cosmetics and other substances like e.g. sunscreens but also for irritancy and toxicity tests as well as for the study of wound healing, cancer research or infection biology. Additionally, skin equivalents offer the possibility to gain more knowledge about the mode of action of (skin) diseases and the according drugs (Ponec, 2002).

2.2.2 Skin barrier function, irritancy and toxicity testing

The skin serves as a barrier and therefore protects us against exogenous harms like environmental hazards, UV-irradiation and pathogenic microbes, but also against endogenous water loss. For the effect of topically applied drugs or cosmetic products, the way of their penetration into the skin is of great importance (Ponec et al, 2001). Here, the stratum corneum serves as the main barrier in the skin and its composition and morphology are major factors in the permeation process of drugs into the skin. Ceramides and lipid composition of the epidermis are important key features with respect to the structure of the epidermis. In this context a model to predict the stratum corneum lipid organization has been developed (Bouwstra et al, 2001). Additionally, the barrier function and organisation of a skin equivalent composed of epidermis reconstructed on de-epidermized dermis (RE-DED) was tested (Ponec et al, 2001). The formation of the stratum corneum barrier in vitro was similar to that in vivo, including all major stratum corneum lipid classes and ceramide fractions, but displaying some differences in the organisation and composition of the fatty acids. Also, the architecture and lipid composition of commercially available skin equivalents (EpiDerm®, Episkin® and SkinEthic®) and the RE-DED skin model were compared (Ponec et al, 2002). The overall ultrastructural appearance of the epidermis in the skin models was similar to that of native skin. Nevertheless, some differences with respect to the differentiation of the keratinocytes and the exact composition of the fatty acids and ceramides were observed. The same skin equivalents were tested in spite of minor variations they were found suitable for the in vitro testing of permeation and percutaneous absorption of topical products like cosmetic ingredients since the reproducibility of such testing was given (Lotte et al, 2002).

On the basis of the aforementioned results, skin equivalents may serve as models for the prediction of human skin irritation, inflammation and toxicity of topically applied substances. Here, single-cell assays under submerged culture conditions, epidermal equivalents, skin equivalents and excised skin under air-liquid-interface culture conditions serve as different kinds of models with different advantages and drawbacks of each (Gibbs, 2009). Now, several commercially available skin equivalents (EpiDerm®, Episkin® and SkinEthic®) are validated as stand-alone test replacements for standard animal experiments (rabbit Draize test) (Macfarlane et al, 2009). But even fifteen years ago, skin models have already been tested for their use in the prediction of skin irritation and for the study of mechanisms of contact irritant dermatitis (Osborne & Perkins, 1994). Three commercially available test systems were analyzed comprising human epidermal keratinocyte cultures (Clonetics), and partially or fully cornified keratinocyte-fibroblast co-cultures (Skin2, Advanced Tissue Sciences and Testskin, Organogenesis). The results of the cell damage measurement in the keratinocyte cultures were not very satisfactory as it did not always correlate with human skin patch data. Different endpoints for the assessment of cytotoxicity and inflammation in response to test formulations were successfully developed in Skin2 and Testskin and proved very useful (Osborne & Perkins, 1994).

Additionally to skin irritations, toxicological testing may be performed on skin equivalents, including phototoxicity, photoprotection and efficacy tests of cosmetic molecules (Damour et al, 1998). The StrataTest® skin model permits the testing of a broad range of test substances. It contains keratinocyte progenitors and forms a fully stratified tissue including epidermal and dermal components and a barrier function of the epidermis (Rasmussen et al, 2010). The skin was exposed to ozone, cigarette smoke or ultraviolet (UV) irradiation, resulting in the formation of reactive oxygen species (ROS). Antioxidants as well as sunscreens could successfully be tested with StrataTest®.

Since nanotechnology has developed very rapidly, humans are exposed to nanoparticles in many different situations. In contrast, the knowledge about their potential harmful effect is still under investigation. As the outer barrier of the body, the skin plays an important role in the nanoparticle penetration and they have been found in different depths and locations in the skin (Smijs & Bouwstra, 2010). The nanoparticles interact with the skin cells and may cause cytotoxicity or undesired immune responses, but the results are often contradicting.

2.2.3 Ultraviolet (UV) irradiation and DNA repair

UV irradiation is present all the time and causes mutations resulting in cancer if the DNA repair system is not functional in the skin cells. Melanin production by melanocytes and sunscreens protect the skin from damage, e.g. DNA changes and tumor formation, and skin equivalents containing a dermis as well as a stratified epidermis can be used to test the effect of sunscreens (Nelson & Gay, 1993). The release of pro-inflammatory mediators was also measured as a response to the UV irradiation.

Skin equivalents may also serve to analyze phenomena like skin photo aging and cancer development (Bernerd, 2005). The effects of different wavelengths of irradiation can be detected in the different layers of the skin. UV-B directly induces DNA lesions and therefore apoptosis in keratinocytes, while UV-A afflicts the dermis through the generation of ROS, fibroblast alterations and extracellular matrix modifications. DNA-repair deficient skin models can be generated by the use of cells (keratinocytes and fibroblasts) from patients with xeroderma pigmentosum. These patients suffer from a severe deficiency in the nucleotide excision repair of UV-induced DNA lesions (Bernerd et al, 2001). These skin equivalents display histological similarities to native skin of patients suffering xeroderma pigementosum and thus may help to achieve a deeper understanding in the fields of photo aging, photo carcinogenesis and tissue therapy. The proliferation of keratinocytes increased while their differentiation was delayed and reduced. Epidermal invasions into the dermis could be shown as seen in native xeroderma pigmentosum tissue.

To achieve a deeper understanding of the mechanisms present in skin, the cellular responses of basal keratinocytes to UV irradiation can be analyzed with the help of skin equivalents comprising a dermis and a differentiated epidermis. The basal keratinocytes can be divided into two subgroups, one of which expressing high levels of $\beta1$ integrin, the other expressing low levels of $\beta1$ integrin. Both populations react differently to UV irradiation with respect to their proliferation and thus representing different subgroups of keratinocytes (Hendrix et al, 1998).

UV irradiation effects are of course dependent on the melanocytes and their pigmentation present in skin. A skin equivalent model was developed by seeding keratinocytes and melanocytes onto a de-epidermized dermis (DED) resulting into a reconstructed epidermis and a physiologic distribution of dendritic melanocytes in the basal layer showing melanosome transfer to keratinocytes (Bessou et al, 1995). UV-B irradiation led to an increase of melanocyte numbers and stimulation of pigmentation as well as an increase of melanosome transfer. In an analogous model, melanin was detected in the melanocytes and the neighbouring keratinocytes. UV-B irradiation resulted in an increase of pigmentation, quantity and dendricity of melanocytes, while the quantity and distribution of melanin appeared to be unchanged at the light microscopic level (Todd et al, 1993).

2.2.4 Cancer models

Cancer can be induced by carcinogenic substances. Therefore, skin equivalents like EpiDerm™ (MatTek Co., MA), which have already been used to study cytotoxicity and irritant potential of cosmetic ingredients and consists of a reconstituted human epidermis, was also employed to evaluate the genotoxicity of carcinogenic agents (topical application of benzo[a]pyrene or UV-A / UV-B irradiation and psoralen-ultraviolet A radiation) (Zhao et al, 1999). The resulting expression of c-fos, p53 and other substances after the treatment of the skin equivalent was similar to that in native skin receiving the same treatment. Thus, this model is a convenient and cost-effective alternative to animal testing for the assessment of genotoxicity and the study of the mode of action of mutagens and carcinogens.

Another great concern with respect to cancer is the invasion and metastatic potential of the cancer cells. Four human melanoma cell lines with different metastatic potentials were analyzed in a skin model containing keratinocytes and melanoma cell lines (Dekker et al, 2000). The cells were either cultured submerged or at the air-liquid-interface (epidermal and dermal part present). In the interface cultures the cancer cells formed tumour cell nests in the epidermis, similar to the situation in vivo. Two of the four cell lines were found to invade into the dermal compartment. Here, a correlation was found between the expression pattern of certain adhesion molecules and the ability for invasive growth. The invasion potential was also analyzed in case of the squamous cell carcinoma (SCC) of the oral cavity (Kataoka et al, 2010) as a model for cancer invasion and metastatic activity. Here, the metastasis involves the destruction of the basement membrane and the invasion into the submucosal tissue. Two SCC (human tongue) cell lines and normal epithelial cells from gingiva as a control were cultured on AlloDerm®, a skin equivalent consisting of allogeneic acellular dermis. One cancer cell line invaded through the basement membrane into the dermis and thus represents an adequate in vitro model for SCC.

Cancer may be caused by human papilloma viruses (HPV). The molecular mechanisms were analyzed using a skin equivalent model with primary adult human epidermal keratinocytes, which were transduced with retroviruses expressing HPV genes (Akgul et al, 2005). They were seeded onto a de-epidermized dermis, previously repopulated with primary dermal fibroblasts. The expression of the HPV E7 gene led to an enhanced terminal differentiation and hyperproliferation of the keratinocytes. E7 uncouples differentiation and proliferation in vivo, such that the differentiating keratinocytes remain in a DNA replication competent stage. Also, E7 caused the keratinocytes to migrate through the basement membrane and thus invade the dermis. An over expression of several metalloproteinases (MMPs) was detected. Thus, the model proved very useful for the study of HPV genes in vitro.

2.2.5 Wound healing and angiogenesis

Wound healing still proves difficult in many situations. Therefore, models for wound repair need to be established and validated giving the opportunity to test new wound healing therapies as well as to optimize dosages. Skin equivalents consisting of DED seeded with either keratinocytes or fibroblasts or both were developed. A full-thickness wound being inserted into the skin model decreased in the course of time, thus representing a wound model with the ability to heal (Xie et al, 2010). The growth factor VNGF was added to the wounds and resulted in an increased and earlier wound closure. Also, the wound model proved useful in the field of mechanistic studies and the assessment of a synthetic biomimetic gel.

The re-epithelialization of a wound is dependent on many factors and another wound model was used to determine the role of fibroblasts in this process and in the formation of the dermal-epidermal junction (DEJ) as well as the analysis of the differential protein expression during the re-epithelialization process (El Ghalbzouri et al, 2004). The fibroblasts facilitate wound closure and affect the deposition of several basement membrane components. Both, keratinocyte growth factor (KGF) and epidermal growth factor (EGF) accelerated the re-epithelialization in full-thickness but not in superficial wounds. The presence of laminin 5 and type IV and VII collagen did not seem to be required for keratinocyte migration.

A more mechanistic study concentrated on the cellular response to injury and the angiogenesis of wound healing (Herman & Leung, 2009). The three-dimensional skin equivalent model comprises several cell types found in normal human skin or chronic wounds. A microvascular component within the dermis-like extracellular matrix mimics the microvasculature of native skin and therefore is used to analyze angiogenesis in response to injury.

2.2.6 *Candida albicans* infections and bacterial contaminations of wounds

Candida albicans is able to colonize the surfaces of certain mucous membranes in humans, e.g. causing cutaneous candidiasis. A skin equivalent model is used to estimate the viability of *C. albicans* based on the quantitative detection of its actin mRNA (Okeke et al, 2001). As after the application of the antimycotic amorolfine the viability of *C. albicans* proved to be reduced, this technique may be useful to evaluate the therapeutic efficacies of antifungal drugs in the treatment of candidiasis. Also, the cytokine expression patterns in cutanous candidosis were investigated (Schaller et al, 2002). Expression of pro-inflammatory cytokines was induced which is important for the recruitment of neutrophils, macrophages and lymphocytes in vivo and the induction of a Th1-type cytokine response.

Infections are feared of in the therapy of wounds and burns since they often lead to complications in the healing process or the rejections of skin substitutes but also resulting in sepsis and death in case of severe infections. Different kinds of skin substitutes (skin equivalent, dermal equivalent, xenograft, control saline gauze) were tested for their effect on wound closure (Fiala et al, 1993). Full-thickness wounds were inserted into rabbits and subsequently inoculated with *Staphylococcus aureus*. Wounds dressed with skin equivalents or dermal substitutes had lower bacterial counts than wounds treated with xenografts. The grafts took well in case of the skin equivalents and dermal equivalents and both are as such more effective as biological dressing materials than xenografts. Furthermore, skin equivalents have been used to analyze the biofilm development of clinical relevant bacterial strains (*Pseudomonas aeruginosa, Staphylococcus aureus*) on wounds (Charles et al, 2009). Those bacteria may also account for the chronicity of wounds. A skin equivalent wound model was developed on the basis of the commercially available Apligraf® / Graftskin, which comprises primary keratinocytes, forming a stratified epidermis, and primary fibroblasts forming a dermis. Full-thickness wounds were inserted and inoculated with the above mentioned bacteria. Biofilm formation is dependent on the inoculation time as well as the bacterial strain, but occurred within some hours. As such, this model is useful for the study of biofilm growth, prevention and eradication.

2.2.7 Psoriasis and (de)pigmentation diseases

Psoriasis is an inflammatory disease of the skin, which is charaterized by hyperproliferation of keratinocytes. TNF-alpha is a pro-inflammatory cytokine and as such implicated as a key cytokine in the pathogenicity of psoriasis. Therefore, its effect on keratinocytes from healthy and psoriatic skin was analyzed (Fransson, 2000). The keratinocytes were combined with fibroblasts from either healthy or psoriatic skin and as such formed a skin equivalent. Nevertheless, no effect of TNF-alpha on proliferation or differentiation of healthy or psoriatic keratinocytes could be found. Further, wound healing in a psoriatic skin may be different from that in normal skin and can be tested in a skin equivalent model (Konstantinova et al, 1998). The nerve system seems to be connected with the psoriasis disease and thus the expression of nerve growth factor was analyzed. While the keratinocytes invaginated into the dermis, it was found under the basal membrane zone, suggesting an influence on the migration of nerves into the regenerated tissue. Another model for psoriasis as well as graft versus host disease (GVHD) is a (mouse) model containing (healthy and psoriatic) keratinocytes, fibroblasts and activated NK cells (Kalish et al, 2009). The isolated, resuspended cells were placed into the chambers in skin of immunodeficient mice, forming skin after several weeks. NK cells were then added for the production of a psoriatic mouse model. Analogously, when T cells were injected, a GVDH model was achieved.

A major disadvantage of the current burn therapies with skin substitutes is the lack of pigmentation, perspiratory glands or hair follicles. Also, pigmentation disorders like hyperpigmentation in café-au-lait macules are the subject of research (Okazaki et al, 2005). A skin equivalent for the research on this disease was developed. It comprises fibroblasts, keratinocytes and melanocytes from café-au-lait macules resulting in a much higher amount of pigment than found in normal skin. Especially the fibroblasts seem to play a major role in this effect. Another approach is the construction of a skin equivalent containing melanocytes to achieve a skin equivalent with normal pigmentation using keratinocytes and melanocytes isolated from hair follicles (Liu et al, 2011). The skin equivalent was able to successfully repair skin defects in nude mice. A further group centred on the questions by which factors the melanocytes are influenced in their proliferation and melanogenesis (Hedley et al, 2002). The basement membrane was found to be necessary for the positional orientation of the melanocytes, i.e. without the basement membrane proteins melanocytes moved to the upper keratinocyte layers. The melanocytes pigmented spontaneously. The addition of fibroblasts led to a decrease of spontaneous pigmentation and neither α-melanocyte-stimulating-hormone nor cholera toxin was followed by pigmentation.

2.3 Gene therapeutic approaches

Transfection of keratinocytes is a promising tool for gene therapy either for temporary production of growth-stimulating factors in wounds (Vogt et al, 1994) or as a bioreactor for systemic expression of genes (Meng et al, 2002). Modification of healing processes by ectopic expression of stimulating polypeptides like cytokines or growth factors has several advantages over direct application of these factors, which are expensive and are restricted in their efficiency by high turn-over rates under systemic conditions.

Transduced keratinocytes are easily accessed, monitored and even removed if necessary, which is all favourable for establishment of gene therapeutic protocols; furthermore, epidermal cells are able to produce and secrete efficient amounts of ectopic protein. Secreted polypeptides have been shown to cross the epidermal-dermal barrier enabling systemic delivery of target proteins (Fenjves et al, 1994). Choice of genetic tools depends on the specific requirements of the therapeutic approach and considerations of safety and reliability. Correction of genetic diseases depends on permanent expression of the target gene e.g. on transgene integration into the host genome - ideally in cells with self-renewal capacity, like stem cells - or on extrachromosomal replication of an episome. Transient gene expression might be adequate for influencing temporal conditions as might occur in wound healing processes. Viral and non-viral gene delivery systems meet these demands to different extents and depend on different conditions for successful gene transfer. While non-viral methods and adenoviruses are essentially transient, viral vectors like retroviruses and lentiviruses might integrate into the host genome.

Most published techniques were performed with viral vectors in order to reach high transfection efficiency (Braun-Falco et al, 1999, Garlick et al, 1991). Keratinocytes have been transfected with several types of viral vectors including adenovirus, adeno-associated virus, retrovirus and lentivirus. Cells were expanded on mouse fibroblast feeder layers and kept under serum to ensure keratinocyte viability and proliferation. Thus, high exposure to virus particles and sufficient transfection rates can be achieved (Aasen & Belmonte, 2010).

These approaches contain several disadvantages, however. Viral vectors bear the risk of uncontrolled immune reactions and provide only limited genomic space for additional genetic material. Many studies focus on the use of retroviruses, e.g. as a corrective transgene for junctional epidermis bullosa; nevertheless, inactivation of gene expression by the host immune response is a serious drawback of this method (Kikuchi et al, 2008). In contrast to retroviruses and lentiviruses adenoviruses do not integrate into the host genome and thus are less prone to arbitrary and possibly harmful activation of host genes. They are able to infect non-dividing cells but are of limited use in gene correction due to their transient expression. Keratinocytes and fibroblasts are transduced by adenoviruses with less efficiency than other cell types due to their low levels of Coxsackie-adenovirus receptor and probably their negative charge of membrane glycoproteins (Kikuchi et al, 2008). As high viral load is needed strong immune response has been observed after treatment with adenovirus (Raper et al, 2003).

Non-viral methods have been developed as an alternative. Keratinocytes have been demonstrated to take up naked plasmid DNA in vivo (Hengge et al, 1995) but this has so far not been shown for an ex vivo setting. Transfection has also been mediated by calcium phosphate precipitation, DEAE-dextran and polybrene treatment followed by a dimethylsulfoxide shock (Jiang et al, 1991). Liposome-mediated transfer yielded about one third of transfected cells (Li et al, 2001). Electroporation can be used in vitro and in vivo (Kikuchi et al, 2008) while nucleofection is an interesting tool for broad transfection of keratinocyte populations because the protocol enables the transferred DNA to directly enter the nucleus. Thus, gene transfer to quiescent and terminally differentiated cells is possible which is important in keratinocyte cultures (Distler et al, 2005). High rates of gene transfer are necessary when functional assays are employed to investigate the success of gene transfer in contrast to the use of reporter genes.

In order to establish a protocol for the enrichment of positive cells we propose magnetic cell separation of transfected cells as described by us previously (Radtke et al, 2009). This enrichment technique has been used for different types of cells intended for gene therapeutic purposes (Kube & Vockerodt, 2001). Essentially, cells were seeded on 10 cm uncoated plastic dishes and grown to 60% confluence. Transfection with pEGFP-C3 using 18 µl Fugene6 (Roche Applied Sciences) complexed with 6 µg DNA was performed 24 hrs after seeding. Transfection reagent was mixed with culture medium and incubated at room temperature for 5 minutes, followed by a 15 minutes incubation period with added DNA to allow for formation of transfection complexes. Importantly, the transfection reagent should not be allowed to attach to the used plastic ware and transfection complexes should be added to the cells in a strict dropwise manner. Fugene6 has been used efficiently in many gene therapeutic contexts (Arnold et al, 2006, Elmadbouh et al, 2004, Young et al, 2002) and has been proposed for generation of induced pluripotent stem cells (Aasen & Belmonte, 2010). It has been used successfully by us and others for keratinocyte transfection (Aasen & Belmonte, 2010, Distler et al, 2005, Radtke et al, 2009). The majority of cells maintained attached and viable. It has been reported that keratinocyte transfection can result in termination of proliferation due to cell-cycle arrest (Jensen et al, 2000). In our approach cells continued to proliferate and grew into a monolayer.

The ectopic expression of the truncated mouse H-2Kk molecule on the cellular surface was used for magnetic labelling via specific antibodies coupled to paramagnetically labelled beads. To this end cells were transfected with pEGFP-C3 (Clontech) and pMACS Kk (Miltenyi). After 24 hours cells were trypsinized until they appeared rounded. The reaction was stopped with 100 µl FCS and the cells were scraped off the dish. Antibodies were added (80 µl anti Kk) and the cell-antibody mixture was incubated at room temperature for 15 min. The volume was adjusted to 2 ml with phosphate buffered saline / ethylenediaminetetraacetic acid. The magnetically labelled cells were separated by MACS as previously described (Wei et al., 2001). Keratinocytes transfected with Fugene6/DNA complexes yielded 35% positive cells under optimized conditions without induction of apoptosis despite growing the cells under serum-free conditions (Radtke et al, 2009).

2.4 Keratinocyte culture and isolation

Keratinocytes can either be maintained under feeder layer-dependent conditions as essentially described by a method developed by Rheinwald and Green or under defined conditions in serum-free, media with a low calcium concentration as proposed by Boyce and Ham in 1983 (Rheinwald & Green, 1975, Boyce & Ham, 1983). Both methods have certain advantages and disadvantages and the users have to decide about their culture strategy based on the specific demands of their application.

For example, in cultures kept in conditions without feeder cells contamination with other cells, growing rapidly under feeder-layer conditions, is suppressed; nevertheless replication of keratinocytes is limited (Krueger et al, 1994, Rochat et al, 1994). In contrast, serum-containing culture medium significantly increases the amount of undesired cells (e.g. fibroblasts and melanocytes) decreasing the amount of attaching keratinocytes at the same time.

Other advantages of serum- and feeder-based techniques include higher resistance to apoptosis, e.g. after adenoviral infection. It has also to be taken into concern that it is possible to switch to serum-free culture conditions at any time point while changing from serum-free medium to serum-based conditions is not recommended (Aasen & Belmonte, 2010). Nevertheless, cell size enlargement has been observed by several authors (Inoue et al, 2006, van Rossum et al, 2004) when serum-containing media were used in contrast to serum-free cultures. Lorenz et al. explain this by stating that keratinocyte stem cell characteristics are better preserved in serum-free media (Lorenz et al, 2009). This is in accordance with the fact that the number of clonogenic cells is increased under appropriate culture conditions. As keratinocytes usually proliferate in low-calcium (0.15 mM $CaCl_2$) and differentiate in high-calcium medium (Daniels et al, 1995) it is of importance to avoid any long-term exposure to high levels of calcium. Compared to some cell types such as fibroblasts, keratinocytes require more care and avoiding apoptosis in low density cultures, and differentiation and senescence when reaching confluence is difficult.

As most commercial products available for keratinocyte culture are optimized for human cells, cultures with cells of non-human organisms are especially difficult to obtain. A method for long-term culture of newborn C57/BL6 mouse epidermal keratinocytes by using highly supplemented rodent fibroblast conditioned medium was described by Hager et al. (Hager et al., 1999). Adult mouse keratinocyte subcultures were established without using fetal bovine serum (FBS), feeder layers, fibroblast conditioned medium (FCM) or bovine pituitary extract (Yano & Okochi, 2005). A detailed description of isolation and culture of keratinocytes from newborn and adult mice was published by Lichti et al. (Lichti et al, 2008). Rodent monocellular protocols are complex, time consuming and the reproducibility of the cell isolation is difficult, but as genetically modified mice are a valuable preclinical tool for understanding pathologies based on genetic disorders, protocols should be optimized and refined as well. Three dimensional skin models with keratinocytes from wildtype or mutant mice might thus profit by the recent progress in protocol modification (Lichti et al, 2008).

We established a simplified method for isolation and maintenance of proliferating human keratinocytes as described before (Radtke et al, 2009). Following this protocol a monoculture of human keratinocytes could be established without the necessity of co-cultures with fibroblasts. From our experience several factors played a role in the preparation of pure, proliferating keratinocyte cultures: 1) donor skin is best from young donors and 2) there are different regions of the body where the probability of harvesting healthy attaching keratinocytes is higher. We suggested that the best skin for preparation of keratinocyte cultures should be taken from anatomical regions without previous mechanical irritation, less cornification and regions without hair to diminish infection rates; while we did not recommend using scar tissue or skin containing striae.

2.4.1 Methods for cell culturing of human keratinocytes

Full thickness human skin has to be cut into small pieces and incubated in a dispase II solution overnight at 37°C. The epidermis should be removed from the dermis with fine forceps and centrifuged at 220g for 5 minutes. The pellet should be resuspended in a 0.1% trypsin/0.02% EDTA solution and incubated at room temperature for 15 minutes. Activity can be stopped by trypsin inhibitor followed by centrifugation. The cells should be resuspended in Waymouth medium and filtered through a 100 µm mesh. Dissociated cells can be seeded on uncoated tissue culture flasks. After 48 hours, cell debris and non-adherent cells should be removed and the culture medium changed to a serum-free keratinocyte growth medium. The plated cells typically reach 70-80% confluence after 5-7 days.

Cells remain in a proliferative state by subculturing in serum-free medium every time before reaching confluence. For passage keratinocytes should be washed with PBS and slightly trypsinized with trypsin (0.05%/0.02% EDTA) at room temperature until the cells start to retract. The trypsinization has to be stopped after 3 to 5 minutes with trypsin neutralizer. Cells should be detached off the ground mechanically and immediately centrifuged at 220g for 5 minutes. After splitting to uncoated cell culture dishes, cells usually adhere the same day and start to divide after 24 to 48 hours. This mild procedure allows passaging vital and proliferative cells for at least 5 passages in serum-free medium (Promocell, Heidelberg, Germany) without the need of a fibroblast feeder layer (Radtke et al, 2009). Expansion of plastic-adherent keratinocytes is achieved without signs of senescence and with doubling times of 5-7 days. This protocol may facilitate the clinical application of keratinocyte based therapies.

We cannot define the exact mechanism for attachment of keratinocytes of different species, but this is one of the key factors in culturing keratinocytes. The attachment of human keratinocytes in our cultures without large contamination of other cell types such as fibroblasts or melanocytes, which have normally a greater proliferation rate and would overgrow the culture in a couple of days, is a clear advantage of this method. The exact mechanism of keratinocyte attachment is not known and various coating matrices (e.g. laminin, poly-L-lysin) do not lead to significant differences. In conclusion, we were able to establish efficient protocols for the handling of keratinocytes for experimental and clinical purposes, including isolation, cultivation, storage and gene therapeutic manipulations (Radtke et al, 2009).

3. Conclusion

Keratinocytes are a useful tool in cellular transplantation studies to improve functional outcome in burn patients and chronic wounds. Although the best clinical outcome might be achieved by transplantation of full-thickness skin grafts, limitations in donor tissue availability - especially in case of large burn wounds - leads to the necessity to use split-thickness grafts as commonly preferred skin replacements. Alternatively, transplantation of autologous keratinocytes - either precultivated to generate confluent keratinocyte sheets or intraoperatively prepared and transplanted in suspension - are used to fulfil special therapeutical requirements such as treatment of faces or when split-thickness grafts of sufficient amount or quality are difficult to obtain.

Beside the urgent need for therapeutical use keratinocyte cultures are an important issue for a number of biological applications. Ex vivo cultivation of skin and primary keratinocytes potentially integrated into different skin equivalents are recommendable model systems to investigate cellular behaviour of epithelial cells, skin diseases and pharmacological kinetics. Culture and subsequent transfection of keratinocytes might also be a promising tool for gene therapeutic approaches either for temporary production of growth-stimulating factors in wounds or as a biological vector for systemic expression of genes.

However, pure keratinocyte cultures are difficult to establish and to maintain for long-term culture. Cultivation in serum-containing media and on a mouse fibroblast feeder layer is not recommended prior to transplantation for safety reasons. We established a protocol for cultivation of keratinocytes under defined, serum-free conditions. From our experience, several factors may play a role in the preparation of a pure, proliferating keratinocyte culture: 1) donor skin is best from young donors and 2) there are different regions of the body with higher probability of harvesting healthy attaching keratinocytes. We suggest that the best skin for preparation and establishment of a pure keratinocyte culture without the need of a fibroblast feeder layer should be taken from anatomical regions without previous mechanical irritation, less cornification and regions without hair, the latter diminishing the infection rate. Skin originating from scar tissue or skin which contains striae is not recommended.

4. Acknowledgment

Skin cell culture in our laboratory is supported by the Deutsche Forschungsgemeinschaft (DFG) within the SFB/TR37 (TP A4).

5. References

Aasen, T. & Belmonte, J. C. (2010). Isolation and cultivation of human keratinocytes from skin or plucked hair for the generation of induced pluripotent stem cells. *Nature protocols,* Vol.5, No.2, 2010), pp. 371-382, ISSN 1750-2799; 1750-2799

Akgul, B.; Garcia-Escudero, R.; Ghali, L.; Pfister, H. J.; Fuchs, P. G.; Navsaria, H. & Storey, A. (2005). The E7 protein of cutaneous human papillomavirus type 8 causes invasion of human keratinocytes into the dermis in organotypic cultures of skin. *Cancer research,* Vol.65, No.6, (Mar 15 2005), pp. 2216-2223, ISSN 0008-5472; 0008-5472

Arnold, A. S.; Laporte, V.; Dumont, S.; Appert-Collin, A.; Erbacher, P.; Coupin, G.; Levy, R.; Poindron, P. & Gies, J. P. (2006). Comparing reagents for efficient transfection of human primary myoblasts: FuGENE 6, Effectene and ExGen 500. *Fundamental & clinical pharmacology,* Vol.20, No.1, (Feb 2006), pp. 81-89, ISSN 0767-3981; 0767-3981

Atiyeh, B. S. & Costagliola, M. (2007). Cultured epithelial autograft (CEA) in burn treatment: three decades later. *Burns : journal of the International Society for Burn Injuries,* Vol.33, No.4, (Jun 2007), pp. 405-413, ISSN 0305-4179; 0305-4179

Bernerd, F. (2005). Human skin reconstructed in vitro as a model to study the keratinocyte, the fibroblast and their interactions: photodamage and repair processes. *Journal de la Societe de biologie,* Vol.199, No.4, 2005), pp. 313-320, ISSN 1295-0661; 1295-0661

Bernerd, F.; Asselineau, D.; Vioux, C.; Chevallier-Lagente, O.; Bouadjar, B.; Sarasin, A. & Magnaldo, T. (2001). Clues to epidermal cancer proneness revealed by reconstruction of DNA repair-deficient xeroderma pigmentosum skin in vitro. *Proceedings of the National Academy of Sciences of the United States of America,* Vol.98, No.14, (Jul 3 2001), pp. 7817-7822, ISSN 0027-8424; 0027-8424

Bessou, S.; Surleve-Bazeille, J. E.; Sorbier, E. & Taieb, A. (1995). Ex vivo reconstruction of the epidermis with melanocytes and the influence of UVB. *Pigment Cell Research / sponsored by the European Society for Pigment Cell Research and the International Pigment Cell Society,* Vol.8, No.5, (Oct 1995), pp. 241-249, ISSN 0893-5785; 0893-5785

Bouwstra, J.; Pilgram, G.; Gooris, G.; Koerten, H. & Ponec, M. (2001). New aspects of the skin barrier organization. *Skin pharmacology and applied skin physiology,* Vol.14 Suppl 1, 2001), pp. 52-62, ISSN 1422-2868; 1422-2868

Boyce, S. T. & Ham, R. G. (1983). Calcium-regulated differentiation of normal human epidermal keratinocytes in chemically defined clonal culture and serum-free serial culture. *The Journal of investigative dermatology,* Vol.81, No.1 Suppl, (Jul 1983), pp. 33s-40s, ISSN 0022-202X; 0022-202X

Braun-Falco, M.; Doenecke, A.; Smola, H. & Hallek, M. (1999). Efficient gene transfer into human keratinocytes with recombinant adeno-associated virus vectors. *Gene therapy,* Vol.6, No.3, (Mar 1999), pp. 432-441, ISSN 0969-7128; 0969-7128

Cervelli, V.; De Angelis, B.; Spallone, D.; Lucarini, L.; Arpino, A. & Balzani, A. (2010). Use of a novel autologous cell-harvesting device to promote epithelialization and enhance appropriate pigmentation in scar reconstruction. *Clinical and experimental dermatology*, Vol.35, No.7, (Oct 2010), pp. 776-780, ISSN 1365-2230; 0307-6938

Charles, C. A.; Ricotti, C. A.; Davis, S. C.; Mertz, P. M. & Kirsner, R. S. (2009). Use of tissue-engineered skin to study in vitro biofilm development. *Dermatologic surgery : official publication for American Society for Dermatologic Surgery [et al.]*, Vol.35, No.9, (Sep 2009), pp. 1334-1341, ISSN 1524-4725; 1076-0512

Coulomb, B.; Friteau, L.; Baruch, J.; Guilbaud, J.; Chretien-Marquet, B.; Glicenstein, J.; Lebreton-Decoster, C.; Bell, E. & Dubertret, L. (1998). Advantage of the presence of living dermal fibroblasts within in vitro reconstructed skin for grafting in humans. *Plastic and Reconstructive Surgery*, Vol.101, No.7, (Jun 1998), pp. 1891-1903, ISSN 0032-1052

Damour, O.; Augustin, C. & Black, A. F. (1998). Applications of reconstructed skin models in pharmaco-toxicological trials. *Medical & biological engineering & computing*, Vol.36, No.6, (Nov 1998), pp. 825-832, ISSN 0140-0118; 0140-0118

Daniels, J. T.; Harris, I. R.; Kearney, J. N. & Ingham, E. (1995). Calcium: a crucial consideration in serum-free keratinocyte culture. *Experimental dermatology*, Vol.4, No.4 Pt 1, (Aug 1995), pp. 183-191, ISSN 0906-6705; 0906-6705

De Corte, P.; Verween, G.; Verbeken, G.; Rose, T.; Jennes, S.; De Coninck, A.; Roseeuw, D.; Vanderkelen, A.; Kets, E.; Haddow, D. & Pirnay, J. P. (2011). Feeder layer- and animal product-free culture of neonatal foreskin keratinocytes: improved performance, usability, quality and safety. *Cell and Tissue Banking*, (Mar 11 2011), ISSN 1573-6814; 1389-9333

Dekker, S. K.; van Doorn, R.; Kempenaar, J.; Gruis, N. A.; Vermeer, B. J. & Ponec, M. (2000). Skin equivalent: an attractive model to evaluate early melanoma metastasis. *Melanoma research*, Vol.10, No.2, (Apr 2000), pp. 127-140, ISSN 0960-8931; 0960-8931

Distler, J. H.; Jungel, A.; Kurowska-Stolarska, M.; Michel, B. A.; Gay, R. E.; Gay, S. & Distler, O. (2005). Nucleofection: a new, highly efficient transfection method for primary human keratinocytes*. *Experimental dermatology*, Vol.14, No.4, (Apr 2005), pp. 315-320, ISSN 0906-6705; 0906-6705

Ebara, M.; Yamato, M.; Hirose, M.; Aoyagi, T.; Kikuchi, A.; Sakai, K. & Okano, T. (2003). Copolymerization of 2-carboxyisopropylacrylamide with N-isopropylacrylamide accelerates cell detachment from grafted surfaces by reducing temperature. *Biomacromolecules*, Vol.4, No.2, (Mar-Apr 2003), pp. 344-349, ISSN 1525-7797; 1525-7797

Ehrlich, H. P. (2004). Understanding experimental biology of skin equivalent: from laboratory to clinical use in patients with burns and chronic wounds. *American Journal of Surgery*, Vol.187, No.5A, (May 2004), pp. 29S-33S, ISSN 0002-9610; 0002-9610

El Ghalbzouri, A.; Hensbergen, P.; Gibbs, S.; Kempenaar, J.; van der Schors, R. & Ponec, M. (2004). Fibroblasts facilitate re-epithelialization in wounded human skin equivalents. *Laboratory investigation; a journal of technical methods and pathology*, Vol.84, No.1, (Jan 2004), pp. 102-112, ISSN 0023-6837; 0023-6837

Elmadbouh, I.; Rossignol, P.; Meilhac, O.; Vranckx, R.; Pichon, C.; Pouzet, B.; Midoux, P. & Michel, J. B. (2004). Optimization of in vitro vascular cell transfection with non-viral vectors for in vivo applications. *The journal of gene medicine,* Vol.6, No.10, (Oct 2004), pp. 1112-1124, ISSN 1099-498X; 1099-498X

Fenjves, E. S.; Smith, J.; Zaradic, S. & Taichman, L. B. (1994). Systemic delivery of secreted protein by grafts of epidermal keratinocytes: prospects for keratinocyte gene therapy. *Human Gene Therapy,* Vol.5, No.10, (Oct 1994), pp. 1241-1248, ISSN 1043-0342; 1043-0342

Fiala, T. G.; Lee, W. P.; Hong, H. Z. & May, J. W.,Jr. (1993). Bacterial clearance capability of living skin equivalent, living dermal equivalent, saline dressing, and xenograft dressing in the rabbit. *Annals of Plastic Surgery,* Vol.30, No.6, (Jun 1993), pp. 516-519, ISSN 0148-7043; 0148-7043

Fransson, J. (2000). Tumour necrosis factor-alpha does not influence proliferation and differentiation of healthy and psoriatic keratinocytes in a skin-equivalent model. *Acta Dermato-Venereologica,* Vol.80, No.6, (Nov-Dec 2000), pp. 416-420, ISSN 0001-5555; 0001-5555

Garlick, J. A.; Katz, A. B.; Fenjves, E. S. & Taichman, L. B. (1991). Retrovirus-mediated transduction of cultured epidermal keratinocytes. *The Journal of investigative dermatology,* Vol.97, No.5, (Nov 1991), pp. 824-829, ISSN 0022-202X; 0022-202X

Gibbs, S. (2009). In vitro irritation models and immune reactions. *Skin pharmacology and physiology,* Vol.22, No.2, 2009), pp. 103-113, ISSN 1660-5535; 1660-5527

Gravante, G.; Di Fede, M. C.; Araco, A.; Grimaldi, M.; De Angelis, B.; Arpino, A.; Cervelli, V. & Montone, A. (2007). A randomized trial comparing ReCell system of epidermal cells delivery versus classic skin grafts for the treatment of deep partial thickness burns. *Burns : journal of the International Society for Burn Injuries,* Vol.33, No.8, (Dec 2007), pp. 966-972, ISSN 0305-4179; 0305-4179

Hedley, S. J.; Layton, C.; Heaton, M.; Chakrabarty, K. H.; Dawson, R. A.; Gawkrodger, D. J. & MacNeil, S. (2002). Fibroblasts play a regulatory role in the control of pigmentation in reconstructed human skin from skin types I and II. *Pigment Cell Research / sponsored by the European Society for Pigment Cell Research and the International Pigment Cell Society,* Vol.15, No.1, (Feb 2002), pp. 49-56, ISSN 0893-5785; 0893-5785

Hendrix, S. W.; Rogers, J. V. & Hull, B. E. (1998). Differential response of basal keratinocytes in a human skin equivalent to ultraviolet irradiation. *Archives of Dermatological Research,* Vol.290, No.8, (Aug 1998), pp. 420-424, ISSN 0340-3696; 0340-3696

Hengge, U. R.; Chan, E. F.; Foster, R. A.; Walker, P. S. & Vogel, J. C. (1995). Cytokine gene expression in epidermis with biological effects following injection of naked DNA. *Nature genetics,* Vol.10, No.2, (Jun 1995), pp. 161-166, ISSN 1061-4036; 1061-4036

Herman, I. M. & Leung, A. (2009). Creation of human skin equivalents for the in vitro study of angiogenesis in wound healing. *Methods in molecular biology (Clifton, N.J.),* Vol.467, 2009), pp. 241-248, ISSN 1064-3745; 1064-3745

Hernon, C. A.; Dawson, R. A.; Freedlander, E.; Short, R.; Haddow, D. B.; Brotherstón, M. & MacNeil, S. (2006). Clinical experience using cultured epithelial autografts leads to an alternative methodology for transferring skin cells from the laboratory to the patient. *Regenerative medicine,* Vol.1, No.6, (Nov 2006), pp. 809-821, ISSN 1746-076X; 1746-0751

Horch, R. E.; Bannasch, H.; Kopp, J.; Andree, C. & Stark, G. B. (1998). Single-cell suspensions of cultured human keratinocytes in fibrin-glue reconstitute the epidermis. *Cell transplantation*, Vol.7, No.3, (May-Jun 1998), pp. 309-317, ISSN 0963-6897; 0963-6897

Inoue, H.; Oshima, H.; Matsuzaki, K. & Kumagai, N. (2006). Application for regenerative medicine of epithelial cell culture-vistas of cultured epithelium. *Congenital anomalies*, Vol.46, No.3, (Sep 2006), pp. 129-134, ISSN 0914-3505; 0914-3505

Ito, M.; Liu, Y.; Yang, Z.; Nguyen, J.; Liang, F.; Morris, R. J. & Cotsarelis, G. (2005). Stem cells in the hair follicle bulge contribute to wound repair but not to homeostasis of the epidermis. *Nature medicine*, Vol.11, No.12, (Dec 2005), pp. 1351-1354, ISSN 1078-8956; 1078-8956

Jensen, U. B.; Petersen, M. S.; Lund, T. B.; Jensen, T. G. & Bolund, L. (2000). Transgene expression in human epidermal keratinocytes: cell cycle arrest of productively transfected cells. *Experimental dermatology*, Vol.9, No.4, (Aug 2000), pp. 298-310, ISSN 0906-6705; 0906-6705

Jiang, C. K.; Connolly, D. & Blumenberg, M. (1991). Comparison of methods for transfection of human epidermal keratinocytes. *The Journal of investigative dermatology*, Vol.97, No.6, (Dec 1991), pp. 969-973, ISSN 0022-202X; 0022-202X

Kalish, R. S.; Simon, M.; Harrington, R.; Gottlieb, A. B. & Gilhar, A. (2009). Skin equivalent and natural killer cells: a new model for psoriasis and GVHD. *The Journal of investigative dermatology*, Vol.129, No.3, (Mar 2009), pp. 773-776, ISSN 1523-1747; 0022-202X

Kataoka, T.; Umeda, M.; Shigeta, T.; Takahashi, H. & Komori, T. (2010). A new in vitro model of cancer invasion using AlloDerm, a human cadaveric dermal equivalent: a preliminary report. *The Kobe journal of medical sciences*, Vol.55, No.5, (Apr 8 2010), pp. E106-15, ISSN 1883-0498; 0023-2513

Kikuchi, Y.; Tamai, K. & Kaneda, Y. (2008). Cutaneous gene delivery. *Journal of dermatological science*, Vol.50, No.2, (May 2008), pp. 87-98, ISSN 0923-1811; 0923-1811

Konstantinova, N. V.; Lemak, N. A. & Duvic, M. (1998). Nerve growth factor in normal and psoriatic skin equivalent models. *Archives of Dermatological Research*, Vol.290, No.11, (Nov 1998), pp. 610-614, ISSN 0340-3696; 0340-3696

Krueger, G. G.; Morgan, J. R.; Jorgensen, C. M.; Schmidt, L.; Li, H. L.; Kwan, M. K.; Boyce, S. T.; Wiley, H. S.; Kaplan, J. & Petersen, M. J. (1994). Genetically modified skin to treat disease: potential and limitations. *The Journal of investigative dermatology*, Vol.103, No.5 Suppl, (Nov 1994), pp. 76S-84S, ISSN 0022-202X; 0022-202X

Kube, D. & Vockerodt, M. (2001). Transient gene expression and MACS enrichment. *Methods in molecular biology (Clifton, N.J.)*, Vol.174, 2001), pp. 155-164, ISSN 1064-3745; 1064-3745

Li, W.; Nadelman, C.; Henry, G.; Fan, J.; Muellenhoff, M.; Medina, E.; Gratch, N. S.; Chen, M.; Han, J. & Woodley, D. (2001). The p38-MAPK/SAPK pathway is required for human keratinocyte migration on dermal collagen. *The Journal of investigative dermatology*, Vol.117, No.6, (Dec 2001), pp. 1601-1611, ISSN 0022-202X; 0022-202X

Lichti, U.; Anders, J. & Yuspa, S. H. (2008). Isolation and short-term culture of primary keratinocytes, hair follicle populations and dermal cells from newborn mice and keratinocytes from adult mice for in vitro analysis and for grafting to immunodeficient mice. *Nature protocols,* Vol.3, No.5, 2008), pp. 799-810, ISSN 1750-2799; 1750-2799

Liu, F.; Luo, X. S.; Shen, H. Y.; Dong, J. S. & Yang, J. (2011). Using human hair follicle-derived keratinocytes and melanocytes for constructing pigmented tissue-engineered skin. *Skin research and technology : official journal of International Society for Bioengineering and the Skin (ISBS) [and] International Society for Digital Imaging of Skin (ISDIS) [and] International Society for Skin Imaging (ISSI),* (Feb 21 2011), ISSN 1600-0846; 0909-752X

Lorenz, K.; Rupf, T.; Salvetter, J. & Bader, A. (2009). Enrichment of human beta 1 bri/alpha 6 bri/CD71 dim keratinocytes after culture in defined media. *Cells, tissues, organs,* Vol.189, No.6, 2009), pp. 382-390, ISSN 1422-6421; 1422-6405

Lotte, C.; Patouillet, C.; Zanini, M.; Messager, A. & Roguet, R. (2002). Permeation and skin absorption: reproducibility of various industrial reconstructed human skin models. *Skin pharmacology and applied skin physiology,* Vol.15 Suppl 1, 2002), pp. 18-30, ISSN 1422-2868; 1422-2868

Macfarlane, M.; Jones, P.; Goebel, C.; Dufour, E.; Rowland, J.; Araki, D.; Costabel-Farkas, M.; Hewitt, N. J.; Hibatallah, J.; Kirst, A.; McNamee, P.; Schellauf, F. & Scheel, J. (2009). A tiered approach to the use of alternatives to animal testing for the safety assessment of cosmetics: skin irritation. *Regulatory toxicology and pharmacology : RTP,* Vol.54, No.2, (Jul 2009), pp. 188-196, ISSN 1096-0295; 0273-2300

Marionnet, C.; Vioux-Chagnoleau, C.; Pierrard, C.; Sok, J.; Asselineau, D. & Bernerd, F. (2006). Morphogenesis of dermal-epidermal junction in a model of reconstructed skin: beneficial effects of vitamin C. *Experimental dermatology,* Vol.15, No.8, (Aug 2006), pp. 625-633, ISSN 0906-6705; 0906-6705

Meng, X.; Sawamura, D.; Ina, S.; Tamai, K.; Hanada, K. & Hashimoto, I. (2002). Keratinocyte gene therapy: cytokine gene expression in local keratinocytes and in circulation by introducing cytokine genes into skin. *Experimental dermatology,* Vol.11, No.5, (Oct 2002), pp. 456-461, ISSN 0906-6705; 0906-6705

Mertsching, H.; Weimer, M.; Kersen, S. & Brunner, H. (2008). Human skin equivalent as an alternative to animal testing. *GMS Krankenhaushygiene interdisziplinar,* Vol.3, No.1, (Mar 11 2008), pp. Doc11, ISSN 1863-5245; 1863-5245

Nelson, D. & Gay, R. J. (1993). Effects of UV irradiation on a living skin equivalent. *Photochemistry and photobiology,* Vol.57, No.5, (May 1993), pp. 830-837, ISSN 0031-8655; 0031-8655

Okazaki, M.; Suzuki, Y.; Yoshimura, K. & Harii, K. (2005). Construction of pigmented skin equivalent and its application to the study of congenital disorders of pigmentation. *Scandinavian journal of plastic and reconstructive surgery and hand surgery / Nordisk plastikkirurgisk forening [and] Nordisk klubb for handkirurgi,* Vol.39, No.6, 2005), pp. 339-343, ISSN 0284-4311; 0284-4311

Okeke, C. N.; Tsuboi, R. & Ogawa, H. (2001). Quantification of Candida albicans actin mRNA by the LightCycler system as a means of assessing viability in a model of cutaneous candidiasis. *Journal of clinical microbiology,* Vol.39, No.10, (Oct 2001), pp. 3491-3494, ISSN 0095-1137; 0095-1137

Osborne, R. & Perkins, M. A. (1994). An approach for development of alternative test methods based on mechanisms of skin irritation. *Food and chemical toxicology : an international journal published for the British Industrial Biological Research Association,* Vol.32, No.2, (Feb 1994), pp. 133-142, ISSN 0278-6915; 0278-6915

Ponec, M. (2002). Skin constructs for replacement of skin tissues for in vitro testing. *Advanced Drug Delivery Reviews,* Vol.54 Suppl 1, (Nov 1 2002), pp. S19-30, ISSN 0169-409X; 0169-409X

Ponec, M.; Boelsma, E.; Gibbs, S. & Mommaas, M. (2002). Characterization of reconstructed skin models. *Skin pharmacology and applied skin physiology,* Vol.15 Suppl 1, 2002), pp. 4-17, ISSN 1422-2868; 1422-2868

Ponec, M.; Gibbs, S.; Pilgram, G.; Boelsma, E.; Koerten, H.; Bouwstra, J. & Mommaas, M. (2001). Barrier function in reconstructed epidermis and its resemblance to native human skin. *Skin pharmacology and applied skin physiology,* Vol.14 Suppl 1, 2001), pp. 63-71, ISSN 1422-2868; 1422-2868

Poumay, Y. & Pittelkow, M. R. (1995). Cell density and culture factors regulate keratinocyte commitment to differentiation and expression of suprabasal K1/K10 keratins. *The Journal of investigative dermatology,* Vol.104, No.2, (Feb 1995), pp. 271-276, ISSN 0022-202X; 0022-202X

Priya, S. G.; Jungvid, H. & Kumar, A. (2008). Skin tissue engineering for tissue repair and regeneration. *Tissue engineering.Part B, Reviews,* Vol.14, No.1, (Mar 2008), pp. 105-118, ISSN 1937-3368; 1937-3368

Radtke, C.; Reimers, K.; Allmeling, C. & Vogt, P. M. (2009). Efficient production of transfected human keratinocytes under serum-free and feeder layer-free conditions. *Handchirurgie, Mikrochirurgie, plastische Chirurgie : Organ der Deutschsprachigen Arbeitsgemeinschaft fur Handchirurgie : Organ der Deutschsprachigen Arbeitsgemeinschaft fur Mikrochirurgie der Peripheren Nerven und Gefasse : Organ der Vereinigun(ABGEKÜRZT),* Vol.41, No.6, (Dec 2009), pp. 333-340, ISSN 1439-3980; 0722-1819

Raper, S. E.; Chirmule, N.; Lee, F. S.; Wivel, N. A.; Bagg, A.; Gao, G. P.; Wilson, J. M. & Batshaw, M. L. (2003). Fatal systemic inflammatory response syndrome in a ornithine transcarbamylase deficient patient following adenoviral gene transfer. *Molecular genetics and metabolism,* Vol.80, No.1-2, (Sep-Oct 2003), pp. 148-158, ISSN 1096-7192; 1096-7192

Rasmussen, C.; Gratz, K.; Liebel, F.; Southall, M.; Garay, M.; Bhattacharyya, S.; Simon, N.; Vander Zanden, M.; Van Winkle, K.; Pirnstill, J.; Pirnstill, S.; Comer, A. & Allen-Hoffmann, B. L. (2010). The StrataTest(R) human skin model, a consistent in vitro alternative for toxicological testing. *Toxicology in vitro : an international journal published in association with BIBRA,* Vol.24, No.7, (Oct 2010), pp. 2021-2029, ISSN 1879-3177; 0887-2333

Rennekampff, H. O.; Hansbrough, J. F.; Woods, V.,Jr & Kiessig, V. (1996). Integrin and matrix molecule expression in cultured skin replacements. *The Journal of burn care & rehabilitation,* Vol.17, No.3, (May-Jun 1996), pp. 213-221, ISSN 0273-8481; 0273-8481

Rheinwald, J. G. & Green, H. (1975). Serial cultivation of strains of human epidermal keratinocytes: the formation of keratinizing colonies from single cells. *Cell,* Vol.6, No.3, (Nov 1975), pp. 331-343, ISSN 0092-8674; 0092-8674

Rochat, A.; Kobayashi, K. & Barrandon, Y. (1994). Location of stem cells of human hair follicles by clonal analysis. *Cell,* Vol.76, No.6, (Mar 25 1994), pp. 1063-1073, ISSN 0092-8674; 0092-8674

Ronfard, V.; Rives, J. M.; Neveux, Y.; Carsin, H. & Barrandon, Y. (2000). Long-term regeneration of human epidermis on third degree burns transplanted with autologous cultured epithelium grown on a fibrin matrix. *Transplantation,* Vol.70, No.11, (Dec 15 2000), pp. 1588-1598, ISSN 0041-1337; 0041-1337

Schaller, M.; Mailhammer, R. & Korting, H. C. (2002). Cytokine expression induced by Candida albicans in a model of cutaneous candidosis based on reconstituted human epidermis. *Journal of medical microbiology,* Vol.51, No.8, (Aug 2002), pp. 672-676, ISSN 0022-2615; 0022-2615

Schoop, V. M.; Mirancea, N. & Fusenig, N. E. (1999). Epidermal organization and differentiation of HaCaT keratinocytes in organotypic coculture with human dermal fibroblasts. *The Journal of investigative dermatology,* Vol.112, No.3, (Mar 1999), pp. 343-353, ISSN 0022-202X; 0022-202X

Seland, H.; Gustafson, C. J.; Johnson, H.; Junker, J. P. & Kratz, G. (2011). Transplantation of acellular dermis and keratinocytes cultured on porous biodegradable microcarriers into full-thickness skin injuries on athymic rats. *Burns : journal of the International Society for Burn Injuries,* Vol.37, No.1, (Feb 2011), pp. 99-108, ISSN 1879-1409; 0305-4179

Smijs, T. G. & Bouwstra, J. A. (2010). Focus on skin as a possible port of entry for solid nanoparticles and the toxicological impact. *Journal of biomedical nanotechnology,* Vol.6, No.5, (Oct 2010), pp. 469-484, ISSN 1550-7033; 1550-7033

Todd, C.; Hewitt, S. D.; Kempenaar, J.; Noz, K.; Thody, A. J. & Ponec, M. (1993). Co-culture of human melanocytes and keratinocytes in a skin equivalent model: effect of ultraviolet radiation. *Archives of Dermatological Research,* Vol.285, No.8, 1993), pp. 455-459, ISSN 0340-3696; 0340-3696

van der Veen, V. C.; van der Wal, M. B.; van Leeuwen, M. C.; Ulrich, M. M. & Middelkoop, E. (2010). Biological background of dermal substitutes. *Burns : journal of the International Society for Burn Injuries,* Vol.36, No.3, (May 2010), pp. 305-321, ISSN 1879-1409; 0305-4179

van Rossum, M. M.; Franssen, M. E.; Cloin, W. A.; van de Bosch, G. J.; Boezeman, J. B.; Schalkwijk, J.; van de Kerkhof, P. C. & van Erp, P. E. (2004). Functional characterization of beta1-integrin-positive epidermal cell populations. *Acta Dermato-Venereologica,* Vol.84, No.4, 2004), pp. 265-270, ISSN 0001-5555; 0001-5555

Vogt, P. M.; Thompson, S.; Andree, C.; Liu, P.; Breuing, K.; Hatzis, D.; Brown, H.; Mulligan, R. C. & Eriksson, E. (1994). Genetically modified keratinocytes transplanted to wounds reconstitute the epidermis. *Proceedings of the National Academy of Sciences of the United States of America,* Vol.91, No.20, (Sep 27 1994), pp. 9307-9311, ISSN 0027-8424; 0027-8424

Williamson, J. S.; Snelling, C. F.; Clugston, P.; Macdonald, I. B. & Germann, E. (1995). Cultured epithelial autograft: five years of clinical experience with twenty-eight patients. *The Journal of trauma,* Vol.39, No.2, (Aug 1995), pp. 309-319, ISSN 0022-5282; 0022-5282

Xie, Y.; Rizzi, S. C.; Dawson, R.; Lynam, E.; Richards, S.; Leavesley, D. I. & Upton, Z. (2010). Development of a three-dimensional human skin equivalent wound model for investigating novel wound healing therapies. *Tissue engineering.Part C, Methods,* Vol.16, No.5, (Oct 2010), pp. 1111-1123, ISSN 1937-3392; 1937-3384

Yano, S. & Okochi, H. (2005). Long-term culture of adult murine epidermal keratinocytes. *The British journal of dermatology*, Vol.153, No.6, (Dec 2005), pp. 1101-1104, ISSN 0007-0963; 0007-0963

Young, A. T.; Lakey, J. R.; Murray, A. G. & Moore, R. B. (2002). Gene therapy: a lipofection approach for gene transfer into primary endothelial cells. *Cell transplantation*, Vol.11, No.6, 2002), pp. 573-582, ISSN 0963-6897; 0963-6897

Zhao, J. F.; Zhang, Y. J.; Kubilus, J.; Jin, X. H.; Santella, R. M.; Athar, M.; Wang, Z. Y. & Bickers, D. R. (1999). Reconstituted 3-dimensional human skin as a novel in vitro model for studies of carcinogenesis. *Biochemical and biophysical research communications*, Vol.254, No.1, (Jan 8 1999), pp. 49-53, ISSN 0006-291X; 0006-291X

14

Bioengineered Skin

María José Escámez[1,2,3] et al.*

[1]*Regenerative Medicine Unit, Epithelial Biomedicine Division, CIEMAT, Madrid,*
[2]*Department of Bioengineering, Universidad Carlos III (UC3M), Madrid,*
[3]*Centro de Investigaciones Biomédicas en Red en Enfermedades Raras (CIBERER), Madrid,*
Spain

1. Introduction

Over the past decades, skin has become an increasingly interesting target for replacement therapies. Easy access plays a pivotal role in its widespread use in this context. Current cell culture techniques have optimized *in vitro* expansion of cells obtained from skin biopsies to be assembled in three-dimensional matrices and engineered skin equivalents that are amenable to clinical use. A wide range of natural scaffolds and synthetic materials are now available as matrices in organotypic skin cultures for skin regeneration (Shevchenko et al., 2010). Patients with severe skin loss require large-scale production of composite skin equivalents. We developed an improved whole autologous bioengineered skin based on the use of a fibrin three-dimensional dermal scaffold in which fibroblasts are embedded (World Patent WO/2002/072800) (Figure 1). We provided evidence that this plasma-based dermal equivalent adequately supports keratinocyte growth (Meana et al., 1998). Immunohistochemical studies over long follow-up periods showed that experimental grafting on immunodeficient mice yielded a healthy and mature skin with human architecture that persisted even after several epidermal turn-overs (Llames et al., 2004). Permanent skin regeneration requires preservation of epidermal cell stemness. The preclinical model fulfils this requirement (Larcher et al., 2007). Bioengineered human skin has been successfully employed in a clinical scenario (Figure 1) for permanent coverage in the case of extensive burns, necrotizing fascitis, removal of giant nevi, and graft-versus-host disease (Llames et al., 2004; 2006; Gómez et al., 2011). Currently, the use of bioengineered skin has spread to a wider range of applications such as the management of injuries of different aetiology including vascular and diabetic wounds and more recently the treatment of wounds associated with genetic rare diseases such as epidermolysis bullosa (EB). EB is characterized by skin blistering following minor friction or mechanical trauma. The condition varies from limited blisters in the skin to a form involving internal epithelial lining. The management of EB is mainly supportive with symptomatic

---

* Lucía Martínez-Santamaría[1,3], Marta García[1,3], Sara Guerrero-Aspizua[1,2], Marta Carretero[1,3], Fernando Larcher[1,3], Álvaro Meana[4] and Marcela Del Río[1,2,3]

1 *Regenerative Medicine Unit, Epthelial Biomedicine Division. CIEMAT, Madrid, Spain,*

2 *Department of Bioengineering. Universidad Carlos III (UC3M) Madrid, Spain,*

3 *Centro de Investigaciones Biomédicas en Red en Enfermedades Raras (CIBERER), Madrid, Spain,*

4 *Centro de Investigaciones Biomédicas en Red en Enfermedades Raras (CIBERER), Oviedo, Spain.*

treatment, since currently no cure exists. Nevertheless, EB patients may benefit from the treatment with new cell-based therapies. In this context, the EMEA awarded the Orphan Drug Designation to a chimerical version of the substitute (orphan designation number EU/306/369). Two additional strategies to treat EB, based on the use of bioengineered skin, are being explored by our team.

Our approach to study the physiopathology of the skin evolved also toward disease modeling. We have established a skin-humanized mouse model system based on bioengineered human skin-engrafted immunodeficient mice (Del Rio et al., 2002b; Llames et al., 2004) (Figure1).

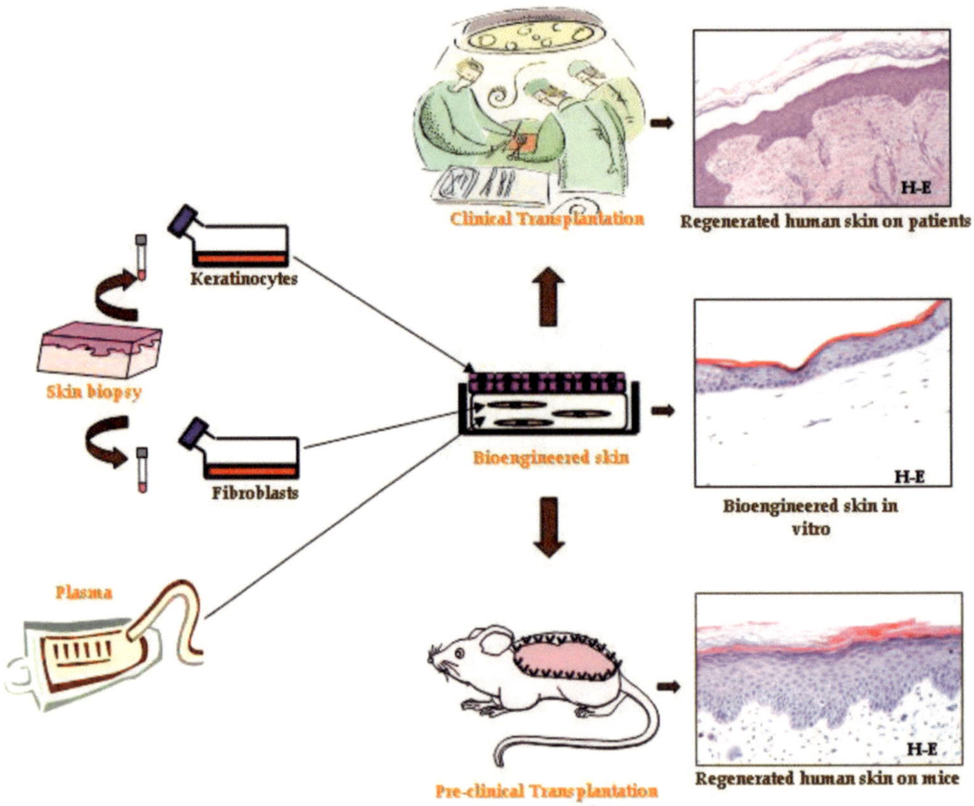

Fig. 1. **Human bioengineered skin.** Human fibroblasts and keratinocytes isolated from a skin biopsy are expanded *in vitro*. The tissue bioengineered skin equivalent is based on a fibrin-based matrix containing live fibroblasts as a dermal component and keratinocytes as the epidermal component. This bioengineered human skin has been successfully transplanted to patients. The skin-humanized mouse model based on the stable engraftment of this setting represents a useful pre-clinical platform to model physiopathological process and to test innovative therapeutic protocols. Histopathological features of the human bioengineered skin *in vitro* and after clinical and preclinical transplantation. H-E: Hematoxylin-Eosin staining.

This chimerical model involves the regeneration of human skin, vascularized and innervated by mouse vessels and nerves. This method allows for the generation of a large number of engrafted mice containing a significant area of homogeneous single donor-derived human skin in a relatively short period of time. We have deconstructed-reconstructed skin disorders using skin cells isolated from healthy donor or patient biopsies. Our work included different rare human monogenic skin diseases, such as the recessive form of dystrophic Epidermolysis Bullosa (RDEB), an inherited mechano-bullous disease (Gache et al., 2004; Spirito et al., 2006), the UV-sensitive cancer-prone disease Xeroderma Pigmentosum (XP) (Garcia et al., 2010), Pachyonychia Congenita (PC) (Garcia et al., 2011) and the Netherton Syndrome (NS) (Di et al., 2011), both debilitating skin disorders. With this model, we have succeeded in reverting the phenotype employing different gene therapy approaches for *ex vivo* correction of cells. We were also able to generate a skin humanized mouse model of acquired conditions such as psoriasis, a common chronic inflammatory disease where the immune component plays a pivotal role (Guerrero-Aspizua et al., 2010). Finally, the model also serves to conduct studies in normal human skin, both in a physiological or pathological context, to gain insight into a process such as wound healing (Escámez et al., 2004, 2008; Martinez-Santamaría et al., 2009 and unpublished results). These wound healing models also allowed the validation of gene and cell therapy approaches to improve impaired wound healing conditions and to favour the efficacy of bioengineered skin substitutes in tissue regeneration.

2. The skin

Skin is the outermost tissue of the body and the largest organ in terms of both weight and surface area. It comprises an area of approximately 1,5-2 m^2 for an adult and represents about 8% of the body weight. The skin has a very complex structure that consists of many components and adnexa including hair follicles, sebaceous glands and sweat glands. The main function of skin is to act as a barrier to the surrounding environment dangers. It protects the body from friction and impact wounds with its flexibility and toughness. It also prevents water loss and regulates body temperature by blood flow and evaporation of sweat. Chemicals, bacteria, viruses and ultraviolet light are also prevented from entering the body by the skin. Furthermore, skin has a large amount of nerves and nerve endings that enable it to act as a sensory organ. When exposed to sunlight, skin can produce vitamin D, a critical molecule for calcium metabolism.

The skin is formed by anatomically, functionally and developmentally distinct tissues: the epidermis and the dermis. These layers are composed of different types of cellular elements. Hence, they are very different in terms of structure and function.

2.1 Epidermis

The epidermis is the outermost component of the skin formed mostly by a particular kind of epithelial cells known as keratinocytes. Other epidermis resident cells also include melanocytes, Merkel and Langerhans cells, responsible for important specialized functions.

The epidermis is morphologically divided into different layers or strata. From the bottom (innermost), these layers are stratum basale (basal cell layer), stratum spinosum (prickle cell layer), stratum granulosum (granular cell layer), stratum lucidum (clear layer) and stratum corneum (horny cell layer). Keratinocytes produced in the basal layer, where cell proliferation is confined, move upward to the outer surface in a process named as epidermal

differentiation. During this turn-over, keratinocytes change their structures and physiological functions. One cycle of this turn-over process takes about 28 days.
The differentiation process involves morphological and biochemical changes with temporal and spatial changes in gene expression. Specific proteins are characteristic of the cells at the different layers of the skin. Thus, the proliferating basal keratinocytes, which express keratin 5 (K5) and keratin 14 (K14), adhere to the basal membrane (BM). Basal keratinocytes mature into suprabasal keratinocytes. This transition is characterized by loss of contact with the BM, proliferation arrest, and downregulation of keratins K5 and K14 accompanied by upregulation of keratins K1 and K10. Finally, suprabasal keratinocytes undergo an apoptosis-related process called terminal differentiation which results in the formation of a layer of dead cornified cells, the stratum corneum. This layer is a main component of the protective skin barrier. The terminal differentiation process is accompanied by the expression of marker proteins such as transglutaminase, involucrin, fillagrin and loricrin among others. The hair follicles (HFs), which together with sweat and sebaceous glands form the epidermal appendages, are formed during embryogenesis as outgrowths of the epidermis.

2.2 Dermis

The dermis is the living layer that acts as a substrate and a support network for the epidermis. The essential dermal cell type is the fibroblast, which is responsible for the production and maintenance of the structural elements of skin. These elements, which include collagen and elastin, combine with non-fibrous substances such as glycosaminoglycans (GAGs) to form the extra-cellular matrix (ECM). The ECM also supports the basement membrane, ensuring the integrity of the dermo-epidermal junction (DEJ). Organized tissue renewal depends on the ECM. Normally, turnover of collagen is low, but occurs at a higher rate during damage repair. The vascular network, which is difficult to replace, is quite critical to skin regeneration. Without an adequate blood supply, repair is impaired, and if revascularization cannot be achieved, undesirable scar tissue formation is enhanced. Adequate regulation of the inflammatory and immunologic responses of the skin also plays a pivotal role in tissue regeneration. Imbalanced inflammation may prevent the progression of the regenerative (Eming et al., 2007; Pierce, 2001)
A complex BM composed by specialized proteins serves as an epidermal and dermal anchoring structure but also clearly establishes a boundary between epithelial and mesenchymal territories. Mutations in the genes coding for the BM proteins (i.e. collagen VII or laminin 5) are responsible for rare inherited mechano-bullous diseases.

2.3 Epidermal stem cells

Early tracing experiments performed in human and mouse epidermis demonstrated that within the basal layer of interfollicular epidermis there was a remarkable proliferative heterogeneity. However, these studies did not lead the way to the identification of *bona fide* functional markers for human epidermal stem cells (ESCs). Markers including, $\alpha6^{bri}$/$CD71^{dim}$, and $Lrig1^{+}$ were suggested to be useful to enrich for highly clonogenic cells (Li et al., 2004; Jensen et al., 2008). However, a criterion established more that 20 years ago, based on the *in vitro* proliferative capacity of keratinocytes remains the most reliable way to identify the putative stem cells of human interfollicular epidermis (Barrandon & Green, 1987). Based on these criterion three populations known as holoclones (clones with high clonogenic capacity and very high proliferative potential), meroclones (clones with less proliferative potential than holoclones, from committed progenitors or transitory amplifying cells) and paraclones (clones with low proliferative capacity near terminal differentiation) were defined. This classification is still valid, and considers the holoclone as strictly derived from the human interfollicular epidermal stem cell. Thus, clonogenic assays appear to be the best predictors of "stemness", at least in terms of extensive proliferative capacity of the putative interfollicular epidermal stem cells (Barrandon & Green, 1987; Mathor et al., 1996). These *in vitro* studies have demonstrated that either wild type or genetically modified cultured human epidermal cell clones named as holoclones, are endowed with an extraordinary replicative potential. One controversial point in the field of human epidermal stem cells in relation to regenerative medicine, is to establish whether there really is a cell subpopulation that has all the attributes of stem cells, or if, conversely, cells with limited proliferative capacity (defined as a population of transitory amplifying cells) can be programmed or reprogrammed to renew the epidermis in the long term (Li et al., 2004). However, neither both the actual proportion and performance, nor dynamics of the human epidermal repopulating clones *in vivo* have been studied in detail as done already with human hematopoietic stem cells. Although previous attempts to assess the putative stem cell behaviour of single genetically modified human clones (holoclones) *in vivo* were unsuccessful (Mathor et al., 1996), recent advances in organotypic cultures and surgical techniques have now made it possible to achive this goal (Larcher et al., 2007).

Much of the current enthusiasm for the study of human embryonic stem cells (hSC) comes from the possible therapeutic use of somatic cells derived from them. While skin biopsies are the regular source of keratinocytes and ESCs, recent studies aim at generating keratinocytes from human embryonic stem cells. By assessing the sequential expression of specific transcription factors, Howard Green and co-workers followed the time- and migration-dependent development of the keratinocyte lineage from human embryonic stem cells in culture (Green et al., 2003). In a recent study these authors also established differences between post-natal keratinocytes and those derived from hSC showing that the latter have much lower proliferative potential in culture implying that hES-derived single keratinocytes cannot be expanded into mass cultures (Iuchi et al., 2006). They also showed that optimization of culture conditions improves the proliferation, but not sufficiently to permit their clonal isolation. However, our group, in collaboration with researchers at INSERM/UEVE U-861 (France) has recently succeeded in obtaining a homogenous population of keratinocytes derived from hSC. Following assembly in a proper scaffold and grafting to immunodeficient mice, these keratinocytes retained their ability to regenerate a fully differentiated self-renewing epidermis (Guenou et al., 2009). In relation with this issue, de-differentiation of adult cells into a pluripotent embryonic stage has been achieved. These cells are known as iPS (induced pluripotent stem cells) (Takahashi et al., 2007). While iPS cells have been generated from somatic cells, optimization of the process is still underway. The obtaining of differentiated cells from iPS or hES is still a major challenge. Recently, iPS cells have been obtained from EB patients (Tolar et al., 2011) and it is expected that iPSs from other skin diseases will soon be generated. So far, iPS cells differentiation to fully functional keratinocytes, as performed with hES, has not been reported. It is, however, a matter of further attempts and time to achieve this major goal.

3. Clinical applications of bioengineered skin

Skin is the most antigenic tissue in the body and it is refractory to currently known tolerance induction regimens. This fact has long precluded the use of allogenic skin grafts for permanent tissue replacement. Allogenic cadaver skin grafts have been shown, however, to be of value as temporary skin replacement (i.e. temporary coverage of burn patients). When used in this context, a rejection of the epidermal layer of the grafted skin is clinically evident within 2-3 weeks post-grafting. Therefore, permanent skin regeneration has only been achieved with autologous ESCs transplantation (either as part of split-thickness grafts or of bioengineered skin equivalents).

The introduction of tissue-engineering in therapeutics opened the debate on the idea that allogenic skin equivalents are better tolerated by the host than the allogenic split-thickness grafts. In fact, allogenic bioengineered skin does not appear to evoke acute clinical rejection (Falanga et al., 1998). Instead, a gradual replacement of the allogenic cells by host cells occurs (silent rejection). This process is probably triggered by a response of the host immune system elicited by HLA-mismatch system (Hohlfeld et al., 2005). During this continuous replacement, cytokine release, structural support and provision of a moist wound environment supplied by the allogenic skin substitute would explain the improvement in the clinical course of wounds treated with allogenic bioengineered skin equivalents. Analysis of donor allogenic cell DNA in biopsies of healed wounds after application of a living skin equivalent (Apligraf®), for example, have demonstrated one-month persistence of allogenic cells in only a minority of venous ulcer patients, and the complete disappearance of these cells by two months post-application (Griffiths et al., 2004; Phillips et al., 2002). It is a widely demonstrated fact that allogenic keratinocytes do not persist and are progressively substituted by autologous keratinocytes of the patient in a process that lasts a few weeks. The fate of allogenic fibroblasts it is less clear. Some studies have reported persistence for up to 2.5 years (Otto et al., 1995). Within this context, it is now clear that allogenic bioengineered skin equivalents have a role only as temporary biological dressings with relevant healing promoting activity. Therefore, allogenic skin substitute transplantation is currently used to improve the healing of both acute and chronic wounds, including EB lesions (Eisenberg & Llewelyn, 1998; Falabella et al., 2000; Fivenson et al., 2003).

3.1 Permanent replacement of skin losses

In the mid seventies, Howard Green and co-workers set up the methods for serial culture and large expansions of human epidermal keratinocytes based on the use of a specific growth factor cocktail and the presence of lethally irradiated mouse fibroblasts acting as a *feeder layer* (Rheinwald & Green, 1975). Although grafting of pure epithelial sheets has helped to save the life of seriously burned patients around the world (Carsin et al., 2000; Compton, 1992; O´Connor et al., 1981), the approach showed various drawbacks including the fragility of the product, a limited engraftment efficacy, abnormal ultrastructure of the dermo-epidermal junction resulting in blistering and contracture leading to poor aesthetic clinical outcome (Mommaas et al., 1992; Woodley et al., 1988). Soon it became evident that a much more robust skin replacement system was needed. A race to develop and market such products started in the 80's and still continues. As a result, bioengineered skin substitutes have emerged as the most carefully studied and proven of the advanced wound management technologies. While the initial impetus for their development was to replace autograft, allograft, and xenograft in acute skin loss applications, they have found even wider application in the treatment of chronic wounds.

Bioengineered skin substitutes represent artificial alternatives to skin grafts that avoid the pain, potential complications and surface limitations of native skin harvesting. They should be easy to manipulate, resistant and always available in any quantity needed. In terms of function, the ideal skin substitute should mimic the physiology of normal skin, being highly effective in achieving tissue regeneration and wound repair. It should be inexpensive, not subject to immune rejection by the host, and should have an extensive shelf-life. Tissue engineering of cultured skin substitutes is largely based on the strategy that the following three components are important in a bioengineered construct: 1) cell source, 2) tissue-regeneration-inducing factors, and 3) matrix or scaffold (Langer & Vacanti, 1993). A variety of cells, soluble mediators, and biopolymers have been tested in various combinations to engineer cultured skin substitutes. As already mentioned, epidermal sheets of cultured keratinocytes have been applied to wounds as allografts or autografts. Later, it was shown that replacing the connective tissue along with keratinocytes may increase mechanical strength of healed wounds and reduce ultimate scarring (Cuono et al., 1987; Desai et al., 1991; Gallico, 1990) so fibroblasts have been included in some artificial skin substitutes (Hansbrough et al., 1989; Llames et al., 2004; Meana et al., 1998). Others have used matrix-cultured dermal fibroblasts alone as a wound healing device (Marston et al., 2003). Due to difficulties in producing and marketing autologous skin equivalents, most current commercial bioengineered skin substitutes consist of sheets of a biomaterial matrix containing allogenic cells (keratinocytes, fibroblasts or both), which are typically derived from neonatal foreskin, a convenient tissue source with the added advantages of a higher content of putative keratinocyte stem cells, robust cell growth and metabolic activity, and reduced antigenicity. The steps in creating and combining the components of bioengineered skin have been comprehensively discussed elsewhere (Boyce and Warden, 2002). Many recent reviews have summarized the history and current status of matrices and skin substitutes (Beele, 2002; Ehrenreich & Ruszczak, 2006; Hansen et al., 2001; Horch et al., 2005).

Although an ideal skin substitute has not yet been developed, we have contributed within this field with the development of a fibroblast-containing fibrin-based bioengineered skin product (WO/2002/072800) that does fulfil many of the clinical requirements. The fibroblast-containing fibrin-based bioengineered skin was devised by carefully looking at the wound healing process. Thus, fibrin was chosen as a matrix suitable to host dermal cells in a bioengineered skin equivalent. Fibrin is the primary and temporary wound healing matrix allowing blood clotting and migration of both, epithelial and mesenchymal cellular elements that, in turn, will repair the damaged tissue. The resistance and flexibility of the fibrin clot are ideally suited for grafting manipulations. In fact, acellular commercial fibrin gels have been used as carriers for human keratinocyte sheets grown, on top, using the standard Rheinwald & Green method. This system, replacing only the epidermal tissue, has been successfully used for grafting of burn patients (Pellegrini et al., 1999; Ronfard et al., 2000).

A major breakthrough was achieved with the demonstration that live human fibroblasts embedded in blood cryoprecipitate-derived fibrin gels were able to support human keratinocyte growth without the need of a *feeder layer* (Meana et al., 1998). Although soluble growth-stimulatory factors provided either by *feeder* cells or live human fibroblasts may be equivalent, the unique mechanical or nesting anti-differentiating signals attributed to *feeder* cells are somehow replaced by survival signals originated as a consequence of keratinocyte-fibroblast-fibrin interactions. However, fibrin (fibrinogen) may not be the only relevant factor since plasma cryoprecipitate also contains additional factors such as fibronectin or thrombospondin that may contribute to keratinocyte adherence and survival. More recently, a fibrin-based dermal matrix was obtained from pure plasma allowing the generation of fully autologous skin equivalents since keratinocytes, fibroblasts and fibrin may come from the same individual (Figure 1) (Llames et al., 2004). A major feature of fibroblast-containing fibrin-based scaffolds is that human keratinocytes can be seeded at low densities, decreasing the amount of primary cells needed to generate a graftable skin equivalent. This is in greater contrast to collagen-based dermal equivalents such as Apligraf® in which keratinocytes are seeded at near confluence densities. Other features of the fibrin-based skin equivalent are its low cost and long shelf life. Moreover, the fibrin-based bioengineered skin developed by our team has been used successfully, in its autologous version, for permanent skin regeneration in different situations such as extensive burns, necrotizing fascitis, removal of giant nevi and graft-versus-host disease (Figure 2) (Llames et al., 2004; Llames et al., 2006; Gómez et al., 2011).

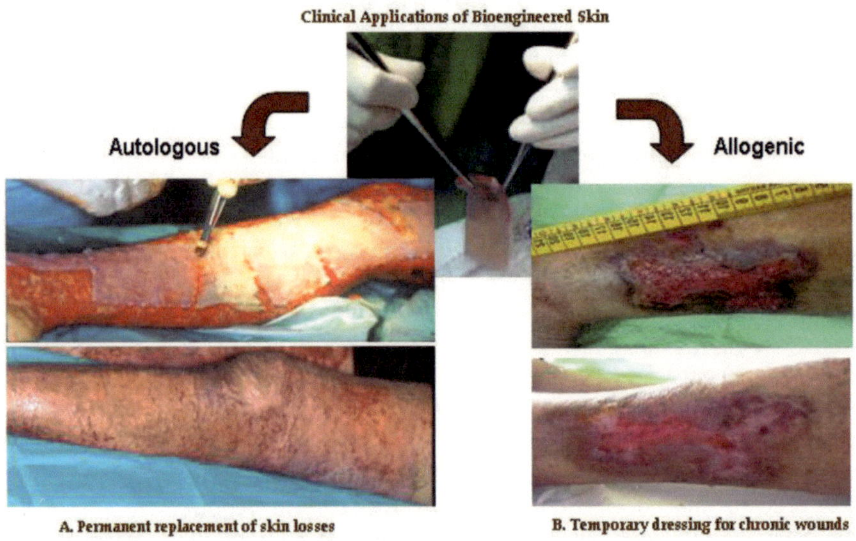

Fig. 2. **Clinical applications of fibrin-based bioengineered skin. (A)** Permanent skin regeneration on burn patients after autologous transplantation. **(B)** Skin regeneration on chronic ulcers by allogenic temporary coverage.

The treatment of more than 100 patients with extensive and severe burns, carried out in several Spanish hospitals, has achieved reasonable cosmetic results and encouraging graft take percentages. Two major causes were disclosed as responsible for cases of poor engraftment: 1) resistant infections of the graft recipient bed and 2) poor vascularised wound beds. These processes jeopardize the viability of bioengineered skin and are significantly affected by wound bed conditioning. Antimicrobial peptides (AMPs) are effective against a broad spectrum of pathogens, have low rates of bacterial resistance and in some cases favour the repair process. As such, they emerge as an alternative to conventional antibiotics. Concerning this issue, our studies support that cutaneous tissue engineering in combination with gene therapies may provide a strategy to promote neoangiogenesis (Lasso et al., 2007; Lugo et al., 2011) and combat infection at the same time (Carretero et al., 2004; Carretero et al., 2008).

3.2 Temporary dressing for chronic wounds

The primary difficulties associated with commercial autologous bioengineering skin substitutes related to high cost and logistics make them relatively unpopular products on the market. However, the use of allogenic skin equivalents for chronic wounds is a different story. The treatment of such hard-to-heal, chronic, open wounds has gained importance as both, the aged segment of the population in the industrialized world and the incidence of comorbid states, such as diabetes mellitus and atherosclerosis have increased. Thus a potential market of 1-2% of the total population in the developed countries led to the development of several competing commercial products struggling to show their benefits in the clinics (Eisenbud et al., 2004; Herschthal & Kirsner, 2011; Límová M., 2010).

Although great advances in terms of molecular mechanisms underlying the process of wound healing are being achieved, the science behind treatment of chronic wounds with skin substitutes is mostly empirical and not well understood. Several beneficial effects range from maintenance of a biochemically balanced moist wound environment to structural support for tissue regeneration and/or the provision of beneficial cytokines and growth factors to the wound bed. The latter is perhaps the best bet as skin substitutes made with younger donor cells appear to work better. In fact, Mansbridge et al. have reported that the viability and metabolic activity of the cellular component of a skin substitute is essential for therapeutic efficacy and have proposed that this is due to the need for ongoing cytokine expression in the wound bed following application (Mansbridge et al., 1998). In this regard, these authors also showed that metabolic activity, but probably not cell proliferative capacity, appears to be the critical event associated with healing efficacy.

As mentioned, allogenic skin substitutes provide cells that do not persist on the recipient site and thus, can be considered safe. In the case of chronic wounds, therefore, the goals of skin substitute therapy have evolved away from providing an immediate new skin (involving graft take) towards the more reasonable goal of providing a temporary biologic dressing that accelerates skin tissue regeneration and wound healing by stimulating the recipient's own wound bed-derived skin cells. Defining the specific, discrete causes of the healing impairment may thus help to develop a combination of cell and gene therapy approaches aimed at providing *a la carte* solutions for the different subsets of chronic wound suffering patients. While the end point of wound closure is the most intensely studied, there is also increasing focus upon the quality of the healed wound and in pain control. Cell-based wound therapies have indeed the potential to reduce both wound contraction and pain. Of note, an allogenic version of the fibroblast-containing fibrin-based skin equivalent has been used as an efficient means for triggering/promoting healing at the patient's own expense and releasing pain (Camblor-Santervas et al., 2003; Coto-Segura et al., 2007, 2008). A great efficacy/recurrence ratio has been achieved by using this allogenic bioengineered skin as a temporary cover. In particular, an 80% healing rate was attained by the weekly application of fresh allogenic bioengineered skin during an average period of 6.6 weeks. Relatively high percentage of ulcer recurrence (25%) is observed since these temporary substitutes do not cure the underlying ischemic or diabetic disease (Llames et al., 2008). As mentioned before, cutaneous tissue engineering in combination with gene therapy may provide strategies that extend the temporal effects at a local level, for example, by producing VEGF or other pro-angiogenic factors that enhance angiogenesis during the healing process (Lasso et al., 2007; Lugo et al., 2011).

3.3 Skin bioengineering for Epidermolysis Bullosa

The skin is the site of a wide variety of inherited diseases. In fact, genes involved in more than 80 skin disorders have been identified some of which are causative of rare diseases. Low prevalence, less than 1 affected in 2000 individuals, is the common feature shared by all rare diseases. Rare diseases are often chronically debilitating or even life-threatening and the impact on the quality of life of affected patients (of whom many are children) and their family members is significant. The limited number of patients and scarcity of relevant knowledge and expertise conferred on them a remarkable research interest on rare diseases. The fact that this low prevalence conditions can serve as models for more common disorders and that their study/management frequently require multidisciplinary innovative approaches add value to the development of this field. To date, a very limited number of so-called orphan drugs are marketed, leaving the majority of rare diseases without any effective treatment. This fact has focused additional attention on new therapeutic approaches such as gene therapy. Cutaneous gene therapy has been one of most intensively explored fields (Del Rio et al., 2002a). In fact, the first successful gene therapy trial for junctional epidermolysis bullosa (JEB), a rare mechano-bullous genodermatosis, has been reported (Mavilio et al., 2006). Mavilio et al. transplanted genetically engineered epidermal stem cells from a JEB adult patient affected by laminin beta3-deficiency modified with a retroviral vector expressing LAMB3 cDNA. Moreover, long-term correction of RDEB using genetically modified human keratinocytes has been also achieved in pre-clinical assays (Del Rio et al., 2004; Spirito et al., 2006). Indeed, permanent correction involves vector-mediated transgene integration into the target-cell genome. Safety concerns related to insertional mutagenesis arose as a consequence of cancer development in two patients undergoing hematopoietic gene therapy for an inherited immunodeficiency (Hacein-Bey-Abina et al., 2003). Therefore, although gene therapy remains the golden standard for genetic disease correction, alternative therapeutic strategies such as cell therapy might be effective. On this regard, the previously mentioned orphan drug chimerical skin (autologous keratinocytes and allogenic fibroblasts) has been proved to be useful for RDEB treatment in the pre-clinical skin humanized mice as discussed further in this chapter. The attempt to improve the healing of EB lesions (including donor sites) by allogenic skin substitute transplantation (Eisenberg & Llewelyn, 1998; Falabella et al., 2000; Fivenson et al., 2003) has shown to report benefit and need to be explored in a systematic manner.

3.3.1 Allogenic bioengineered skin

Mitten deformities of the hands and feet occur in nearly every patient with the most severe form of RDEB (RDEB sev gen), and in at least 40–50% of all other RDEB patients. Hand deformities include adduction contractures of the first web space, pseudosyndactyly, and flexion contractures of the interphalangeal, metacarpophalangeal, and wrist joints. Surgical intervention is commonly performed to correct these deformities, but recurrence and the need for repeated surgery are common. Life-table analyses emphasize the need for early surveillance and intervention, since musculoskeletal complications may occur within the first year of life. The severity of the deformity worsens with age, and surgical correction becomes more difficult. Standard surgical procedures for the management of hand deformities in DEB includes incisional release of contracture and digits follow by autologous partial-thickness skin grafts transplantation to cover secondary wounds. Partial-thickness skin grafts are taken from patient's own skin (e.g. the top segment of the leg), thus creating an additional open wound (a donor site).

Figure 3 shows a surgically created donor site during the standard programmed treatment for pseudosyndactyly and contracture. The skin obtained from the patient's donor site (Figure 3F) is used to cover the wounds that result from incisional release of contracture and digits (Figure 3B-C). In the literature there is no consensus on the management of the split-thickness donor sites secondary to reconstructive surgery (Demirtas et al., 2010; Pan et al., 2011). On the other hand, allogenic bioengineered skin transplantation has proven to be of clinical value when used as a healing device aiming at tissue repair/regeneration for chronic wounds (Camblor-Santervas et al., 2003; Coto-Segura et al., 2007, 2008; Eisenbud et al., 2004; Herschthal & Kirsner, 2011; Límová M., 2010) such as vascular ulcers and for full thickness excisional surgical wounds for skin cancer treatment (Donohue et al., 2005; Gohari et al., 2002). As previously discussed, this strategy provides a temporary biologic dressing that accelerates skin tissue regeneration promoting re-epithelialization from patient wound edges and release pain. On that basis, we are currently testing the clinical benefits of allogenic bioengineered skin transplantation on DEB patient donor sites to reduce pain and accelerate healing (Figure 3G-I).

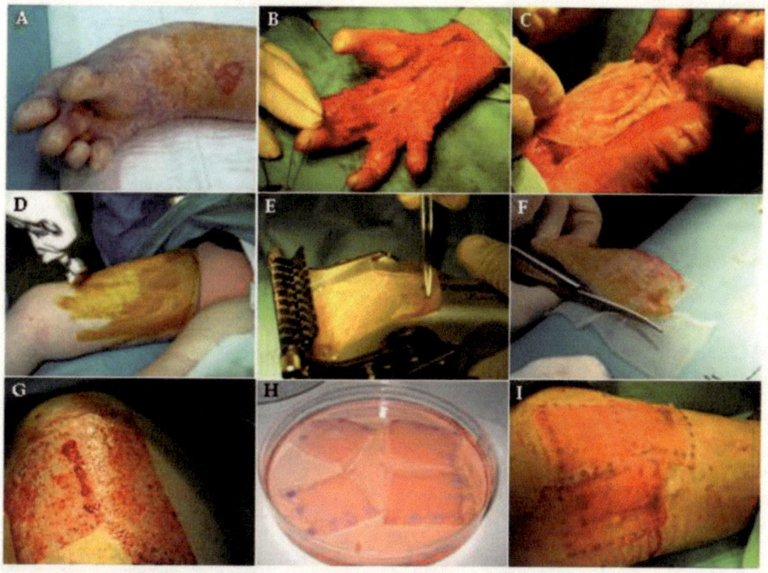

Fig. 3. **Surgical management of hand contractures and pseudosyndactyly in RDEB.** **(A)** Typical pseudosyndactyly and contracture of the thumb and fingers developed by RDEB patients. **(B)** Standard surgical procedure for the correction of these deformities by incisional release. **(C)** Autograft of secondary wounds with split-thickness skin from donor site. **(D-E)** Surgical generation of a donor site on the patient's upper-leg using a dermatome. **(F)** Split-thickness skin from donor site. **(G-I)** Donor site transplantation using allogenic bioengineered skin (panel H). Courtesy of Dr. Mir, Plato Clinic (Barcelona). The clinical images have been taken and reproduced with the signed consent of the patient.

3.3.2 Autologous "revertant" bioengineered skin

The term somatic revertant mosaicism refers to the occurrence of a natural phenomenon involving spontaneous genetic correction of a first pathogenic mutation in a somatic cell (Davis & Candotti, 2010). Different molecular mechanisms such as back mutation, intragenic crossover, mitotic gene conversion, and/or second-site mutation might underlie the *in vivo* reversion. Somatic mosaicism has also been reported in genodermatoses, including EB. In the skin of these patients, revertant mosaicism is manifested as small patches of clinically "better than expected" skin surrounded by easily blistering tissue (Jonkman & Pasmooij, 2009; Pasmooij et al., 2010). The incidence of this phenomenon of genetic reversion, thought to be rare for years, appears to be more common than imagined (Lai-Cheong et al., 2011; May, 2011). As a matter of fact, to date the phenomenon of revertant mosaicism has already been found in three Spanish RDEB patients. These patients display patches of non-blistering unaffected skin (Figure 4A). The clinical reversion on these long-term persistent patches was further confirmed by the presence of type VII collagen that was almost absent in the non revertant skin (Figure 4B). *COL7A1* pathogenic mutations leading to premature termination codons caused this blistering condition in all three patients. In one of these patients, a second-site mutation, present in revertant keratinocytes, resulted in reading frame correction and wild-type type VII collagen expression leading to restoration of skin function (Pasmooij et al., 2010).

Transplantation of autologous "revertant" bioengineered skin may be a tailored EB therapy for patients with somatic mosaicism and is currently being explored in our laboratory in collaboration with Marcel Jonkman's team in the Netherlands. The ultimate goal of this strategy is the production of sufficient collagen VII from revertant epidermal stem cells to ensure adequate and long-term formation of the anchoring fibrils.

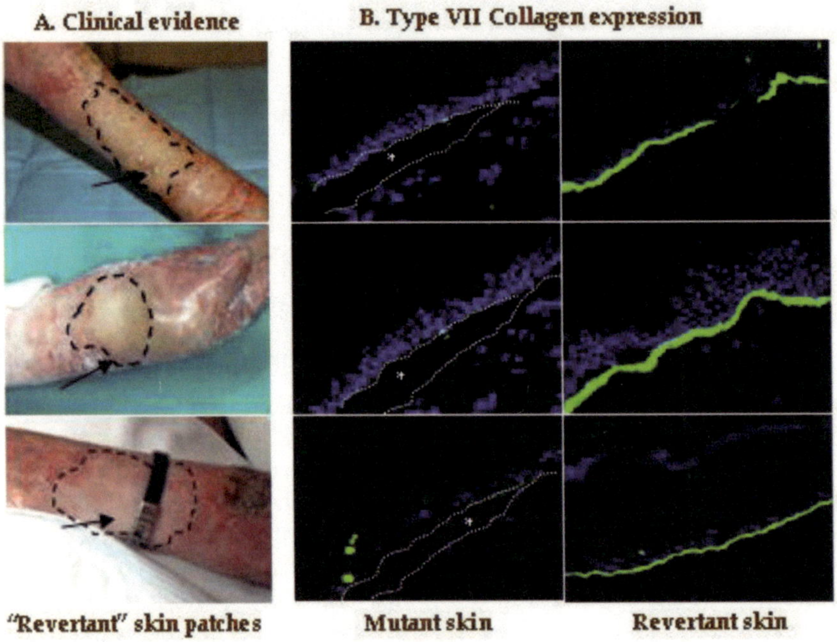

Fig. 4. **Revertant mosaicism in RDEB Spanish patients. (A)** Clinical evidence of "revertant" skin patches (black dashed lines). **(B)** Type VII collagen expression detected by immunofluorescence shows almost complete absence of labelling at the dermal–epidermal junction in mutant skin but bright linear labelling in the revertant samples. White dashed line indicates dermal–epidermal junction. Asterisk depict sub-epidermal blistering.

4. The skin-humanized mouse

In vivo studies in the skin of human beings are obviously limited by ethical and practical constraints. Current knowledge mainly stems from the use of murine models, including knockout and transgenic strategies. However, based on the significant differences existing between human and murine skin architecture and physiology, the question remains as to how far the results can be extrapolated to the human scenario. As an example, animal models such as the two-stage carcinogenesis model in the mouse are valuable tools to unravel critical mechanisms of disease, but do not faithfully recapitulate the human illness counterpart (Garlick, 2007). Studies in large animals such as pigs, whose skin architecture and dynamics resemble that of humans, are an alternative, but troublesome and expensive (Sullivan et al., 2001). Skin organotypic cultures represent a valid alternative to native skin *in vivo* studies (Bernerd et al., 2001; Egles et al., 2010; Harrison et al., 2006). However, they are restricted, among other constraints, by their short culture life span and the absence or faulty pivotal mesenchymal responses such as angiogenesis. To circumvent these problems, researchers have often used xenogenic transplantation of donor/patient cutaneous biopsies to immunocompromised mice to perform relevant *in vivo* experimentation in a human context. However, in addition to difficulties in sourcing, a major concern for this type of experiments is the marked heterogeneity of the graftable skin samples. In fact, differences in genetic background, body site or patient's sun exposure history, among other factors, may severely hamper the outcome of the study. A possibility to overcome these drawbacks involves the stable regeneration of normal or diseased human skin in appropriate hosts by means of tissue engineering (Khavari, 2006). This approach, although realistic, represents a significant challenge that involves adequate human epidermal stem cell manipulation *in vitro*, a technique that only a limited number of laboratories can handle. Hence, stable engraftment and regeneration of enough human skin for *in vivo* studies upon grafting of skin substitutes to immunodeficient mice need to be standardized. Our group has developed a methodology enabling the generation of large numbers of mice engrafted with a significant area of single donor-derived human skin. The system, named as the skin-humanized mouse, is based on the optimized grafting of a fibrin-based bioengineered human skin (Del Rio et al., 2002b; Escámez et al., 2004; Llames et al., 2004). Using this setting, a mature, quiescent, homogeneous human skin is achieved avoiding the need for volunteers and overcoming major differences in tissue architecture and kinetics with mouse skin.

The technical procedure involves the deconstruction-reconstruction of the skin of healthy donors or patients suffering from the different diseases (Figure 1). That is, *in vitro* isolation and amplification of cells (fibroblasts and keratinocytes, including the population of epidermal stem cells) from biopsies and their assembly as a bioengineered skin that is subsequently transplanted to immunodeficient mice (Del Rio et al., 2002b; Llames et al., 2004) (Figure 5).

The human regenerated skin showed the restoration of both epidermal and dermal skin compartments (Figure 6; Llames et al., 2004) indicating functional epidermal stem-cell preservation as further confirmed by the analysis of the regenerated skin after a secondary transplant protocol (Larcher et al., 2007). The secondary transplant protocol on immunodeficient mice is conducted by purifying epidermal and dermal cells from the regenerated skin after primary transplantation. These cells are secondary transplanted to immunodeficient mice as part of a human bioengineered skin. Stable regeneration of skin displaying a well-stratified and differentiated epithelium 40 weeks post-grafting is achieved, which is only possible with epidermal stem cells whose stemness has been preserved.

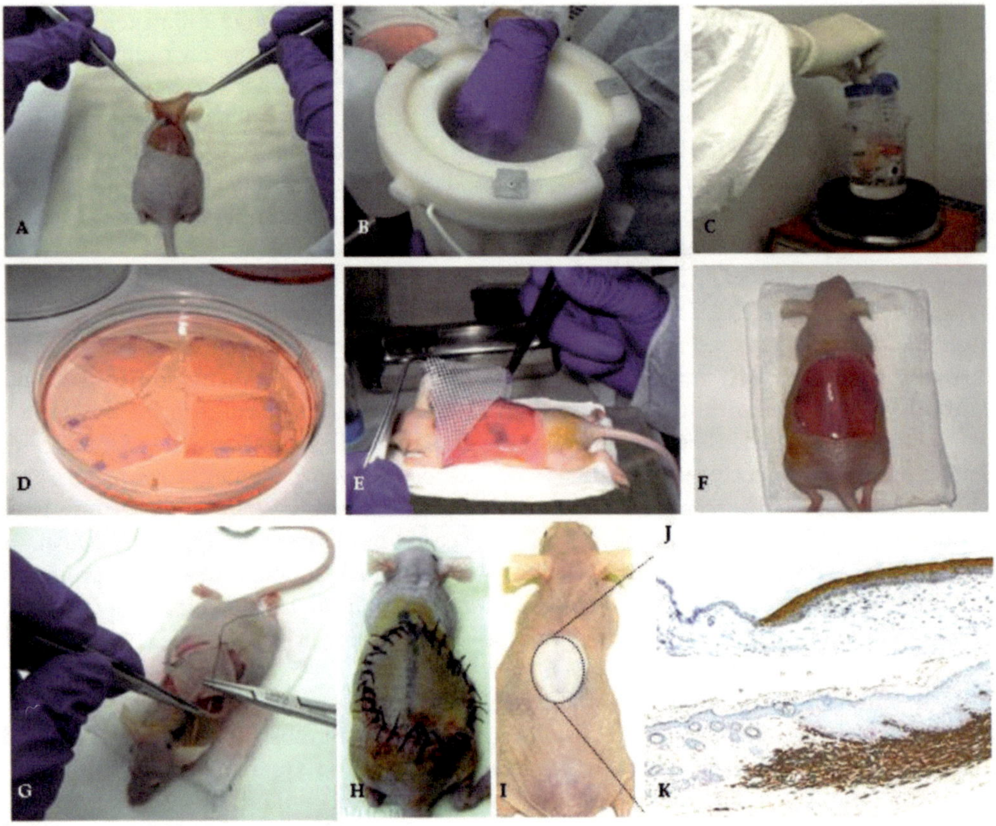

Fig. 5. **Bioengineered skin orthotopical transplantation procedure. (A)** Full thickness 12 mm circular wounds are created on the dorsum of a 6-week old nude mouse. **(B-C)** Mouse skin is de-vitalized by three frozen and thaw cycles. **(D-F)** The bioengineered skin is placed covering the wound. **(G-H)** De-vitalized mouse skin is used as a biological bandage and held in place by suture. **(I)** Human and mouse skin boundaries are outlined by a dashed line. **(J)** Immunostaining of human involucrin at the junction of regenerated human skin and murine host denoting the human origin of the regenerated epidermis. **(K)** Immunostaining of human vimentin at the junction of regenerated human skin and murine host denoting the human origin of the regenerated dermis.

Moreover, regenerated human skin retains the main physio-pathological characteristics of the donor/patient opening a range of possibilities for faithful recreation of different human skin pathologies *in vivo* (Gache et al., 2004; Spirito et al., 2006). The skin-humanized mouse model also offers the possibility of using genetically modified human keratinocytes and/or fibroblasts. These humanized models have been a unique platform on which to evaluate innovative therapeutic strategies in dermatology such as cell therapy using ESCs derived from both adult and embryonic stem cells (Escámez et al., 2009; Guenou et al., 2009; Larcher et al., 2008; Larcher et al., 2009) and gene therapy (Bergoglio et al., 2007; Del Rio et al., 2002b; Di Nunzio et al., 2008; Escámez et al., 2008; Escámez et al., 2004; Larcher et al., 2001; Larcher et al., 2007; Lasso et al., 2007). In this chapter, we summarized our experience with the system in modeling various normal and pathologic skin processes.

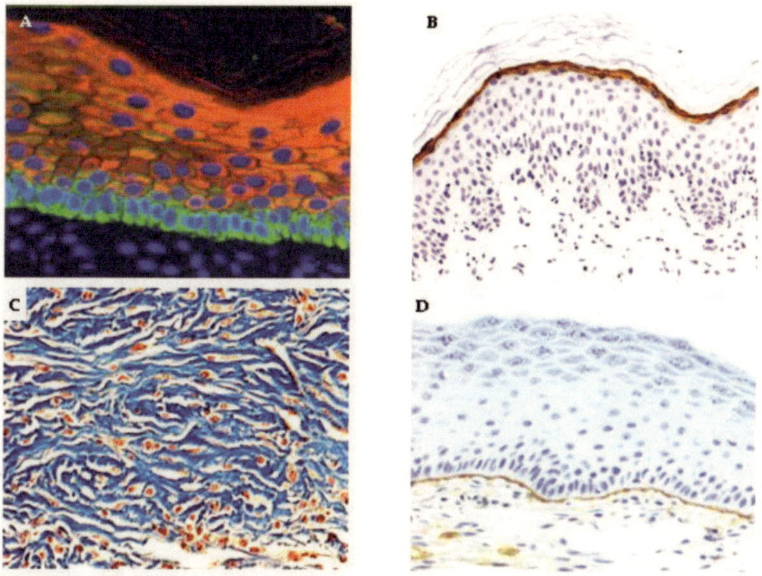

Fig. 6. **The skin humanized model recapitulates the main anatomo-pathological features of human skin.** Presence of a stratified well-differentiated epithelium. **(A)** Keratin K5 immunostaining (green) and keratin K10 immunostaining (red) on the regenerated human skin. **(B)** Loricrin immunostaining on the regenerated human skin. **(C)** Masson's trichrome staining showing a well-vascularized, mature, collagen-rich dermis on the regenerated human skin. **(D)** Laminin immunostaining of the dermo-epidermal junction denoting basal membrane restoration on the regenerated human skin.

4.1 Modeling rare monogenic skin diseases

The European Commission on Rare Diseases estimated that between 6000 and 8000 different rare diseases affect or will affect 29 million people in the European Union. In Spain, around 3 million people are affected by a rare disease. Poor availability of diagnostic and therapeutic options is a major consequence of the limited funding dedicated to research on rare diseases. Recently, a great effort is being made by the worldwide scientific community to optimize human and financial resources for the study of these diseases. In Spain, as an initiative of the Instituto Nacional de Salud Carlos III, the Centre for Biomedical Network Research on Rare Diseases (CIBERER), a network structure has been set up to pool and promote excellence in research devoted to the diagnosis and therapies of rare diseases. Within this picture, development of rare disease models, especially in a human context, would contribute to the basic and translational research toward individualized medicine by making patients and their families more immediately aware of potential medical interventions. Moreover, rare diseases can serve as models for more common diseases and the complexity of rare diseases often requires multidisciplinary innovative approaches. Based on our solid background in the field of dermatology and our consubstantiation with the objectives of CIBERER, our interest in translational research has grown over the years.

As a result, we have model a wide range of different rare genodermatosis including photosensitive conditions, some of which are described in the present chapter.

4.1.1 Mechano-Bullous genodermatosis: Recessive Dystrophic Epidermolysis Bullosa (RDEB)

As already mentioned, Epidermolysis Bullosa (EB) comprises a clinically and genetically heterogeneous group of rare skin disease characterized by skin blistering, either spontaneous or induced by minimal trauma. Based on the level of blister disruption, three types of EB are defined: Simplex (EBS), junctional (JEB) and dystrophic (DEB) (Fine et al., 2008). The prevalence of EB in Europe is estimated to be 0.60 per 10,000 individuals (Bruckner-Tuderman, 2008). In Spain the prevalence remains unknown because the genetic diagnosis has been recently settled by our team since 2006 with the scientific support of

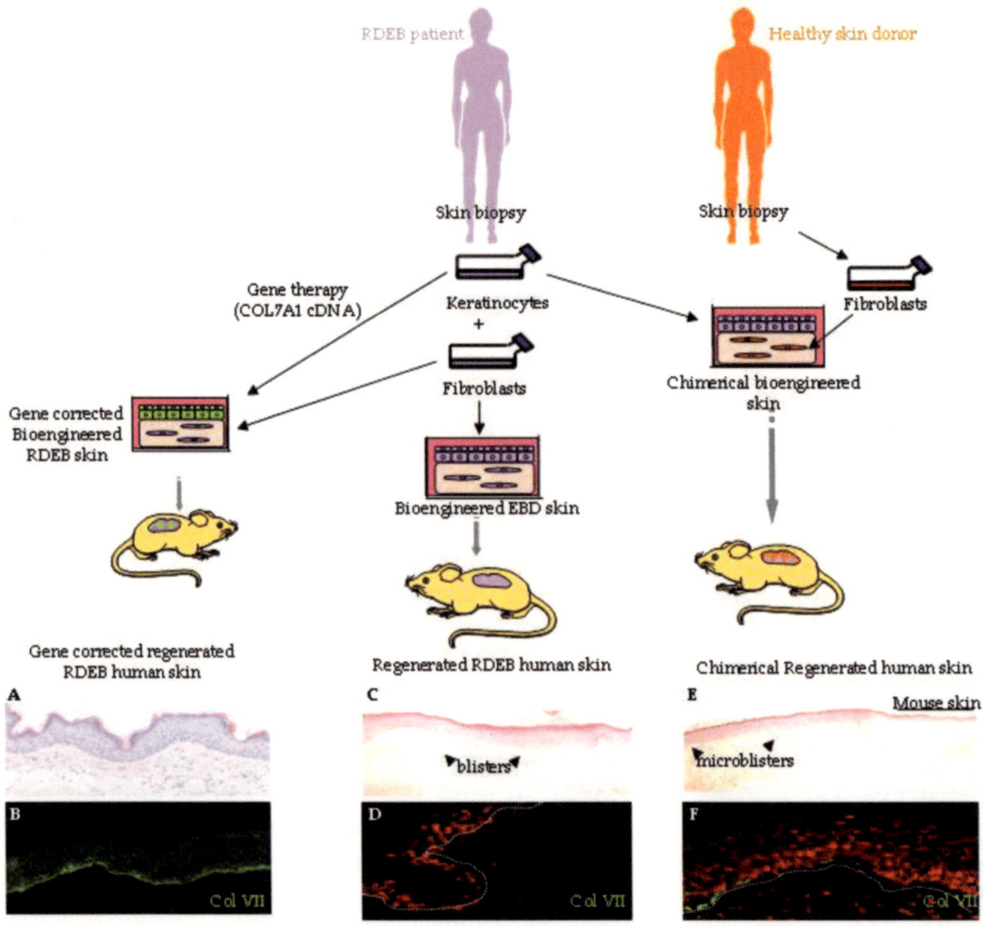

Fig. 7. **Schematic diagram of the experimental design for *in vivo* RDEB keratinocyte correction in a humanized mouse model by gene therapy and chimerical bioengineered skin.** Histological and immunofluorescence staining for Col VII appearance of a **(A,B)** genetically corrected, **(C,D)** non-corrected and **(E,F)** chimerical bioengineered EBD engrafted mice.

European Diagnosis Reference Centres[1] and as part of the CIBERER network (Cuadrado-Corrales et al., 2010; Escámez et al., 2010; García et al., 2011). Studies carried out by our research team in collaboration with Dr. Meneguzzi team showed the possibility of achieving a lasting recapitulation of monogenic hereditary skin diseases of different subtypes of EB (Del Rio et al., 2004; Gache et al., 2004; Garcia et al., 2007). For instance, the recessive subtype of DEB (RDEB; OMIM: 120120), the most severe form of EB, is due to mutations in the gene encoding type VII collagen (*COL7A1*). In particular, null mutations leading to complete absence of collagen VII entail physical deformities and increased risk of developing skin cancer which reduces their life expectancy dramatically. Extensive blistering of regenerated human skin obtained by orthotopic grafting of bioengineered cutaneous equivalents containing collagen VII-null RDEB keratinocytes was observed at a histological level, similarly to skin biopsies from RDEB patients (Figure 7C-D). Genetic modification of RDEB epidermal stem cells by retroviral vectors encoding human collagen type VII used in the generation of the skin equivalents (Figure 7A-B) resulted in a complete and permanent reversion of this phenotype. Phenothypic correction was also attained by a cell-based therapy based on the use of a chimerical bioengineered skin (Figure 7E-F).

4.1.2 Xeroderma Pigmentosum (XP): A photosensitive condition

UV radiation is the main noxious and carcinogenic agent for human skin (Brash et al., 1996; Kraemer, 1997; Matsumura & Ananthaswamy, 2002; Mudgil et al., 2003; Setlow, 1974). There is compelling evidence that each of the three main types of skin cancer, basal cell carcinoma (BCC), squamous cell carcinoma (SCC) and melanoma, is caused by sun exposure. As commented above, studies of UVB effects on the skin of volunteers are precluded by ethical and technical restraints and are inconceivable in cancer-prone patients. Molecular changes associated to UVB irradiation have been extensively characterized *in vitro* in keratinocytes in culture (Li et al., 2001; Sesto et al., 2002). Although highly informative, these transcriptional profiling and other biochemical analyses are somewhat skewed by the fact that cultured keratinocytes represent only a mitotically activated basal cell compartment. The presence of differentiated cell layers of the epidermis achieved in 3D organotypic cultures allows for more accurate *in vitro* models to study UV effects. However, the organotypic systems often maintain a (hyper) proliferative basal stratum as compared with quiescent native human epidermis and only allow for relatively short-term studies. Reliable *in vivo* studies lack behind due to the ethical or practical constraints of using human volunteers or inaccurate animal models. We therefore challenged our system to assess whether it was capable of adequately responding to UV irradiation. To that end, we examined the effect of one biological efficient dose (BED) of UVB light in terms of sunburn cell formation and p53 induction, two well-described surrogate markers of UV action. As predicted, both effects were readily detected after irradiation (Figure 8).

Moreover, by using Caucasian or African-descent donor keratinocytes we were able to confirm the well known modulation of the UVB responses by the degree of skin pigmentation (Del Bino et al., 2006; Kobayashi et al., 1998). The model also proved satisfactory to test topic photoprotective agents as well as DNA damage repair kinetics after UVB irradiation in terms of epidermal hyperplasia and keratin K6 induction (Del Bino et al., 2004; Lee et al., 2002). Based on those results we have also established a photosensitive humanized skin models by grafting bioengineered skin containing Xeroderma

[1] Dr. Zambruno (IDI, Italy), Dr. Meneguzzi (INSERM, France) and Dr. Batty (Ninewells Hospital, UK)

Pigmentosum (XP) patient cells (Figure 8). Xeroderma Pigmentosum (XP) is an autosomal and recessive disorder characterized by a severe deficiency in the most versatile DNA-repair mechanism in charge of the removal of bulky DNA adducts including UV-induced cyclobutane pyrimidine dimmers (CPDs) and pyrimidine pyrimidone photoproducts (6-4PPs). The first *in vivo* evidence of XP keratinocyte deficiency in nucleotide excision repair (NER) was obtained after acute UVB irradiation (Garcia et al., 2010). Our model recapitulated the findings of CPD persistence as previously described using XP-C organotypic skin cultures (Li et al., 2001) (Figure 8) and appears suitable to study chronic effects including mutagenesis and carcinogenesis.

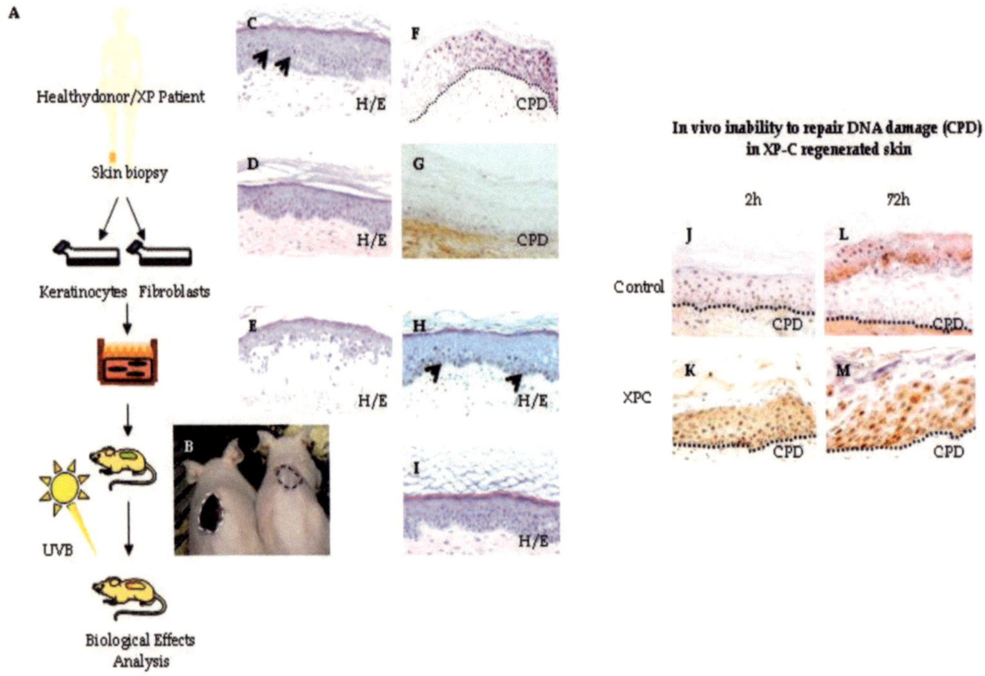

Fig. 8. **Skin humanized mice as a model to study UV responses and carcinogenesis-prone inherited cutaneous disorders. (A)** Schematic diagram of the experimental design. **(B)** Macroscopic appearance of Caucasian (right) and African (left) descent-derived regenerated skins. **(C)** Histological appearance of a 1 BED irradiated Caucasian and **(D)** African descent derived skin 24 hours after irradiation. **(F)** CPD immunostaining of 1 BED-irradiated Caucasian and **(G)** African human regenerated skin 24 hours after irradiation. **(E)** Histological appearance of a 4 BED irradiated Caucasian- and **(H)** African descent-derived skin 24 hours after irradiation. (Arrows indicate sunburn cells). **(I)** Histological appearance of a representative section of a photoprotected (SPF 90), UVB-irradiated (4 BED) Caucasian-derived skin 24 hours after irradiation. Note the absence of acanthosis, epidermolysis, and sunburn cells. ***In vivo* inability to repair DNA damage (CPD) in XP-C regenerated skin.** CPD immunostaining of 4 BED-irradiated normal African-derived skin (control) section at **(J)** 2 and **(L)** 72 hours after irradiation. CPD immunostaining of 4 BED-irradiated XP-C regenerated skin section at **(K)** 2 and **(M)** 72 hours after irradiation. Note the persistence of CPD labeled cells in all epidermal strata indicating a DNA damage repair defect.

4.1.3 Pachyonychia Congenita (PC)

Pachyonychia congenita (PC) is a rare autosomal dominant keratin disorder characterized by thickened and dystrophic nails as well as painful palmoplantar keratoderma and blisters on or near the pressure points of the feet (Leachman et al., 2005; Smith et al., 2006).

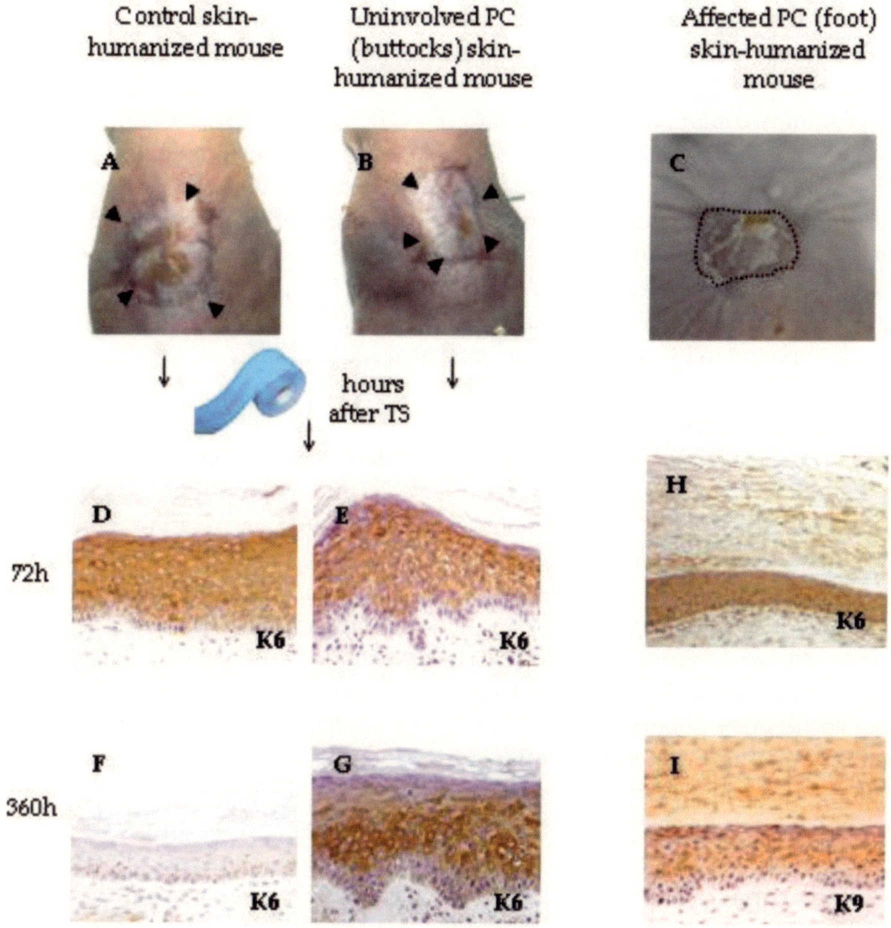

Fig. 9. **Clinical and histopathological features of human pachyonychia congenita (PC) skin. (A-C)** Clinical appearance of engrafted mice. **(A)** Normal, **(B)** PC-regenerated skin from non-affected (buttocks) area and **(C)** PC-regenerated skin from affected foot sole-derived PC cells on immunodeficient mice. **Development of a hyperplastic response in normal and pachyonychia congenita (PC)-regenerated human skin after tape stripping:** Keratin K6 immunoperoxidase staining of **(D,F)** normal and **(E,G)** involved PC-regenerated skin sections at 72 and 360 hours after tape stripping (TS). **(H)** Constitutive expression of K6 in the foot sole-derived PC graft. **(I)** Expression of K9, which is characteristic and exclusively expressed in the palmoplantar suprabasal keratinocytes.

PC is caused by dominant-acting mutations in any one of the genes encoding the differentiation-specific and stress-inducible keratins, K6a, K6b, K16, or K17 (Smith et al., 2005; Wilson et al., 2011). The dominant-negative mutations on these keratins lead to defective intermediate filament formation responsible for all of the epithelial fragility symptoms associated with PC. Mouse models involving the PC-related keratin genes elicit only a subset of minor PC-specific epithelial lesions (Chen et al., 2008; Chen & Roop, 2005; Wong et al., 2005). Importantly, mouse models of PC are recessive, carrying loss-of-function alleles whereas, as mentioned, the human PC mutations are dominant negative (Smith et al., 2005; Wilson et al., 2011). Within this context, our group has contributed with the establishment of two skin-humanized models of PC (Figure 9). First model involves the use of bioengineered skin from an uninvolved area of PC patients carrying the same K6a mutation, displayed epidermal phenotypic changes consistent with a hyperproliferative response. Moreover, the use of keratinocytes from affected skin from another patient carrying a different mutation in the same codon of the keratin K6a gene resulted in the development of a constitutively expressed, *bona fide* PC phenotype. Currently we are evaluating the amenability of these humanized PC models to genetic intervention similar to that recently reported in PC patients (Leachman et al., 2010).

4.1.4 Netherton Syndrome (NS)

Netherton syndrome (NS) is a congenital skin disorder caused by mutations in the SPINK5 gene encoding the lymphoepithelial Kazal-type-related inhibitor (LEKTI) (Bitoun et al., 2003; Chavanas et al., 2000). It is characterized by defective keratinization, recurrent infections, and hypernatremic dehydration with a mortality rate of about 10% in the first year of life (Borgoño et al., 2007; Descargues et al., 2006; Ishida-Yamamoto et al., 2005). Grafting of human NS bioengineered skin onto immunodeficient mice made it possible to recapitulate the characteristic histological features of NS (Di et al., 2011), including psoriasiform changes and hypergranulosis with a parakeratotic stratum corneum and exfoliated corneocytes (Figure 10B). An *ex vivo* approach using a lentiviral vector to direct SPINK5 expression in keratinocytes resulted in reversal of skin abnormalities (Figure 10A) (Di et al., 2011). In this study we found that limited numbers of LEKTI-expressing cells mediate valuable beneficial effects likely through paracrine effects.

4.2 Modeling psoriasis, an inflammatory skin disease

Inflammatory and autoimmune cutaneous disorders are a major health and social concern worldwide. They can be disfiguring and disabling and take a toll in terms of the patient's psychological distress. Skin infiltrating T lymphocytes play a pivotal role in triggering and maintaining common chronic inflammatory skin diseases such as psoriasis and atopic dermatitis, where an unequivocal deregulation in the Th1/Th2/Th17 balance accounts for the pathogenesis. In psoriasis this equilibrium is skewed towards Th1, whereas a Th2 phenotype is predominant in atopic dermatitis. Th17 cells are more abundant in both disorders (Di Cesare et al., 2008).

Reliable animal models for inflammatory cutaneous pathologies will contribute to the comprehensive knowledge of the basic mechanisms underlying the epidermal-immune cell interactions and the development of new therapeutic strategies. The adequacy of the animal model and its robustness to predict outcome will condition clinical success.

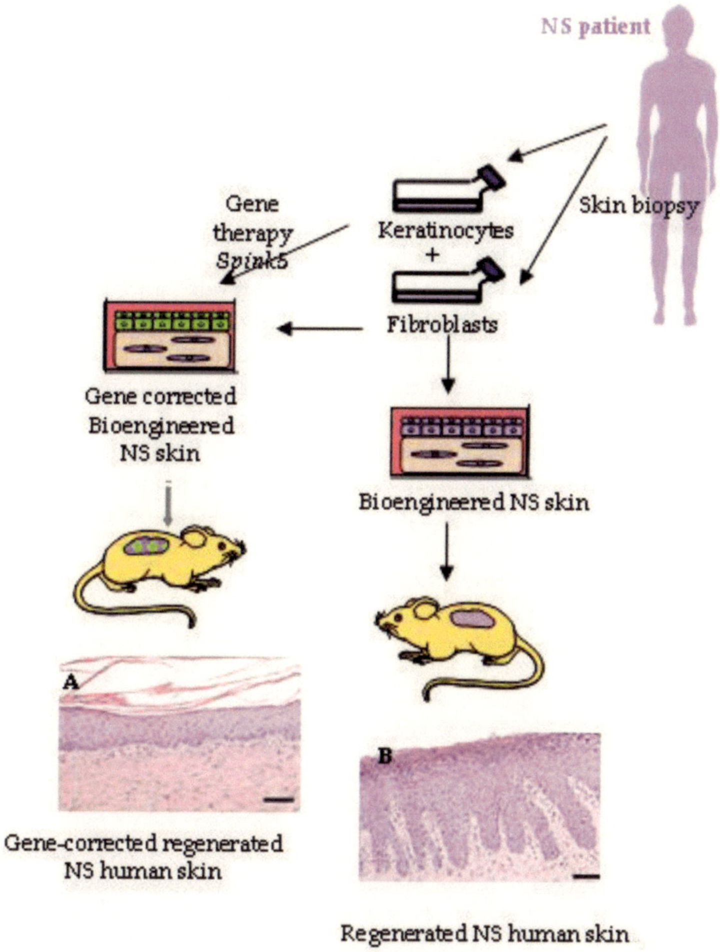

Fig. 10. ***In vivo* assessment of Netherton syndrome (NS) keratinocyte correction in a humanized mouse model by gene therapy.** Schematic diagram of the experimental design for the generation of skin-humanized mouse model: Histological appearance of a gene corrected **(A)** and non-corrected **(B)** NS engrafted mice.

Several transgenic and knockout animal models gave rise to psoriasis- or atopic dermatitis-like phenotypes (Danilenko, 2008; Nestle & Nickoloff, 2005; Schon, 1999; Shiohara et al., 2004; Zheng & Zhu, 2005). Although the differences in both architecture and function between mouse and human skin impose constraints on these models, nonetheless they contribute to elucidate the role of certain molecules in the underlying pathological processes. Xenotransplantation models of psoriasis closely mimic human disorders and have been used extensively (Gilhar et al., 1997; Nickoloff et al., 1995; Wrone-Smith & Nickoloff, 1996). However, the number of grafted mice that can be obtained from a single patient has ethical and practical limitations. Within this context, the bioengineered-skin humanized mouse model emerges as a powerful tool. One of the several potential advantages over other genetically modified or xenotrasplantation animal models is the feasibility of performing studies in a human context on homogeneous and large samples. This approach was recently used to generate a *bona fide* skin-humanized mouse model for psoriasis (Figure 11) (Guerrero-Aspizua et al., 2010). Activated specific lymphocyte subpopulations from the same patients (autologous approach) re-introduced by subcutaneous injection, coupled to tape stripping and the ensuing mild alteration of the epidermal barrier, triggered the psoriatic response. We demonstrated that a healthy normal human skin regenerated in immunodeficient mice using bioengineering technology, might give rise to a psoriasiform phenotype if the appropriate signals are present, i.e. a wounding stimulus and the appropriate cytokines produced by specific lymphocyte subpopulations (Th1/Th17) obtained from unrelated healthy donors (allogeneic approach). These signals play a pivotal role in the formation of the psoriatic plaque. This approach has contributed to elucidate the immunopathogenesis of psoriasis. Several genetic association studies revealed that a large range of susceptibility factors are paramount in the acquisition and/or severity of the disease (Roberson & Bowcock, 2010). However, a specific spatiotemporal combination of cytokines/factors can act directly on the normal lymphocyte-keratinocyte interacting pathways and produce the disease. Furthermore, accessible genetic manipulation of the individual cellular components of the bioengineered humanized skin will make it possible to assess the contribution of potential susceptibility factors to the pathogenesis of psoriasis using this model. Finally, the combined use of these technologies will allow for evaluation of the potential therapeutic effectiveness of novel compounds.

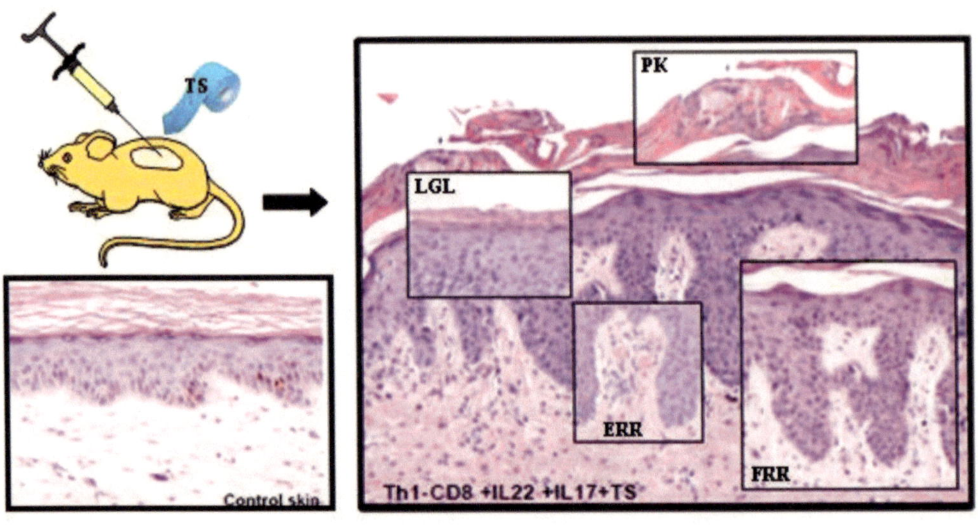

Fig. 11. **The skin humanized model develops a psoriasiform phenotype (A)** after cytokine injection and tape stripping (TS). **(B)** Psoriatic phenotypic hallmarks included elongation (ERR) and fusion of rete ridges (FRR), parakeratosis (PK), and partial loss of the granular layer (LGL).

4.3 Modeling a physiological process: Wound healing

Human cutaneous wound healing is a complex process not completely understood (Coulombe, 2003; Martin, 1997; Singer & Clark, 1999). Development of chronic ulcers associated to a variety of diseases with a prevalence of 1% in the population are major problems of the health care system and carry a high social cost (Ramsey et al., 1999; Stockl et al., 2004). Even more importantly, those clinical situations may not only have severe effects on life quality but also condition the survival of patients, mainly due to the loss of the barrier function of the skin. Despite the absence of effective therapies, palliative treatments are available. Effective treatment of chronic ulcers is one of the greatest medical challenges (Langer & Rogowski, 2009). Currently around 100 clinical trials designed for this purpose are ongoing (Margolis et al., 2004; Senet et al., 2003). Within this context, the search for reliable human wound-healing models that allow us to address both mechanistic and therapeutic matters is warranted. To this end, our team developed an *in vivo* wound-healing model by creating excision wounds on the skin humanized mouse model that faithfully recapitulates all major features of cutaneous wound healing (Figure 12). A careful characterization of the healing process by monitoring the expression of various epidermal and mesenchymal markers showed that re-epithelialization, dermal matrix remodeling and basal membrane reorganization accurately mimic the process in humans (Escámez et al., 2004). This model also allows for the use of *in vitro* genetically manipulated human keratinocytes and/or fibroblasts during the amplification procedure, either to overexpress or silence specific genes, generating transgenic or KO humanized-skin respectively.

A central aim of regenerative medicine is to optimize healing and improve cosmetic outcome. In this sense, one of the main challenges is to create smart bioengineered products that can deliver growth factors and/or cytokines in a time-controlled fashion, promoting scar-free regeneration of embryonic or fetal skin. The combination of cell- and genetic-based therapy has made it possible to evaluate the promoting or detrimental wound-healing activities of specific factors using different model systems, such as transgenic mice, KO-mice or xenograft models (Davidson, 2001; Demarchez et al., 1986; Werner & Grose, 2003). As a proof of concept, we selected KGF, a well-characterized factor that is differentially regulated in normal and impaired healing, to compare the efficacy of different transient gene transfer strategies aimed at delivering smart factors to promote cutaneous repair in the wound healing skin-humanized model (Escámez et al., 2008). In the first approach, hKGF was delivered to wounds by intradermal injection of an adenoviral suspension. Although wound acceleration was achieved, the effect of hKGF was unreliable both in terms of the number of successfully targeted animals (*versus* the total number of treated animals) and re-epithelialization efficiency. In the second approach, KGF-encoding adenoviral vectors were immobilized in a fibrin gel carrier and applied immediately after wounding. In this case, the proportion of successfully targeted animals was higher than that achieved with the adenoviral injection method, and wound closure rose significantly. A third strategy was explored consisting in delivering hKGF protein from *ex vivo* adenoviral transduced fibroblasts that were, in turn, embedded in a fibrin matrix and used to treat the wound. In contrast to the two previous methods based on direct adenovirus delivery, this cell-mediated system did not depend on *in vivo* cell transduction. This method depends on the direct transfer of exogenous KGF therapeutic protein from gene targeted fibroblasts that was, in fact, achieved in all treated wounds, leading to a significant improvement in wound closure. Although all delivery systems achieved KGF protein overproduction at the wound site, with a concomitant re-epithelialization enhancement, only the use of genetically modified fibroblast-containing matrix as an *in situ* protein bioreactor was highly reproducible. This method appears the most reliable means to deliver growth factors to wounds avoiding the potential danger of scoring cases of faulty administration as therapeutic failures and direct exposure to viral vectors. The bioengineered skin humanized mouse model of wound healing emerges as a unique platform for evaluating pharmacological, cell and gene therapy strategies for wound healing (Davidson, 2008).

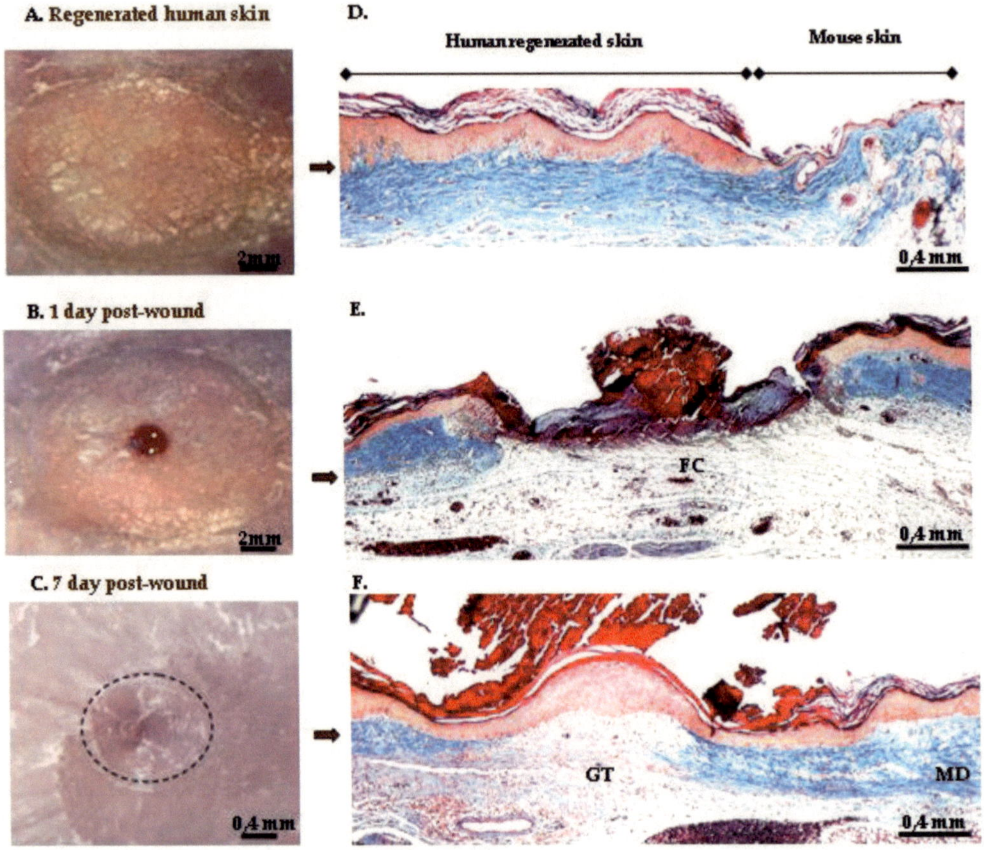

Fig. 12. **The skin humanized model truly recreates the human wound healing process.** **(A-C)** Clinical and **(D-F)** histological features of the healing process of a wound until complete closure. **(A)** Non-wounded regenerated skin showing a multilayered human epithelium easily distinguish from the mouse epithelium. **(D)** Differences in the collagen deposition are also observed. **(B)** 1 day-wound plugged with a fibrin-rich clot (FC) **(F)** gradually populated by endothelial cells and fibroblasts (granulation tissue: GT) that by remodeling generates a mature dermis (MD) as observed on the older areas of a 7day wound. The epithelial tongue observed in **(E)** migrates along the time until completely cover the damaged area by a neoepithelium.

Diabetes is a systemic disorder with a high and continuously increasing incidence, affecting approximately 4% of the world population in developed countries. This index increases in relation to current lifestyle (Ramsey et al., 1999; Wild et al., 2004). Despite recent advances in the diagnosis and treatment of diabetes, its complications still represent a challenge for public health, since approximately 15% of diabetic patients develop a lower extremity ulcer during the course of their illness. In fact, over 25% of hospital admissions of diabetic patients are connected to problems with ulcers, particularly on the feet, which if not properly treated will result in the amputation of the affected limb (Moulik et al., 2003; Widatalla et al., 2009; Wu & Armstrong, 2005). Employing the widely used model of diabetes impaired-wound healing, i.e. leptin-deficient *ob/ob* mice, we examined the repair-promoting activities of the pleiotropic factor LL-37 antimicrobial peptide. This peptide has been shown to play a role in defense and favour repair as previously mentioned. We used adenoviral-mediated gene transfer to overexpress this factor around wound margins of full-thickness wounds generated in this animal model. We showed that LL-37 enhanced the re-epithelialization rate and granulation tissue formation in a healing-impaired context (Carretero et al., 2008). Although this and other animal models have been extensively useful in diabetes research (Frank et al., 2000; Michaels et al., 2007), the need to design appropriate models in a humanized context has become mandatory as previously discussed. To this end, our studies are mainly devoted to develop a humanized animal model of impaired wound healing (Martínez-Santamaría et al., 2009 and unpublished results).

5. Conclusion

Skin bioengineering has become a bright star in the field of regenerative medicine. The original feeble sheet of keratinocytes developed by Green and coworkers (Gallico et al., 1984) driven by the urgent need to cover a severe burn patient in the mid eighties has evolved into complex tridimensional products combining epithelial and mesenchymal cells together with a variety of matrices and scaffold materials. The spectrum of applications has also grown remarkably counting not only big skin losses (e.g. severe buns) but also various forms of chronic wounds including those of genetic origin. Recently, skin bioengineering has met gene therapy (Mavilio et al., 2006) and that couple is here to stay as new combined therapy protocols are foreseen not only with genetically manipulated keratinocytes but also with revertant, spontaneously corrected cells.

Major challenges remain. At the experimental level, human skin bioengineering has allowed the development of faithful skin disease models amenable to the screening of therapeutic approaches and mechanistic studies. Some but not all of the skin functions can be restored with existing autologous skin substitutes. In fact, bioengineered constructs offering the complete regeneration of functional skin, including all the skin appendages (hair follicles, sweat glands and sensory organs) are still awaiting development. Establishment of a functional vascular and nerve network and scar-free integration of current bioengineered products with the surrounding host tissue has neither fully achieved. New basic knowledge about epidermal stem cells and their interaction with neighboring mesenchyma will be a key to developing new enhanced tissue-engineered skin substitutes. We certainly cannot leave iPS cells out of any regenerative medicine equation. Attainable and safe production of genetically stable, truly iPS cells together with reliable procedures to obtain specific differentiated cell lineages, including epidermis, is conceivable and a door to an unlimited source of autologous cells. A smart combination of all these new advances to come hold the promise to fulfill the dream of perfect skin regeneration through off-the-shelf, next generation skin bioengineering.

6. Acknowledgment

We wish to thank all patients and their families from who we have learned so much over the past years. They are the genuine driving force behind our work. We thank IPCC

(International Pachyonychia Congenita Consortium) and DEBRA (Dystrophic Epidermolysis Bullosa Research Association) for its constant support and motivation. We kindly acknowledge the indispensable collaboration of dermatologists, surgeons, nurses and other health professionals. We especially thank our technicians Almudena Holguín, Nuria Illera, María Luisa Retamosa, Blanca Duarte, Isabel de los Santos, Federico Sanchez, Jesús Martínez and Edilia Almeida for their meticulous work and professional dedication.
Thanks to Aurora de la Cal, Sergio Losada, Mª Angeles Acevedo and Soledad Moreno for making our daily work easier. Finally, we would like to acknowledge the invaluable contribution to our co-workers at CIEMAT-CIBERER-u714 and our collaborators from INSERM (Nice, France), IDI (Rome, Italy) and Ninewells Hospital (Dundee, UK) in the development of this work
This work was supported by grants from the Science and Innovation Ministry of Spain (SAF-2004-07717, SAF2007-61019, SAF2010-16976 and PSE-010000-2008-7), from the Biomedical Network Research Centre on Rare Diseases (CIBERER; INTRA/08/714.1 and INTRA/09/758.2), from the Spanish Ministry of Health (Advanced Therapies, TRA049 and TRA0160) and from the European Union (LSHB-CT-503447, LSHB-CT-512073, LSHB-CT-512102, AFM project N°13746 and E-Rare JTC 2009-091).

7. References

Barrandon, Y., and H. Green, 1987, Three clonal types of keratinocyte with different capacities for multiplication: Proc Natl Acad Sci U S A, v. 84, p. 2302-6.

Beele, H., 2002, Artificial skin: past, present and future: Int J Artif Organs, v. 25, p. 163-73.

Bergoglio, V., F. Larcher, O. Chevallier-Lagente, A. Bernheim, O. Danos, A. Sarasin, M. D. Rio, and T. Magnaldo, 2007, Safe selection of genetically manipulated human primary keratinocytes with very high growth potential using CD24: Mol Ther, v. 15, p. 2186-93.

Bernerd, F., D. Asselineau, C. Vioux, O. Chevallier-Lagente, B. Bouadjar, A. Sarasin, and T. Magnaldo, 2001, Clues to epidermal cancer proneness revealed by reconstruction of DNA repair-deficient xeroderma pigmentosum skin *in vitro*: Proc Natl Acad Sci U S A, v. 98, p. 7817-22.

Bitoun, E., A. Micheloni, L. Lamant, C. Bonnart, A. Tartaglia-Polcini, C. Cobbold, T. Al Saati, F. Mariotti, J. Mazereeuw-Hautier, F. Boralevi, D. Hohl, J. Harper, C. Bodemer, M. D'Alessio, and A. Hovnanian, 2003, LEKTI proteolytic processing in human primary keratinocytes, tissue distribution and defective expression in Netherton syndrome: Hum Mol Genet, v. 12, p. 2417-30.

Borgoño, C. A., I. P. Michael, N. Komatsu, A. Jayakumar, R. Kapadia, G. L. Clayman, G. Sotiropoulou, and E. P. Diamandis, 2007, A potential role for multiple tissue kallikrein serine proteases in epidermal desquamation: J Biol Chem, v. 282, p. 3640-52.

Boyce, S. T. & G. D. Warden, 2002, Principles and practices for treatment of cutaneous wounds with cultured skin substitutes: Am J Surg, v. 183, p. 445-56.

Brash, D. E., A. Ziegler, A. S. Jonason, J. A. Simon, S. Kunala, and D. J. Leffell, 1996, Sunlight and sunburn in human skin cancer: p53, apoptosis, and tumor promotion: J Investig Dermatol Symp Proc, v. 1, p. 136-42.

Bruckner-Tuderman, L., 2008, European Dermatology Forum: skin diseases in Europe. Skin diseases with a high public health impact: Epidermolysis bullosa.: Eur J Dermatol., v. 18, p. 214-6.

Camblor-Santervas, L., A. Mena-Infiesta, J. Llanesa-Coto, F. Vaquero-Lorenzo, S. Gómez-Llanes, D. López-García, H. Cubillas-Martín, M. J. Ramos-Gallo, J. A. Carreño-Morrondo, J. Álvarez-Fernández, and J. M. Gutiérrez-Julián, 2003, Tratamiento de úlceras vasculares crónicas con equivalentes cutáneos obtenidos mediante ingeniería tisular.: Angiología, v. 55, p. 21-33.

Carretero, M., M. Del Rio, M. Garcia, M. J. Escámez, I. Mirones, L. Rivas, C. Balague, J. L. Jorcano, and F. Larcher, 2004, A cutaneous gene therapy approach to treat infection through keratinocyte-targeted overexpression of antimicrobial peptides: Faseb J, v. 18, p. 1931-3.

Carretero, M., M. J. Escámez, M. Garcia, B. Duarte, A. Holguin, L. Retamosa, J. L. Jorcano, M. D. Rio, and F. Larcher, 2008, *In vitro* and *in vivo* wound healing-promoting activities of human cathelicidin LL-37: J Invest Dermatol, v. 128, p. 223-36.

Carretero, M., S. Guerrero-Aspizua, and M. Del Rio, 2011, Applicability of bioengineered human skin: from preclinical skin humanized mouse models to clinical replacement therapies: Bioeng Bugs. 2(4).

Carsin, H., P. Ainaud, H. Le Bever, J. Rives, A. Lakhel, J. Stephanazzi, F. Lambert, and J. Perrot, 2000, Cultured epithelial autografts in extensive burn coverage of severely traumatized patients: a five year single-center experience with 30 patients: Burns, v. 26, p. 379-87.

Chavanas, S., C. Bodemer, A. Rochat, D. Hamel-Teillac, M. Ali, A. D. Irvine, J. L. Bonafe, J. Wilkinson, A. Taieb, Y. Barrandon, J. I. Harper, Y. de Prost, and A. Hovnanian, 2000, Mutations in SPINK5, encoding a serine protease inhibitor, cause Netherton syndrome: Nat Genet, v. 25, p. 141-2.

Chen, J., K. Jaeger, Z. Den, P. J. Koch, J. P. Sundberg, and D. R. Roop, 2008, Mice expressing a mutant Krt75 (K6hf) allele develop hair and nail defects resembling pachyonychia congenita: J Invest Dermatol, v. 128, p. 270-9.

Chen, J., and D. R. Roop, 2005, Mouse models in preclinical studies for pachyonychia congenita: J Investig Dermatol Symp Proc, v. 10, p. 37-46.

Compton, C. C., 1992, Current concepts in pediatric burn care: the biology of cultured epithelial autografts: an eight-year study in pediatric burn patients: Eur J Pediatr Surg, v. 2, p. 216-22.

Coto-Segura P, García E, García V, Fueyo-Casado A, Vázquez-López F, Pérez-Oliva N, Meana-Infiesta A, 2007, Letter: efficacy of a self-made artificial skin in the treatment of chronic ulcers. Dermatol Surg 33(3):392-4.

Coto-Segura P, Vazquez-Lopez F, Garcia-Perez E, Garcia V, Meana-Infiesta A, Perez-Oliva N. 2008. Potent analgesic effect of tissue-engineered skin in a terminal patient with severe leg ulcer pain. Dermatol Surg. 34(10):1414-6.

Coulombe, P. A., 2003, Wound epithelialization: accelerating the pace of discovery: J Invest Dermatol, v. 121, p. 219-30.

Cuadrado-Corrales, N., C. Sanchez-Jimeno, M. Garcia, M. J. Escámez, N. Illera, A. Hernandez-Martin, M. J. Trujillo-Tiebas, C. Ayuso, & M. Del Rio, 2010, A prevalent mutation with founder effect in Spanish Recessive Dystrophic Epidermolysis Bullosa families: BMC Med Genet, v. 11, p. 139.

Cuono, C. B., R. Langdon, N. Birchall, S. Barttelbort, & J. McGuire, 1987, Composite autologous-allogeneic skin replacement: development and clinical application: Plast Reconstr Surg, v. 80, p. 626-37.

Danilenko, D. M., 2008, Review paper: preclinical models of psoriasis: Vet Pathol, v. 45, p. 563-75.

Davidson, J., 2001, Experimental animal wounds models: Wounds, v. 13, p. 9-23.

Davidson, J., 2008, First-class delivery: getting growth factors to their destination: J Invest Dermatol, v. 128, p. 1360-2.

Davis, B. R., & F. Candotti, 2010, Genetics. Mosaicism--switch or spectrum?: Science, v. 330, p. 46-7.

Del Bino, S., J. Sok, E. Bessac, & F. Bernerd, 2006, Relationship between skin response to ultraviolet exposure and skin color type: Pigment Cell Res, v. 19, p. 606-14.

Del Bino, S., C. Vioux, P. Rossio-Pasquier, A. Jomard, M. Demarchez, D. Asselineau, & F. Bernerd, 2004, Ultraviolet B induces hyperproliferation and modification of epidermal differentiation in normal human skin grafted on to nude mice: Br J Dermatol, v. 150, p. 658-67.

Del Rio, M., Y. Gache, J. L. Jorcano, G. Meneguzzi, & F. Larcher, 2004, Current approaches and perspectives in human keratinocyte-based gene therapies: Gene Ther, v. 11 Suppl 1, p. S57-63.

Del Rio, M., F. Larcher, & J. Jorcano, 2002a, Recent advances in gene therapy with skin cells: European Reviews, v. 10, p. 369-388.

Del Rio, M., F. Larcher, F. Serrano, A. Meana, M. Munoz, M. Garcia, E. Munoz, C. Martin, A. Bernad, & J. L. Jorcano, 2002b, A preclinical model for the analysis of genetically modified human skin *in vivo*: Hum Gene Ther, v. 13, p. 959-68.

Demarchez, M., P. Sengel, & M. Prunieras, 1986, Wound healing of human skin transplanted onto the nude mouse. I. An immunohistological study of the reepithelialization process: Dev Biol, v. 113, p. 90-6.

Demirtas Y, Yagmur C, Soylemez F, Ozturk N, Demir A, 2010, Management of split-thickness skin graft donor site: a prospective clinical trial for comparison of five different dressing materials. Burns. 36(7):999-1005

Desai, M. H., J. M. Mlakar, R. L. McCauley, K. M. Abdullah, R. L. Rutan, J. P. Waymack, M. C. Robson, & D. N. Herndon, 1991, Lack of long-term durability of cultured keratinocyte burn-wound coverage: a case report: J Burn Care Rehabil, v. 12, p. 540-5.

Descargues, P., C. Deraison, C. Prost, S. Fraitag, J. Mazereeuw-Hautier, M. D'Alessio, A. Ishida-Yamamoto, C. Bodemer, G. Zambruno, & A. Hovnanian, 2006, Corneodesmosomal cadherins are preferential targets of stratum corneum trypsin- and chymotrypsin-like hyperactivity in Netherton syndrome: J Invest Dermatol, v. 126, p. 1622-32.

Di Cesare, A., P. Di Meglio, & F. O. Nestle, 2008, A role for Th17 cells in the immunopathogenesis of atopic dermatitis?: J Invest Dermatol, v. 128, p. 2569-71.

Di Nunzio, F., G. Maruggi, S. Ferrari, E. Di Iorio, V. Poletti, M. Garcia, M. Del Rio, M. De Luca, F. Larcher, G. Pellegrini, & F. Mavilio, 2008, Correction of laminin-5 deficiency in human epidermal stem cells by transcriptionally targeted lentiviral vectors: Mol Ther, v. 16, p. 1977-85.

Di, W. L., F. Larcher, E. Semenova, G. E. Talbot, J. I. Harper, M. Del Rio, A. J. Thrasher, & W. Qasim, 2011, Ex-vivo gene therapy restores LEKTI activity and corrects the architecture of Netherton syndrome-derived skin grafts: Mol Ther, v. 19, p. 408-16.

Donohue KG, Carson P, Iriondo M, Zhou L, Saap L, Gibson K, Falanga V, 2005, Safety and efficacy of a bilayered skin construct in full-thickness surgical wounds. J Dermatol. 32(8):626-31.

Egles, C., J. A. Garlick, & Y. Shamis, 2010, Three-dimensional human tissue models of wounded skin: Methods Mol Biol, v. 585, p. 345-59.

Ehrenreich, M., & Z. Ruszczak, 2006, Update on tissue-engineered biological dressings: Tissue Eng, v. 12, p. 2407-24.

Eisenberg, M., & D. Llewelyn, 1998, Surgical management of hands in children with recessive dystrophic epidermolysis bullosa: use of allogeneic composite cultured skin grafts: Br J Plast Surg, v. 51, p. 608-13.

Eisenbud, D., N. Huang, S. Luke, & M. Silberklang, 2004, Skin substitutes and wound healing: Current status and challenges: Wounds, v. 16, p. 2-17.

Eming, S. A., T. Krieg, & J. M. Davidson, 2007, Inflammation in wound repair: molecular and cellular mechanisms: J Invest Dermatol, v. 127, p. 514-25.

Escámez, M., M. Carretero, M. García, A. Meana, F. Larcher, & M. Del Río, 2009, Terapia génica y celular como estrategias de intervención en enfermedades dermatológicas huérfanas, *in* A. K. a. J. M. Mascaró, ed., Monografías de Dermatología: Enfermedades huérfanas, v. 22: Madrid, Aula médica Ediciones, p. 69-77.

Escámez, M. J., M. Carretero, M. Garcia, L. Martinez-Santamaria, I. Mirones, B. Duarte, A. Holguin, E. Garcia, V. Garcia, A. Meana, J. L. Jorcano, F. Larcher, & M. Del Rio, 2008, Assessment of optimal virus-mediated growth factor gene delivery for human cutaneous wound healing enhancement: J Invest Dermatol, v. 128, p. 1565-75.

Escámez, M. J., M. Garcia, N. Cuadrado-Corrales, S. G. Llames, A. Charlesworth, N. De Luca, N. Illera, C. Sanchez-Jimeno, A. Holguin, B. Duarte, M. J. Trujillo-Tiebas, J. L. Vicario, J. L. Santiago, A. Hernandez-Martin, A. Torrelo, D. Castiglia, C. Ayuso, F. Larcher, J. L. Jorcano, A. Meana, G. Meneguzzi, G. Zambruno, & M. Del Rio, 2010, The first COL7A1 mutation survey in a large Spanish dystrophic epidermolysis bullosa cohort: c.6527insC disclosed as an unusually recurrent mutation: Br J Dermatol, v. 163, p. 155-61.

Escámez, M. J., M. Garcia, F. Larcher, A. Meana, E. Munoz, J. L. Jorcano, & M. Del Rio, 2004, An *in vivo* model of wound healing in genetically modified skin-humanized mice: J Invest Dermatol, v. 123, p. 1182-91.

Falabella, A. F., I. C. Valencia, W. H. Eaglstein, & L. A. Schachner, 2000, Tissue-engineered skin (Apligraf) in the healing of patients with epidermolysis bullosa wounds: Arch Dermatol, v. 136, p. 1225-30.

Falanga, V., D. Margolis, O. Alvarez, M. Auletta, F. Maggiacomo, M. Altman, J. Jensen, M. Sabolinski, & J. Hardin-Young, 1998, Rapid healing of venous ulcers and lack of clinical rejection with an allogeneic cultured human skin equivalent.: Arch Dermatol, v. 134, p. 293-300.

Fine, J. D., R. A. Eady, E. A. Bauer, J. W. Bauer, L. Bruckner-Tuderman, A. Heagerty, H. Hintner, A. Hovnanian, M. F. Jonkman, I. Leigh, J. A. McGrath, J. E. Mellerio, D. F. Murrell, H. Shimizu, J. Uitto, A. Vahlquist, D. Woodley, & G. Zambruno, 2008, The classification of inherited epidermolysis bullosa (EB): Report of the Third International Consensus Meeting on Diagnosis and Classification of EB: J Am Acad Dermatol, v. 58, p. 931-50.

Fivenson, D. P., L. Scherschun, M. Choucair, D. Kukuruga, J. Young, & T. Shwayder, 2003, Graftskin therapy in epidermolysis bullosa: J Am Acad Dermatol, v. 48, p. 886-92.

Frank, S., B. Stallmeyer, H. Kampfer, N. Kolb, & J. Pfeilschifter, 2000, Leptin enhances wound re-epithelialization and constitutes a direct function of leptin in skin repair: J Clin Invest, v. 106, p. 501-9.

Gache, Y., C. Baldeschi, M. Del Rio, L. Gagnoux-Palacios, F. Larcher, J. P. Lacour, & G. Meneguzzi, 2004, Construction of skin equivalents for gene therapy of recessive dystrophic epidermolysis bullosa: Hum Gene Ther, v. 15, p. 921-33.

Gallico GG 3rd, O'Connor NE, Compton CC, Kehinde O, Green H. Permanent coverage of large burn wounds with autologous cultured human epithelium. N Engl J Med. 1984.

Gallico, G. G., 3rd, 1990, Biologic skin substitutes: Clin Plast Surg, v. 17, p. 519-26.

Garcia, M., M. J. Escámez, M. Carretero, I. Mirones, L. Martinez-Santamaria, M. Navarro, J. L. Jorcano, A. Meana, M. Del Rio, & F. Larcher, 2007, Modeling normal and pathological processes through skin tissue engineering: Mol Carcinog, v. 46, p. 741-5.

Garcia, M., F. Larcher, R. P. Hickerson, E. Baselga, S. A. Leachman, R. L. Kaspar, & M. Del Rio, 2011, Development of skin-humanized mouse models of pachyonychia congenita: J Invest Dermatol, v. 131, p. 1053-60.

Garcia, M., S. Llames, E. Garcia, A. Meana, N. Cuadrado, M. Recasens, S. Puig, E. Nagore, N. Illera, J. L. Jorcano, M. Del Rio, & F. Larcher, 2010, *In vivo* assessment of acute UVB responses in normal and Xeroderma Pigmentosum (XP-C) skin-humanized mouse models: Am J Pathol, v. 177, p. 865-72.

García, M., J. Santiago, A. Terrón, A. Hernández-Martín, A. Vicente, C. Fortuny, De Lucas, J. López, N. Cuadrado-Corrales, A. Holguín, N. Illera, B. Duarte, C. Sánchez-Jimeno, S. Llames, E. García, C. Ayuso, L. Martínez-Santamaría, D. Castiglia, N. De Luca, A. Torrelo, D. Mechan, D. Baty, G. Zambruno, M. Escámez, & M. Del Río, 2011, Two novel recessive mutations in KRT14 identified in a cohort of 21 Spanish families with epidermolysis bullosa simplex: Br J Dermatol, v. In press.

Garlick, J. A., 2007, Engineering skin to study human disease--tissue models for cancer biology and wound repair: Adv Biochem Eng Biotechnol, v. 103, p. 207-39.

Gilhar, A., M. David, Y. Ullmann, T. Berkutski, & R. S. Kalish, 1997, T-lymphocyte dependence of psoriatic pathology in human psoriatic skin grafted to SCID mice: J Invest Dermatol, v. 109, p. 283-8.

Gohari, S., C. Gambla, M. Healey, G. Spaulding, K. B. Gordon, J. Swan, B. Cook, D. P. West, & J. C. Lapiere, 2002, Evaluation of tissue-engineered skin (human skin substitute) and secondary intention healing in the treatment of full thickness wounds after Mohs micrographic or excisional surgery: Dermatol Surg, v. 28, p. 1107-14; discussion 1114.

Gómez, C., J. Galán, V. Torrero, I. Ferreiro, D. Pérez, R. Palao, E. Martínez, S. Llames, A. Meana, & P. Holguín, 2011, Use of an autologous bioengineered composite skin in extensive burns: Clinical and functional outcomes. A multicentric study.: Burns. 2011; 37(4):580-9.

Green, H., K. Easley, & S. Iuchi, 2003, Marker succession during the development of keratinocytes from cultured human embryonic stem cells: Proc Natl Acad Sci U S A, v. 100, p. 15625-30.

Griffiths, M., N. Ojeh, R. Livingstone, R. Price, & H. Navsaria, 2004, Survival of Apligraf in acute human wounds: Tissue Eng, v. 10, p. 1180-95.

Guenou, H., X. Nissan, F. Larcher, J. Feteira, G. Lemaitre, M. Saidani, M. Del Rio, C. C. Barrault, F. X. Bernard, M. Peschanski, C. Baldeschi, & G. Waksman, 2009, Human embryonic stem-cell derivatives for full reconstruction of the pluristratified epidermis: a preclinical study: Lancet, v. 374, p. 1745-53.

Guerrero-Aspizua, S., M. Garcia, R. Murillas, L. Retamosa, N. Illera, B. Duarte, A. Holguin, S. Puig, M. Hernandez, A. Meana, J. Jorcano, F. Larcher, M. Carretero, & M. Del Rio, 2010, Development of a bioengineered skin-humanized mouse model for psoriasis: dissecting epidermal-lymphocyte interacting pathways: Am J Pathol. 177(6), p 3112-24.

Hacein-Bey-Abina, S., C. Von Kalle, M. Schmidt, M. P. McCormack, N. Wulffraat, P. Leboulch, A. Lim, C. S. Osborne, R. Pawliuk, E. Morillon, R. Sorensen, A. Forster, P. Fraser, J. I. Cohen, G. de Saint Basile, I. Alexander, U. Wintergerst, T. Frebourg, A. Aurias, D. Stoppa-Lyonnet, S. Romana, I. Radford-Weiss, F. Gross, F. Valensi, E. Delabesse, E. Macintyre, F. Sigaux, J. Soulier, L. E. Leiva, M. Wissler, C. Prinz, T. H. Rabbitts, F. Le Deist, A. Fischer, & M. Cavazzana-Calvo, 2003, LMO2-associated clonal T cell proliferation in two patients after gene therapy for SCID-X1: Science, v. 302, p. 415-9.

Hammond, E. J., R. L. Ng, M. A. Stanley, & A. J. Munro, 1987, Prolonged survival of cultured keratinocyte allografts in the nonimmunosuppressed mouse: Transplantation, v. 44, p. 106-12.

Hansbrough, J. F., S. T. Boyce, M. L. Cooper, & T. J. Foreman, 1989, Burn wound closure with cultured autologous keratinocytes and fibroblasts attached to a collagen-glycosaminoglycan substrate: Jama, v. 262, p. 2125-30.

Hansen, S. L., D. W. Voigt, P. Wiebelhaus, & C. N. Paul, 2001, Using skin replacement products to treat burns and wounds: Adv Skin Wound Care, v. 14, p. 37-44; quiz 45-6.

Harrison, C. A., F. Gossiel, C. M. Layton, A. J. Bullock, T. Johnson, A. Blumsohn, and S. MacNeil, 2006, Use of an *in vitro* model of tissue-engineered skin to investigate the mechanism of skin graft contraction: Tissue Eng, v. 12, p. 3119-33.

Herschthal J, Kirsner RS. Current management of venous ulcers: an evidence-based review. Surg Technol Int. 2008;17:77-83.

Hohlfeld, J., A. de Buys Roessingh, N. Hirt-Burri, P. Chaubert, S. Gerber, C. Scaletta, P. Hohlfeld, & L. A. Applegate, 2005, Tissue engineered fetal skin constructs for paediatric burns: Lancet, v. 366, p. 840-2.

Horch, R. E., J. Kopp, U. Kneser, J. Beier, & A. D. Bach, 2005, Tissue engineering of cultured skin substitutes: J Cell Mol Med, v. 9, p. 592-608.

Ishida-Yamamoto, A., C. Deraison, C. Bonnart, E. Bitoun, R. Robinson, T. J. O'Brien, K. Wakamatsu, S. Ohtsubo, H. Takahashi, Y. Hashimoto, P. J. Dopping-Hepenstal, J. A. McGrath, H. Iizuka, G. Richard, & A. Hovnanian, 2005, LEKTI is localized in lamellar granules, separated from KLK5 and KLK7, and is secreted in the extracellular spaces of the superficial stratum granulosum: J Invest Dermatol, v. 124, p. 360-6.

Iuchi, S., S. Dabelsteen, K. Easley, J. G. Rheinwald, & H. Green, 2006, Immortalized keratinocyte lines derived from human embryonic stem cells: Proc Natl Acad Sci U S A, v. 103, p. 1792-7.

Jensen KB, Watt FM. Single-cell expression profiling of human epidermal stem and transit-amplifying cells: Lrig1 is a regulator of stem cell quiescence. Proc Natl Acad Sci U S A. 2006 Aug 8;103(32):11958-63.

Jonkman, M. F., 1999, Revertant mosaicism in human genetic disorders: Am J Med Genet, v. 85, p. 361-4.

Jonkman, M. F., & A. M. Pasmooij, 2009, Revertant mosaicism--patchwork in the skin: N Engl J Med, v. 360, p. 1680-2.

Khavari, P. A., 2006, Modeling cancer in human skin tissue: Nat Rev Cancer, v. 6, p. 270-80.

Kobayashi, N., A. Nakagawa, T. Muramatsu, Y. Yamashina, T. Shirai, M. W. Hashimoto, Y. Ishigaki, T. Ohnishi, & T. Mori, 1998, Supranuclear melanin caps reduce ultraviolet induced DNA photoproducts in human epidermis: J Invest Dermatol, v. 110, p. 806-10.

Kraemer, K. H., 1997, Sunlight and skin cancer: another link revealed: Proc Natl Acad Sci U S A, v. 94, p. 11-4.

Lai-Cheong, J. E., J. A. McGrath, & J. Uitto, 2011, Revertant mosaicism in skin: natural gene therapy: Trends Mol Med, v. 17, p. 140-8.

Langer, A., & W. Rogowski, 2009, Systematic review of economic evaluations of human cell-derived wound care products for the treatment of venous leg and diabetic foot ulcers: BMC Health Serv Res, v. 9, p. 115.

Langer, R., & J. P. Vacanti, 1993, Tissue engineering: Science, v. 260, p. 920-6.

Larcher, F., M. Del Rio, F. Serrano, J. C. Segovia, A. Ramirez, A. Meana, A. Page, J. L. Abad, M. A. Gonzalez, J. Bueren, A. Bernad, & J. L. Jorcano, 2001, A cutaneous gene therapy approach to human leptin deficiencies: correction of the murine ob/ob phenotype using leptin-targeted keratinocyte grafts: Faseb J, v. 15, p. 1529-38.

Larcher, F., E. Dellambra, L. Rico, S. Bondanza, R. Murillas, C. Cattoglio, F. Mavilio, J. L. Jorcano, G. Zambruno, & M. Del Rio, 2007, Long-term engraftment of single genetically modified human epidermal holoclones enables safety pre-assessment of cutaneous gene therapy: Mol Ther, v. 15, p. 1670-6.

Larcher, F., J. Jorcano, A. Meana, & M. Del Rio, 2008, Skin Regeneration, *in* J. M. G. V. Damián García Olmo, Jorge Alemany & José A. Gutiérrez Fuentes., ed., Cell Therapy, v. 17, Editorial McGraw Hill, p. 209-223.

Larcher, F., A. Meana, J. Jorcano, & M. Del Río, 2009, Equivalentes cutáneos desarrollados mediante ingeniería tisular, *in* A. Ediciones, ed., Medicina regenerativa e ingeniería tisular. Del laboratorio a la clínica, v. 12: México, G.D. Ascencio, p. 165-184.

Lasso, J. M., M. Del Rio, M. Garcia, V. Martinez Calleja, P. Nava, M. A. Munoz-Fernandez, & R. Perez Cano, 2007, Improving flap survival by transplantation of a VEGF-secreting endothelised scaffold during distal pedicle flap creation: J Plast Reconstr Aesthet Surg, v. 60, p. 279-86.

Leachman, S. A., R. P. Hickerson, M. E. Schwartz, E. E. Bullough, S. L. Hutcherson, K. M. Boucher, C. D. Hansen, M. J. Eliason, G. S. Srivatsa, D. J. Kornbrust, F. J. Smith, W. I. McLean, L. M. Milstone, & R. L. Kaspar, 2010, First-in-human mutation-targeted siRNA phase Ib trial of an inherited skin disorder: Mol Ther, v. 18, p. 442-6.

Leachman, S. A., R. L. Kaspar, P. Fleckman, S. R. Florell, F. J. Smith, W. H. McLean, D. P. Lunny, L. M. Milstone, M. A. van Steensel, C. S. Munro, E. A. O'Toole, J. T. Celebi, A. Kansky, & E. B. Lane, 2005, Clinical and pathological features of pachyonychia congenita: J Investig Dermatol Symp Proc, v. 10, p. 3-17.

Lee, J. H., H. T. An, J. H. Chung, K. H. Kim, H. C. Eun, & K. H. Cho, 2002, Acute effects of UVB radiation on the proliferation and differentiation of keratinocytes: Photodermatol Photoimmunol Photomed, v. 18, p. 253-61.

Li, A., N. Pouliot, R. Redvers, & P. Kaur, 2004, Extensive tissue-regenerative capacity of neonatal human keratinocyte stem cells and their progeny: J Clin Invest, v. 113, p. 390-400.

Li, D., T. G. Turi, A. Schuck, I. M. Freedberg, G. Khitrov, & M. Blumenberg, 2001, Rays and arrays: the transcriptional program in the response of human epidermal keratinocytes to UVB illumination: Faseb J, v. 15, p. 2533-5.

Límová M. Active wound coverings: bioengineered skin and dermal substitutes. Surg Clin North Am. 2010 90(6) p. 1237-55.

Lugo LM, Lei P, Andreadis ST. Vascularization of the dermal support enhances wound re-epithelialization by *in situ* delivery of epidermal keratinocytes. Tissue Eng Part A. 2011 (5-6) p. 665-75.

Llames, S., E. Garcia, V. Garcia, M. del Rio, F. Larcher, J. L. Jorcano, E. Lopez, P. Holguin, F. Miralles, J. Otero, & A. Meana, 2006, Clinical results of an autologous engineered skin: Cell Tissue Bank, v. 7, p. 47-53.

Llames, S., E. Garcia-Perez, V. Garcia, M. Pevida, L. Camblor, J. Llaneza, R. Martinez, P. Cañal, F. Menendez-Tevar, & A. Meana, 2008, Treatment of diabetic foot trophic lesions using a tissue-engineered dermal graft: Tissue Engineering: Part A, v. 14, p. 924.

Llames, S. G., M. Del Rio, F. Larcher, E. Garcia, M. Garcia, M. J. Escámez, J. L. Jorcano, P. Holguin, & A. Meana, 2004, Human plasma as a dermal scaffold for the generation of a completely autologous bioengineered skin: Transplantation, v. 77, p. 350-5.

Mansbridge, J., K. Liu, R. Patch, K. Symons, & E. Pinney, 1998, Three-dimensional fibroblast culture implant for the treatment of diabetic foot ulcers: metabolic activity and therapeutic range: Tissue Eng, v. 4, p. 403-14.

Margolis, D. J., T. Cromblehome, M. Herlyn, P. Cross, L. Weinberg, J. Filip, & K. Propert, 2004, Clinical protocol. Phase I trial to evaluate the safety of H5.020CMV.PDGF-b and limb compression bandage for the treatment of venous leg ulcer: trial A: Hum Gene Ther, v. 15, p. 1003-19.

Marston, W. A., J. Hanft, P. Norwood, & R. Pollak, 2003, The efficacy and safety of Dermagraft in improving the healing of chronic diabetic foot ulcers: results of a prospective randomized trial: Diabetes Care, v. 26, p. 1701-5.

Martin, P., 1997, Wound healing--aiming for perfect skin regeneration: Science, v. 276, p. 75-81.

Martínez-Santamaría, L., M. Escámez, M. Carretero, S. Llames, E. García, M. Pevida, B. Duarte, L. Retamosa, A. Holguin, N. Illera, F. Larcher, J. Jorcano, A. Meana, & M. Del Río, 2009, A new diabetic skin-humanized mouse model unravels the regenerative potential of fibroblasts in impaired healing process.: Human Gene Therapy, v. 20, p. 1048-93.

Martínez-Santamaría, L., M. Escámez, S. Llames, E. García, M. Pevida, B. Duarte, L. Retamosa, A. Holguin, N. Illera, F. Larcher, A. Meana, C. Conti, J. Jorcano, & M. Del Río, 2011a, Characterization of diabetic wound healing in a new skin -humanized mouse model: Manuscript in preparation.

Martínez-Santamaría, L., S. Guerrero-Aspizua, & M. Del Rio, 2011b, Bioingeniería cutánea: Aplicaciones preclínicas y clínicas. Skin bioengineering: pre-clinical and clinical applications: Actas Dermosifiliogr. In press.

Mathor, M. B., G. Ferrari, E. Dellambra, M. Cilli, F. Mavilio, R. Cancedda, & M. De Luca, 1996, Clonal analysis of stably transduced human epidermal stem cells in culture: Proc Natl Acad Sci U S A, v. 93, p. 10371-6.

Matsumura, Y., & H. N. Ananthaswamy, 2002, Molecular mechanisms of photocarcinogenesis: Front Biosci, v. 7, p. d765-83.

Mavilio, F., G. Pellegrini, S. Ferrari, F. Di Nunzio, E. Di Iorio, A. Recchia, G. Maruggi, G. Ferrari, E. Provasi, C. Bonini, S. Capurro, A. Conti, C. Magnoni, A. Giannetti, & M. De Luca, 2006, Correction of junctional epidermolysis bullosa by transplantation of genetically modified epidermal stem cells: Nat Med, v. 12, p. 1397-402.

May, M., 2011, Mutations to the rescue: Nat Med, v. 17, p. 405-7.

Meana, A., J. Iglesias, M. Del Rio, F. Larcher, B. Madrigal, M. F. Fresno, C. Martin, F. San Roman, & F. Tevar, 1998, Large surface of cultured human epithelium obtained on a dermal matrix based on live fibroblast-containing fibrin gels: Burns, v. 24, p. 621-30.

Michaels, J. t., S. S. Churgin, K. M. Blechman, M. R. Greives, S. Aarabi, R. D. Galiano, & G. C. Gurtner, 2007, db/db mice exhibit severe wound-healing impairments compared with other murine diabetic strains in a silicone-splinted excisional wound model: Wound Repair Regen, v. 15, p. 665-70.

Mommaas, A. M., R. G. Teepe, I. M. Leigh, A. A. Mulder, E. J. Koebrugge, & B. J. Vermeer, 1992, Ontogenesis of the basement membrane zone after grafting cultured human epithelium: a morphologic and immunoelectron microscopic study: J Invest Dermatol, v. 99, p. 71-7.

Moulik, P. K., R. Mtonga, & G. V. Gill, 2003, Amputation and mortality in new-onset diabetic foot ulcers stratified by etiology: Diabetes Care, v. 26, p. 491-4.

Mudgil, A. V., N. Segal, F. Andriani, Y. Wang, N. E. Fusenig, & J. A. Garlick, 2003, Ultraviolet B irradiation induces expansion of intraepithelial tumor cells in a tissue model of early cancer progression: J Invest Dermatol, v. 121, p. 191-7.

Nestle, F. O., & B. J. Nickoloff, 2005, From classical mouse models of psoriasis to a spontaneous xenograft model featuring use of AGR mice: Ernst Schering Res Found Workshop, p. 203-12.

Nickoloff, B. J., S. L. Kunkel, M. Burdick, & R. M. Strieter, 1995, Severe combined immunodeficiency mouse and human psoriatic skin chimeras. Validation of a new animal model: Am J Pathol, v. 146, p. 580-8.

O'Connor, N., J. Mulliken, S. Banks-Schlegel, O. Kehinde, & H. Green, 1981, Grafting of burns with cultured epithelium prepared from autologous epidermal cells: Lancet, v. 1, p. 75-8.

Otto, W. R., J. Nanchahal, Q. L. Lu, N. Boddy, & R. Dover, 1995, Survival of allogeneic cells in cultured organotypic skin grafts: Plast Reconstr Surg, v. 96, p. 166-76.

Pan Y, Liang Z, Yuan S, Xu J, Wang J, Chen S, 2011, A long-term follow-up study of acellular dermal matrix with thin autograft in burns patients. Ann Plast Surg.

Pasmooij, A., M. Garcia, M. Escámez, A. Nijenhuis, A. Azon, N. Cuadrado-Corrales, M. Jonkman, & M. Del Rio, 2010, Revertant mosaicism due to a second-site mutation in COL7A1 in a patient with recessive dystrophic epidermolysis bullosa.: J Invest Dermatol., v. 130, p. 2407-11.

Pellegrini, G., R. Ranno, G. Stracuzzi, S. Bondanza, L. Guerra, G. Zambruno, G. Micali, & M. De Luca, 1999, The control of epidermal stem cells (holoclones) in the treatment of massive full-thickness burns with autologous keratinocytes cultured on fibrin: Transplantation, v. 68, p. 868-79.

Phillips, T. J., J. Manzoor, A. Rojas, C. Isaacs, P. Carson, M. Sabolinski, J. Young, & V. Falanga, 2002, The longevity of a bilayered skin substitute after application to venous ulcers: Arch Dermatol, v. 138, p. 1079-81.

Pierce, G. F., 2001, Inflammation in nonhealing diabetic wounds: the space-time continuum does matter: Am J Pathol, v. 159, p. 399-403.

Ramsey, S. D., K. Newton, D. Blough, D. K. McCulloch, N. Sandhu, G. E. Reiber, & E. H. Wagner, 1999, Incidence, outcomes, and cost of foot ulcers in patients with diabetes: Diabetes Care, v. 22, p. 382-7.

Regauer, S., G. R. Seiler, Y. Barrandon, K. W. Easley, & C. C. Compton, 1990, Epithelial origin of cutaneous anchoring fibrils: J Cell Biol, v. 111, p. 2109-15.

Rheinwald, J. G., & H. Green, 1975, Serial cultivation of strains of human epidermal keratinocytes: the formation of keratinizing colonies from single cells: Cell, v. 6, p. 331-43.

Roberson, E. D., & A. M. Bowcock, 2010, Psoriasis genetics: breaking the barrier: Trends Genet, v. 26, p. 415-23.

Ronfard, V., J. M. Rives, Y. Neveux, H. Carsin, & Y. Barrandon, 2000, Long-term regeneration of human epidermis on third degree burns transplanted with autologous cultured epithelium grown on a fibrin matrix: Transplantation, v. 70, p. 1588-98.

Rouabhia, M., L. Germain, F. Belanger, & F. A. Auger, 1993, Cultured epithelium allografts: Langerhans cell and Thy-1+ dendritic epidermal cell depletion effects on allograft rejection: Transplantation, v. 56, p. 259-64.

Schon, M. P., 1999, Animal models of psoriasis - what can we learn from them?: J Invest Dermatol, v. 112, p. 405-10.

Senet, P., F. X. Bon, M. Benbunan, A. Bussel, R. Traineau, F. Calvo, L. Dubertret, & C. Dosquet, 2003, Randomized trial and local biological effect of autologous platelets used as adjuvant therapy for chronic venous leg ulcers: J Vasc Surg, v. 38, p. 1342-8.

Sesto, A., M. Navarro, F. Burslem, & J. L. Jorcano, 2002, Analysis of the ultraviolet B response in primary human keratinocytes using oligonucleotide microarrays: Proc Natl Acad Sci U S A, v. 99, p. 2965-70.

Setlow, R. B., 1974, The wavelengths in sunlight effective in producing skin cancer: a theoretical analysis: Proc Natl Acad Sci U S A, v. 71, p. 3363-6.

Shevchenko, R. V., S. L. James, & S. E. James, 2010, A review of tissue-engineered skin bioconstructs available for skin reconstruction: J R Soc Interface, v. 7, p. 229-58.

Shiohara, T., J. Hayakawa, & Y. Mizukawa, 2004, Animal models for atopic dermatitis: are they relevant to human disease?: J Dermatol Sci, v. 36, p. 1-9.

Singer, A. J., & R. A. Clark, 1999, Cutaneous wound healing: N Engl J Med, v. 341, p. 738-46.

Smith, F., R. Kaspar, M. Schwartz, W. McLean, & S. Leachman, 2006, Pachyonychia congenita: Gene Rev.

Smith, F. J., H. Liao, A. J. Cassidy, A. Stewart, K. J. Hamill, P. Wood, I. Joval, M. A. van Steensel, E. Bjorck, F. Callif-Daley, G. Pals, P. Collins, S. A. Leachman, C. S. Munro, & W. H. McLean, 2005, The genetic basis of pachyonychia congenita: J Investig Dermatol Symp Proc, v. 10, p. 21-30.

Spirito, F., A. Capt, M. Del Rio, F. Larcher, E. Guaguere, O. Danos, & G. Meneguzzi, 2006, Sustained phenotypic reversion of junctional epidermolysis bullosa dog keratinocytes: Establishment of an immunocompetent animal model for cutaneous gene therapy: Biochem Biophys Res Commun, v. 339, p. 769-78.

Stockl, K., A. Vanderplas, E. Tafesse, & E. Chang, 2004, Costs of lower-extremity ulcers among patients with diabetes: Diabetes Care, v. 27, p. 2129-34.

Sullivan, T. P., W. H. Eaglstein, S. C. Davis, & P. Mertz, 2001, The pig as a model for human wound healing: Wound Repair Regen, v. 9, p. 66-76.

Takahashi, K., K. Tanabe, M. Ohnuki, M. Narita, T. Ichisaka, K. Tomoda, & S. Yamanaka, 2007, Induction of pluripotent stem cells from adult human fibroblasts by defined factors: Cell, v. 131, p. 861-72.

Tolar, J., L. Xia, M. J. Riddle, C. J. Lees, C. R. Eide, R. T. McElmurry, M. Titeux, M. J. Osborn, T. C. Lund, A. Hovnanian, J. E. Wagner, & B. R. Blazar, 2011, Induced pluripotent stem cells from individuals with recessive dystrophic epidermolysis bullosa: J Invest Dermatol, 131(4), p.848-56

Verplancke, P., H. Beele, S. Monstrey, & J. M. Naeyaert, 1997, Treatment of dystrophic epidermolysis bullosa with autologous meshed split-thickness skin grafts and allogeneic cultured keratinocytes: Dermatology, v. 194, p. 380-2.

Wada, T., & F. Candotti, 2008, Somatic mosaicism in primary immune deficiencies: Curr Opin Allergy Clin Immunol, v. 8, p. 510-4.

Werner, S., & R. Grose, 2003, Regulation of wound healing by growth factors and cytokines: Physiol Rev, v. 83, p. 835-70.

Widatalla, A. H., S. E. Mahadi, M. A. Shawer, H. A. Elsayem, & M. E. Ahmed, 2009, Implementation of diabetic foot ulcer classification system for research purposes to predict lower extremity amputation: Int J Diabetes Dev Ctries, v. 29, p. 1-5.

Wild, S., G. Roglic, A. Green, R. Sicree, & H. King, 2004, Global prevalence of diabetes: estimates for the year 2000 and projections for 2030: Diabetes Care, v. 27, p. 1047-53.

Wilson, N. J., S. A. Leachman, C. D. Hansen, A. C. McMullan, L. M. Milstone, M. E. Schwartz, W. H. McLean, P. R. Hull, & F. J. Smith, 2011, A large mutational study in pachyonychia congenita: J Invest Dermatol, v. 131, p. 1018-24.

Wollina, U., H. Konrad, & T. Fischer, 2001, Recessive epidermolysis bullosa dystrophicans (Hallopeau-Siemens)--improvement of wound healing by autologous epidermal grafts on an esterified hyaluronic acid membrane: J Dermatol, v. 28, p. 217-20.

Wong, P., R. Domergue, & P. A. Coulombe, 2005, Overcoming functional redundancy to elicit pachyonychia congenita-like nail lesions in transgenic mice: Mol Cell Biol, v. 25, p. 197-205.

Wong, T., L. Gammon, L. Liu, J. E. Mellerio, P. J. Dopping-Hepenstal, J. Pacy, G. Elia, R. Jeffery, I. M. Leigh, H. Navsaria, & J. A. McGrath, 2008, Potential of fibroblast cell therapy for recessive dystrophic epidermolysis bullosa: J Invest Dermatol, v. 128, p. 2179-89.

Woodley, D., H. Peterson, S. Herzog, G. Stricklin, R. Burgeson, R. Briggaman, D. Cronce, & E. O'Keefe, 1988, Burn wounds resurfaced by cultured epidermal auto-grafts show abnormal reconstitution of anchoring fibrils: JAMA, v. 259, p. 2566-71.

Woodley, D. T., G. G. Krueger, C. M. Jorgensen, J. A. Fairley, T. Atha, Y. Huang, L. Chan, D. R. Keene, & M. Chen, 2003, Normal and gene-corrected dystrophic epidermolysis bullosa fibroblasts alone can produce type VII collagen at the basement membrane zone: J Invest Dermatol, v. 121, p. 1021-8.

Wrone-Smith, T., & B. J. Nickoloff, 1996, Dermal injection of immunocytes induces psoriasis: J Clin Invest, v. 98, p. 1878-87.

Wu, S., & D. G. Armstrong, 2005, Risk assessment of the diabetic foot and wound: Int Wound J, v. 2, p. 17-24.

Zheng, T., & Z. Zhu, 2005, Lessons from murine models of atopic dermatitis: Curr Allergy Asthma Rep, v. 5, p. 291-7.

Part 4

Skin Biopsy as a Tool to Environmental Research

15

Skin Biopsies as Tools to Measure Fish Coloration and Colour Change

P. Andreas Svensson[1] and Helen Nilsson Sköld[2]
[1]*Deakin University, School of Life and Environmental Sciences*
[2]*University of Gothenburg, Marine Ecology-Kristineberg*
[1]*Australia*
[2]*Sweden*

1. Introduction

1.1 Preliminaries

A biopsy is a link between the whole organism and its cells. Many recent advances in the field of fish coloration have been gained through experimentation on skin biopsies. In particular, this strategy has allowed the in-depth knowledge from pigment cell physiology to be applied to wider topics, such as behavioral ecology. Moreover, melanophores from fish and frogs have long served as models for a general understanding of intracellular transport and organelle positioning. For this purpose, fish skin biopsies have frequently been used for isolation of pigment cells but also for isolation of fibroblasts. In fish pigmentation research, skin biopsies have also been used to understand what causes changes in the skin's overall appearance, especially in the context of short or long-term modulation of tissue coloration. Examples of this are how many fishes rapidly change their colour during courtship or aggressive displays. Here, we review our methodology for the use of skin biopsies in research on fish coloration - from pigment cell physiology to animal behavior. We also highlight some of the most significant findings from this research, and present unsolved issues and suggestions for future directions. In this chapter, we will provide a description of the experimental procedures we have used to manipulate and analyze fish skin biopsies in the context of fish coloration - from chromatophores to animal behavior. Since our research has mainly focused on marine fishes, the protocols (e.g. the choice of buffers) were chosen to suit such animals. However, with minor modifications, these methods will likely work also on most fresh water species. Many of the experimental procedures are fast to assess and easy to perform, and we therefore encourage the experimentation on fish biopsies for use in education. The protocols described in this chapter are also suitable for such exercises.

1.2 Overview

Body colour patterns are important for animals because they can function in inter- and intra species communication and provide camouflage, thermoregulation and protection against solar radiation. In many taxa, colour patterns are caused by large star-shaped pigment containing cells, chromatophores, which are located in the skin. The chromatophores are grouped into subclasses based on the colour of their pigment containing organelles: xanthophores (yellow), erythrophores (red/orange), iridophores (reflective/iridescent), leucophores (white), melanophores (black/brown) and the more rare cyanophores (blue).

As opposed to birds and mammals, where feathers and fur merely absorb pigment from pigment producing cells, fish, amphibians, reptiles and certain invertebrates display the pigment that reside inside chromatophores in the skin itself (Figure1).
Fish chromatophores are found in dermis, epidermis and on the scales that cover the skin. Interestingly, chromatophores and especially melanophores are also located in the peritoneum, the epithelium that covers the abdominal cavity at the inside of the fish. The belly of the fish is typically whitish, both at the outside and the inside of the fish, as a result of large densities of leucophores in these areas. The dorsal areas are on the other hand typically dark as a result of high densities of melanophores. As a result of sexual selection, males and females may display different body colours and patterns. Often juveniles have distinctive colours that differ from the adults of the same species or gender. In adults, particularly in males, the colour patterns can change over the year to be cryptic in winter and more conspicuous during the breeding season. Such a relatively slow and long term change in coloration, is caused by changes in the number of chromatophores in the skin, and called morphological colour change. Skin patterns and colours can also be modified within minutes by reflective changes in iridophores as well as through the aggregation or dispersion of the pigment-containing organelles inside the chromatophores. Both these more rapid changes are referred to as physiological colour change. Vision, direct light, hormones and neurotransmittors can all be used in the regulation of physiological colour change. Dispersal of the pigment inside the chromatophores will increase body pigmentation while pigment aggregation causes reduced pigmentation. A reduced coloration due to chromatophore pigment aggregation will typically also result in increased skin transparency.

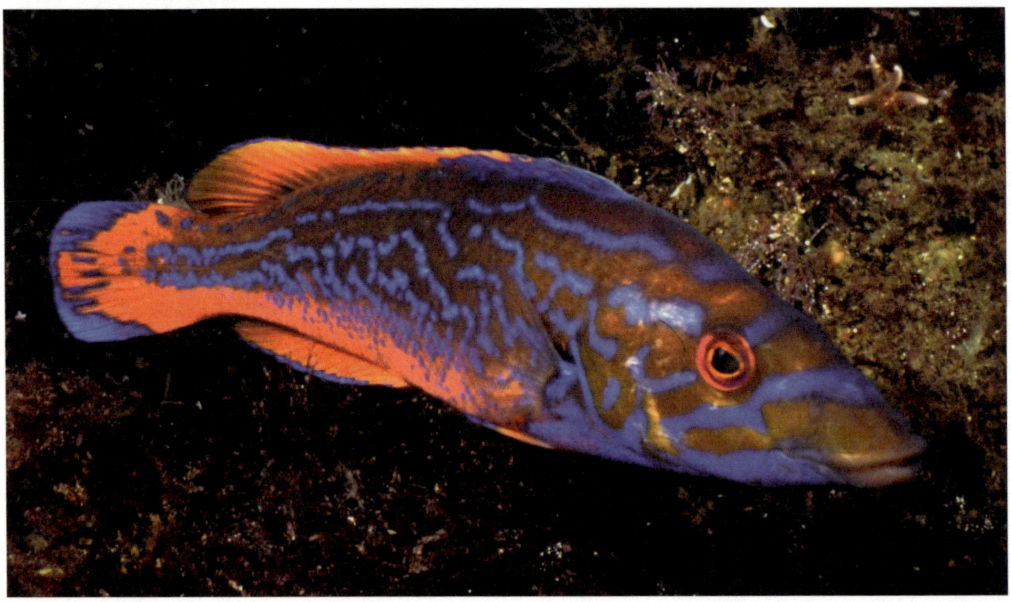

Fig. 1. An adult male cuckoo wrasse, *Labrus bimaculatus*, displaying its characteristic red and blue skin pattern in the wild. This fish does not have blue pigment cells but the blue colour of the skin is instead an effect of chromatic interactions between melanophores and iridophores. Females of this species lack the blue colours (not shown). The photograph was kindly provided by Dr Mattias Sköld.

On a cellular level, melanophores, with their distinctive dark melanin-containing organelles, melanosomes, are relatively well studies compared to the other chromatophore types. The cellular regulation of melanophores is therefore rather well understood. To achieve maximum lightness of the skin, the melanosomes are tightly aggregated to a spherical pigment mass in the center of each melanophore. A common observation is that fish often appear pale during sleep at night. The melanophore pigment aggregating effect of melatonin, which is released at night, causes this body paling. Both aggregation of pigment and the maintenance of the pigment within the spherical central pigment mass (CPM) depend on the molecular motor dynein and the presence of low levels of intracellular cAMP. Dyneins carry the melanosomes while they move along the microtubule tracks towards the center of the melanophore. On the other hand, to achieve maximum darkness of the skin, the pigment needs to be evenly dispersed throughout the cells. Such dispersion depends on a kinesin-like motor that moves along microtubules in the opposite direction of the dynein motor, and on high levels of cAMP. Dynein is inactivated during dispersion to allow rapid dispersal from the cell centre. The pigment do however not all move all the way to the periphery of the cells, but they stop at different position to become evenly dispersed throughout the cells. This even distribution is achived by movements of both dynein and the kinesin, together with actin and the actin-dependent motor myosin V, also located on the melanin pigment organelles. How the degree of dispersion is coordinated and maintained at the intracellular level is not yet fully understood.

Chromatophore-based pigment patterns are used by animals in a variety of behavioral contexts. In fishes, the regulation of physiological colour change has been mostly studied in the context of crypsis (i.e. camouflage). Recently, studies have been conducted on the often more complex nuptial colour patterns that are used for courtship and aggression. For a more comprehensive overview of fish coloration and patterns, including regulation and mechanisms behind the different types of colour changes, we refer to recent and classic reviews as well as some particularly relevant original publications (Kasukawa et al., 1987; Fujii and Oshima, 1994; Fujii 2000; Amundsen and Forsgren 2001; Nilsson Sköld et al., 2002; Siebeck 2004; Nilsson Sköld et al., 2008; Aspengren et al., 2008; 2009; Mills and Patterson 2009; Leclercq et al., 2010).

To fully understand short-term regulation of fish coloration one needs to address a wide range of phenomena: from the very fine details of the intracellular motile machineries to the complex chromatic interaction between tissue types and the signalling behaviours of the animals. We believe the use of skin biopsies work as a link between these traditionally disparate scientific disciplines. Skin biopsies can therefore become a bridge between physiology at cellular and organismal levels to animal behaviour and ecology.

2. Methodology for assessing fish coloration and colour change

2.1 Assays for analysis of rapid colour change

2.1.1 Skin biopsies

Skin biopsies can be excised from various parts of the fish body depending of purpose and area of interest. We have recently used biopsies from the abdomen (Nilsson Sköld et al., 2008; 2010) because these contain both epidermal (external) and peritoneal (internal) chromatophores (Figure 2). Melanophores, erythrophores, xanthophores, leucophores and iridophores are the most common chromatophore types found in the skin of fish.

Although blue cyanophores have been described, most blue and green skin colors are the result of chromatic interactions between melanophores, xanthophores and the reflective iridophores.

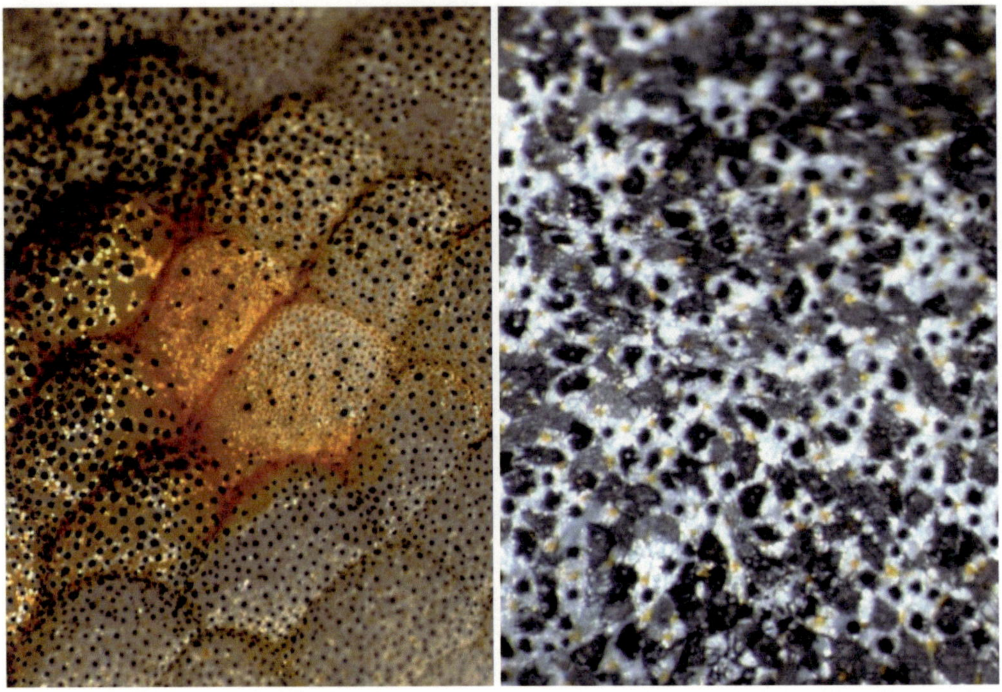

Fig. 2. Example of how the skin (left) and peritoneum (right) of a fish, *Pleuronectes platessa*, appears on close up photographs of an abdominal biopsy. In both photographs, examples of chromatophores with either aggregated or dispersed pigment can be observed.

In order to better understand the roles of different chromatophores on skin coloration or to test possible effects of certain hormones, the rapid color change reaction can be manipulated and monitored using skin biopsies excised from the fish of interest. A list of extracellular hormones and effectors reported to regulate skin coloration in various fish species is listed in Table 1. In principle, the biopsies are immersed in such hormones and the colour effect monitored. In our studies, we used abdominal biopsies which were excised so that they included the ventral and some of the lateral skin. Cutting the biopsy down the middle allows it to be used in both treatment and control. The biopsies were placed in saltwater or in Atlantic cod Ringer´s saline at pH7.5 (150 mM NaCl, 5.2 mM KCl, 1.8 mM $MgSO_4$, 7.0 mM NaHCO, 1.9 mM NaH_2PO_4 and 1 mg/ml glucose). In saltwater, melanophores, erythrophores and xanthophores become fully dispersed. In the Ringer's saline, the chromatphores are more or less dispersed. In order to trigger the pigment aggregation response, the biopsies can then be transferred into Nunc plastic wells (VWR International AB Stockholm) containing either Atlantic cod Ringer´s saline as a control, or freshly diluted 10 μM melatonin or norepinephrine (Sigma Aldrich, St. Louis, MO, USA), to induce pigment aggregation (Nilsson Sköld et al., 2008). Norephinephrine appears to be a general pigment aggregating agents across species, but melatonin varies in effectiveness among species. We had often problems with the consistency of the effect of epinephrine or melatonin in natural saltwater, but defined solutions such as Atlantic cod Ringer's saline were more reliable. The biopsies should be incubated in dark during the treatments since chromatophores in many (but not all) fish species are light sensitive. The light intensity also needs to be standardized during microscopy. It is advisable to do paired treatments where each fish produces both the control and the treatment biopsy. Both the epidermal and peritoneal side of the abdominal biopsies can be tested at the same time, if of interest. Cutting and pinching with forceps can cause cell damage, so the cell morphology and response to treatments are not representative in those parts of the biopsy. Soft insect forceps are advisable to use when handling the biopsies or scales.

The rate of colour change can be categorized subjectively under an inverted brightfield microscope using the Melanophore Index, MI (Hogben and Slome 1931), where fully aggregated melanosomes give MI = 1 and fully dispersed melanosomes give MI = 5. Occasionally, a hyperdispersed state can occur where the pigment is located only at the extremities of the cells, and this is given MI = 6 (Nilsson 2000). See figure 3 for illustration of the melanophore index. The MI shall be monitored just prior to applying the treatments, and at regular intervals thereafter; for example at 5, 10, 15, 20, 25, 30, 60, 120 and 180 minutes. Sometimes it is sufficient to use longer time intervals. In some species, the reaction occurs within minutes but in others it is slower. However, in most species the response is complete within one hour. Pilot observations testing a suitable timing of observations and hormone concentrations, is advisable when investigating a new species for the first time. The MI index works best for melanophores and erythrophores. For skin xanthophores, the aggregated state is easily identifiable but the different levels of dispersal are less distinct. MI is also less applicable when analysing whitish chromatophores. An alternative to MI scores is to quantify the coloration of the biopsy (see 2.2). However, a hyperdispered state will not then be distinguishable from MI 2-3. Although we have not ourselves investigated the rapid colour change of iridophores and its effects on the skin coloration, detailed information of the technical procedures for such investigations is given in an excellent study on the spectacular blue damselfish (Kasukawa et al., 1987).

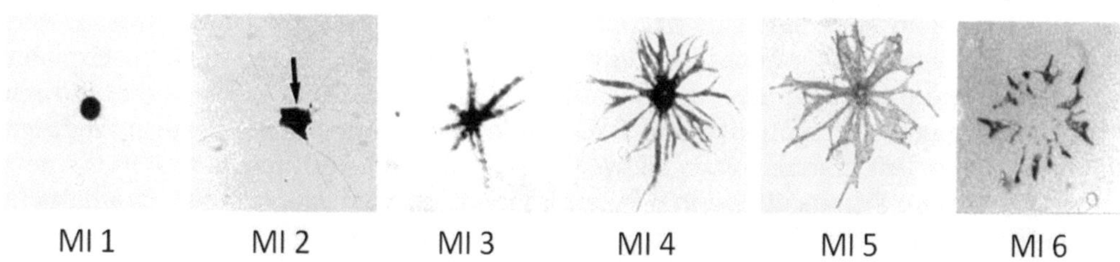

Fig. 3. Description of the Melanophore Index (MI) used to manually score the degree of pigment dispersal in fish melanophores. Arrow points at MI 2 which is similar to the shape of a deformed central pigment mass. MI 6 is normally a reversible state after a fast dispersal or an artefact seen after inhibition of dynein (in this case) or after modulation of the actin network. Damaged cells in the periphery of biopsies can also be hyperdispered. The depicted cells are primary cultures of cod skin melanophores.

Aggregation :	Colour response	Dispersion :	Colour response
Melatonin	pale	Adrenalin	dark
Noradrenalin	pale	Nitic Oxide	dark
Endothelins	pale	MSH	dark/red/yellow
MCH	pale	Prolactin	(dark)red/yellow
Light	pale	ACTH	dark/red/yellow
		UV	dark
		Light	dark
		*T/11kT	dark/red/yellow
		*E2	dark/red/yellow

Summarized from Fuji and Oshima, 1994; Fujii, 2000; Nilsson Sköld et al., 2008

Table 1. Extracellular signals reported to mediate fast or slow colour change in skin of fish. The colour response refers to the appearance of the skin. *The steroid hormones regulate morphological but not physiological colour changes directly. The other signals and hormones listed mediate both physiological and morphological colour change.

Skin explants in cultures have successfully been used for treatments with non-cell permeable agents to investigate intracellular mechanisms behind maintenance of the circular central pigment mass (CPM) and melanosome movements (Nilsson and Wallin 1997). The culture procedure makes the melanophores more exposed to the agents compared to the original biopsy, and the colour change reaction therefore occurs much faster. We here describe our own procedures for testing the aggregation inhibitory effects of the phosphatase inhibitor and putative dynein inhibitor vanadate. The same experimental principles can be used to assess effects of other agents, cell permeable or non-cell permeable. Skin pieces of about 1 mm^2 were prepared from Atlantic cod dorsal fins and allowed to adhere to the bottom of sterile plastic culture dishes in one drop of medium for about 1 hr before addition of a cell culture medium (medium 199 with Hank's salts supplemented with 10% fetal calf serum, 1% antibiotic/antimycotic solution, and 1% L-glutamine, all from Life Technologies, Renfrewshire, Scotland) and further incubation at 12°C. To facilitate permeabilization of cell membranes to the otherwise non-cell permeable agent vanadate, 0.02% of the mild detergent saponin was included in the lysis buffer during subsequent experiments, as described below. The experiments were performed the day after at 12°C in medium 199, or in lysis buffer at pH 7.0 made according to Grundström et al. (1985). Pigment aggregation was induced by addition of norepinephrine to the medium. Explants were tested before the treatments for the aggregation capacity, and explants that did not respond by pigment aggregation within 3 minutes were discarded. If the treatment induced aggregation, pigment granules were allowed to redisperse in fresh medium until the next day. Explants were then incubated in different concentrations of vanadate for 10 minutes in lysis buffer with saponin. The time of treatment was standardized to 10 min, as longer time in 0.02% saponin was found to inhibit the norepinephrine-induced pigment aggregation. Controls were treated with lysis buffer with or without saponin. Norepinephrine was added and the rate of aggregation monitored every 30 seconds for 6 minutes.

To investigate if the cytoskeleton is involved in maintenance of the spherical shape of the CPM (i.e. maximal aggregation), we tested the effects of microtubule and actin inhibitors in the shape of the CPM. For these experiments, the melanophores on the biopsy cultures were induced to aggregate pigment completely by addition of norepinephrine. After this, microtubule or actin disrupting agents were added for 2 hours of incubation in the presence

of norepinephrine. Controls were incubated in norepinephrine only. The skin explants were then fixed in ice-cold methanol for 6 minutes and rinsed in phosphate buffered saline for subsequent scoring of the amount of deformed versus spherical CMP´s on each explant. The results showed that microtubules, but not actin (not shown), maintain the spherical shape of the CPM (Nilsson and Wallin, 1997). Also here, the non-cell membrane permeable agent vanadate was added at different concentrations, now together with norepinephrine in the saponin containing lysis buffer. Controls were treated with lysis buffer with or without saponin. The treated explants were fixed after 10 minutes of treatment and the degree of aggregation (MI) evaluated as described above.
To investigate possible effects of vanadate on dispersion, melanophores were first induced to aggregate pigment for 4 minutes and then incubated for 10 minutes in vanadate together with epinephrine in lysis buffer with saponin, or in lysis buffer only with or without saponin together with 1 µM NA as controls. Measurements of dispersion were performed after removing the NA by rinsing the explants with lysis buffer including only vanadate, or lysis buffer without vanadate for the controls. The MI was scored every following minute until controls were fully dispersed (after approximately 20 minutes). We then statistically compared both time for onset of dispersion, which was faster in presence of vanadate, and the rate of dispersion, which did not differ from controls. Other ways to initiate dispersion than rinsing off norepinephrine, is to add agents that elevate intracellular cAMP levels such as the cell-membrane permeable forskolin or the melanocyte stimulating hormone (MSH) to the buffer. This speeds up dispersion to be completed within 5-10 minutes.

2.1.2 Scales

Scales have been widely used to investigate regulation of rapid colour change using both melanophores and erythrophores. Many scales can be collected from each fish, which allows multiple treatments and controls to be applied while also controlling for inter-individual differences. This is very useful when analyzing dose response effects. In our studies (Nilsson 2000; Andersson et al., 2003) scales from the area of interest were collected with fine forceps and placed in either Atlantic cod Ringer's saline or in phosphate buffered saline (136.9 mM NaCl, 2.7 mM KCl, 1.5 mM KH_2PO_4, 8.0 mM Na_2HPO_4 at pH 7.3). Fish scales can also be collected into culture medium for weeks of storage, but this has reported to create some response artifacts (Mårtensson and Andersson, 1997). In either condition, melanosomes and erythrosomes become fully dispersed within the chromatophores. Aggregation, shape of the CPM and dispersion can be tested using different hormones and inhibitors, as for the biopsies described above, and distribution of pigment scored under microscopy using the MI index. The reactions are slightly faster on scales than when using biopsies. As with the biopsies, care shall be taken to standardize the light intensity and the time of light exposure. Not all chromatophores within a scale will start translocation of pigment organelles simultaneously. The cells around the edges will often react first, so for reliable results, score either only the cells around the edges or use an average MI of the entire scale.

2.1.3 Melanophore primary cultures

For a direct assessment on the role of different molecular motors, second messengers, receptors or extracellular signals on the chromatophores, these cells need to be isolated. For this purpose, we developed and refined a procedure to obtain primary cultures of cod (*Gadus morhua*) skin melanophores (Townsley et al. 1963; Nilsson et al., 1996; Nilsson and Wallin, 2007). We here describe the final protocol and some of the experiments we did.

A slice of a dorsal fin is removed and placed in a sterile glass dish with cell culture medium 199 with Hank's salts and the supplements described above for the biopsies. Tissue pieces of about 1 mm^2 are cut and placed in a drop of the medium on sterile glass or plastic coverslips in a sterile culture dish. The explants are kept at 12°C for about an hour without drying in order to enhance the adhesion before further addition of medium. The cultures are incubated in darkness at 12°C and medium changed twice a week. A monolayer of skin cells including melanophores are under these conditions formed around the fin explants. In order to obtain more isolated and free melanophores, the medium is changed to serum-free CO_2-independent medium supplied with 1% antibiotic/antimycotic solution and 1% L-glutamine (Life Technologies), 5 µg/ml insulin, 5 µg/ml transferrin, and 5 ng/ml sodium selenite (Boehringer Mannheim, Mannheim, Germany) and 1 mg/ml glucose. After a few days in this medium, most cells except melanophores will detach from the coverslips. Isolated melanophores could be kept for weeks under these conditions if the medium was changed twice weekly. In both mediums, pigment was evenly dispersed in the melanophores. Pigment aggregation is then induced with micromolar concentrations of noradrenaline and pigment dispersal by removal of the noradrenaline by adding fresh culture medium. For a faster dispersal, the cAMP elevating agent forskolin could be added. Melanophores isolated by this procedure were used for immunocytochemistry, microinjections of anti-dynein antibodies, melanosome trackings and various other manipulations. Altogether, melanophore primary cultures have experimentally been a very powerful system for the present theory of the intracellular transport mechanisms in these cells - from the cytoskeleton to second messengers and receptors (Nilsson et al., 1996; Nilsson and Wallin 1997, 1998; Aspengren et al., 2003; Nilsson Sköld et al., 2003).

2.1.4 A fixed-time in vitro melanosome motility assay

As a complemental method to microinjections and other cell based methods for investigating intracellular aspects of melanophore colour change, we developed fixed-time in vitro melanosome motility assay that mimics the cellular situation. The preparation and application of melanophore lysate, including the MI scoring and photography, can all be done within one working day. The method is originally described in Nilsson et al. (2001).
Melanophores from dorsal scales of *Fundulus heteroclitus* were used to prepare melanophore lysates. These lysates were then used for the fixed-time in vitro melanosome motility assay. The scales were liberated from several individuals according to a method described in detail by Haimo (1998). In brief, the scales were rinsed three times in Marine Ringer's containing 50 mM ethylenediaminetetraacetic acid (EDTA), transferred into 15-ml falcon tubes with 5 ml of Marine Ringer's containing 5 mg/ml collagenase type 2 and 10 mg/ml bovine serum albumin and mixed slowly with a rotary shaker for 40 minutes at room temperature. Scales were allowed to settle, the supernatant collected and the melanophores pelleted by centrifugation at 500*g* for 5 minutes at room temperature. The supernatant was collected and added back to the scales. The melanophore pellet was carefully resuspended in cold freshwater Ringer's (Haimo, 1998) containing protease inhibitors (leupeptin, pepstatin A, aprotinin, and chymostatin each at 10 mg/ml and 1 mM phenylmethylsulphonyl fluoride). Solutions were prepared once a week and oxygenated 15 minutes before use. At this stage, the isolated melanophores contained dispersed pigment. In some treatments, cells were treated with isobutylmethylxanthine or forskolin (agents known to increase intracellular cAMP levels and thus facilitate dispersion) for 15 minutes before lysis. Aggregation was induced by incubation of the cells with norepinephrine for 30 minutes. Aggregation was not

always successful after liberation. Only preparations where 80% of cells aggregated their pigment within 30 min were used for the subsequent fixed-time in vitro motility assay. In the next step, the liberated melanophores were pelleted and resuspended in a small volyme of ice cold IMB50 buffer containing protease inhibitors, a buffer previously developed for an in vitro motility assay with frog melanosomes (Rogers et al., 1998). In our case either norepinephrin to induce aggregation or the combination of IBMX and forskolin to induce dispersion, were added to the buffer. Melanophores were then lysed in the buffer by 5-10 passes through a 22s gauge syringe. Cell fragments and remaining dermis were pelleted by centrifugation at 500*g*, for 5 minutes. The supernatant containing the melanosome solution was handled carefully to avoid bubbles and 100 µl pipetted using a tip with a cut end. Everything was kept cold during the procedure.

KCl activated oocytes of the clam, *Spisula solidissima* were used to produce lysates with microtubule asters for the motility assay (Palazzo et al., 1988) and kept as aliquots at -80 °C. Such oocyte lysates contain centrosomes that spontaneously nucleate microtubules arrays when warmed. For visualization of the asters, 0.1 mg/ml of rhodamine-labeled bovine tubulin (Cytoskeleton, Inc., Denver, CO) was added to 20 µl of ice-cold activated lysate. The mixture was then warmed to room temperature for 15 min to allow aster formation. The mixture was then diluted 1:5 into IMB50 buffer containing 10 mM of the microtubule-stabilizing agent taxol (Sigma Chem Co.) and the antifade agent oxyrace (Oxyrace, Inc., Mansfield, OH) at 1:100, and placed on ice. The mixture was then diluted 1:2 into the freshly prepared melanophore lysate and this mixture was then divided into aliquots for each subsequent treatment, for example addition of an inhibitory anti dynein antibody. For the in vitro pigment translocation to start, ATP was added to 2 mM. The total assay volume for each treatment was 10 µl. Each reaction mixture were then placed on a glass cover slip, incubated as a droplet at room temperature for 30 min in a humid chamber, and then overlaid with a glass slide. No pre-coating of the glass was necessary. The distribution of pigment on the asters in the different samples was immediately scored and recorded using a microscope with a 63x magnification. With this procedure, more than 50 asters could be scored on each slide. Melanophore lysates prepared from dispersed melanophores induced dispersal of pigment in vitro, and melanophore lysates prepared from aggregated melanophores induced aggregation of pigment in vitro. Addition of an inhibitory anti dynein antibody blocked the in vitro aggregation and pigment ended up in the periphery of the aster (Nilsson et al., 2001), similar to what happened after microinjection of the antibody into cultured cod melanophores (Nilsson and Wallin, 1997; Nilsson Sköld et al., 2002).

2.2 Measuring biopsy coloration and transparency

In this section, we will describe how to measure coloration and colour change with digital photography and computer-aided image analysis. The methods described have been used by us in the following papers: Svensson et al. (2005), Sköld et al. (2008), Svensson et al. (2009a,b) and Nilsson-Sköld et al. (2010), but also by others (Heflin et al., 2009). They are applicable to both biopsies and whole (living) fish.

2.2.1 Digital photography and colour

To quantify the degree of pigmentation in fish tissues, we developed methods to analyse the transparency and colour intensity of biopsies as well as whole animals. Many different approaches are possible for this task, all with their own limitations. Spectrometry and microspectrometry have long been the colorimetric methods of choice for many biologists because of their objectivity and wide spectral range. However, carefully standardized digital photography has been put forward as a strong alternative (Stevens et al., 2007). After much experimenting, our choice fell on digital photography coupled with image analyses in the CIE Lab colour space (Svensson et al., 2005; Sköld et al., 2008; Nilsson Sköld et al., 2010). Importantly, photography is much faster than spectrometry, which is advantageous when dealing with tissues prone to rapid colour change. To obtain a photograph takes only a few seconds, but to take multiple readings with a spectrometer can be very time consuming. Photographs can also easily be taken without having to remove the biopsy from a reagent solution. This can be important in repeated measures and time-series designs. Furthermore, digital photography allows measurements of pre-defined areas by using anatomical landmarks on the biopsy/animal. Another benefit is that images can be analysed and re-analysed at a later date, allowing the researcher to decouple, in space and time, colour quantifiaction from the experimental work. Photographs also offer superior spatial resolution, which is crucial for analysis of complex colour patterns (Stevens et al., 2007). By using all the pixels inside the selected area, rather than a few point samples, one can obtain very precise estimates of colour parameters. It is important to point out that digital cameras have potential issues with non-linearity and spectral bias, which may affect the measurements. In many situations this may not be a great concern, for example when the degree of colour difference is relatively small. However, non-linearity and spectral bias can be formally addressed through calibration procedures, making the colorimetric data equal in quality to spectrometry, as described by Stevens et al. (2007). A potential disadvantage of photography is a limitation to the wavelengths of human colour vision. Importantly, certain fish colour patterns are only observable in the UV. However, cameras that can detect UV and IR light are now commercially available (e.g. the Fujifilm FinePix S3 Pro UV IR and a range of specialist cameras). For examples and methodologies for assessing the little studied UV-aspects of fish coloration, we refer to the excellent work by Siebeck (2004).

When measuring coloration it is important to realize that colour is not a physical property of an object but a property of the visual system of the observer (Grether et al, 2004). Quantifying colour in a way that is relevant to the animal in question may therefore be non-trivial. It is important to choose a method that is suitable for the question and study species at hand. Consequently, the methods described here may not be appropriate in all circumstances; they should rather be seen as a starting point for method development. The painstaking process of finding the best way to quantify coloration will ultimately have to be done anew for any new study system (Dawson, 2006). The aim should be to arrive at a method that maximizes relevance, accuracy and precision of the measurements. In other words, the obtained data should have both high within-specimen repeatability and high between-specimen variation.

2.2.2 Image analysis

After digital photographs have been taken, the information contained in them has to be converted to data. The simplest method is to let a panel of people score the photographs. However, digital image analysis provides a finer discrimination than human observers (Villafuerte & Negro, 1998). The next question is what to measure. There are several different colour parameters in various colour spaces available. For example, some early studies quantified red-orange colour intensity using a red index, $Ri = R / (R+G+B)$, based on the RGB (Red, Green, Blue) colour space (Frischknecht, 1993; Barber et al., 2000; Pelabon et al., 2003). Other studies have used cylindrical representations of the RGB colour space, such as HSL,

HSB and HSV (Hue, Saturation and Lightness/Brightness/Value) (Hatlen et al., 1998; Nordeide, 2002). The RGB-colour space is device dependent and countless versions exist, even within the same software (e.g. Adobe RGB, apple RGB and sRGB IEC61966-2.1). In contrast, CIE L*a*b* is a standardized, perceptually uniform and device independent colour space (Chen *et al*, 2004), designed in 1976 by the International Lighting Commission (Commission International de l'Eclairage, CIE). CIE Lab measurements based on spectrometry have become standard in the field of animal coloration (e.g. Skrede & Storebakken, 1986; Smith et al., 1992; Craig & Foote, 2001), but few studies have applied CIE Lab to quantify animal coloration from digital photographs. Adobe Photoshop™ has a colour space called "Lab colour mode" which is based on CIE Lab. As it name suggests, it consists of three parameters: L*, a* and b*. In Photoshop, the asterisks have been dropped, but for clarity, we have chosen to retain them. The L* channel stands for lightness (or luminosity) and describes the relative lightness from total black to total white. In an 8 bit/channel image, L* will range from 0 (black) to 255 (white). The a* channel is the balance between green and magenta (Margulis, 2006). Thus, a* ranges from 0 (pure green) to 255 (pure magenta), while a* = 128 (or, more specifically 127.5) describes a neutral grey. The b* channel describes the balance between blue and yellow, where 0 is pure blue, and 255 is pure yellow, while b* = 128 (127.5) describes a neutral grey. Typically, however, Lab values are expressed differently. L* is often described as ranging from 0 to 100, while a* and b* range from -100 to 100, with zero corresponding to neutral grey. It is easy to convert 8-bit a* and b* values to this scale by the following formula: $a^* = (a^*_{8bit} - 127.5) / 1.275$. This conversion is important if one aims to use a* and b* values to calculate chroma or hue (Little, 1975):

$$\text{chroma} = \sqrt{a^{*2} + b^{*2}} \quad (1)$$

$$\text{hue} = \text{atan}\,(b^* / a^*) \quad (2)$$

A major advantage of Lab colour is that it separates colour from contrast (lightness), as opposed to RGB where all three channels affect both these parameters. Thus, a* and b* affects only colour while L* affects only contrast. In theory, the a* and b* channels are therefore completely insensitive to variations in light intensity. However, even when analysis takes place in Lab, the image capture does not, because all digital cameras use a RGB sensor to capture the image. Differences in the light intensity of the image can therefore affect both contrast and colour information. This is a major reason why the photographic conditions must be highly standardized if one is to accurately quantify biopsy coloration. A second source of concern is that the algorithms used to convert RGB to Lab may differ between software versions. For example, an a* value obtained from Photoshop 4.0 will not exactly match a value from Photoshop 5.0. In more recent software versions, however, ICE colour management can be used to control the RGB-Lab conversion.

When choosing how to quantify colour, it is important to select colour parameters that maximize relevance, accuracy and precision for the investigation at hand. For example, we found untransformed values of the a* channel to be superior in describing the orange belly ornament in female *G. flavescens*, as verified by a strong relationship between a* and actual pigment concentration (measured by HPLC, Svensson et al., 2005; Svensson et al., 2006). For blue and yellow hues, the b* channel may be more relevant. In other circumstances, parameters like chroma and hue (which take both a* and b* into account) may prove a better option. When quantifying the transparency of biopsies and/or the effect of melanophores, the L* channel is typically the most relevant parameter (see below).

2.2.3 Standardization and setup

As already mentioned, it is important that the entire photographic procedure is standardized. For example, one should minimize variation in the handling time of the biopsies when taking the photographs. It is also vital that all camera settings are kept constant. This includes the light conditions, the lens zoom setting, flash settings and, on the camera itself: shutter speed, aperture, ISO, white balance and image file storage settings. The exposure should be set so that it maximizes the dynamic range of the image file. This means that the lightest area (typically the background) should be close to 100% exposure, without being overexposed. Likewise, the darkest area (typically the zero-light reference) should be close to 0% exposure. In other words, the tonal histogram of the biopsy should not be cut off at either end. Ideally, images should be saved without any in-camera processing (i.e. saving in "camera raw" format), and subjected to a standardized conversion to the target format (e.g. tiff or jpeg) before analysis. The image analysis should, if possible, be done blindly so that the person analysing images is unaware from which treatment they originate.

We have used two camera setups, either a Canon D30 dSLR camera with Canon 50 mm f/2.5 EF Compact Macro lens (Svensson et al., 2005; Sköld et al., 2008) or a Nikon D80 dSLR camera with a Nikon 105 mm AF Micro Nikkor lens (Nilsson Sköld et al., 2010). If dealing with small biopsies it is important to choose a camera/lens with good macro capabilities. Alternatively, cameras can be mounted on a dissecting microscope.

2.2.4 Method to quantify biopsy transparency

To measure the transparency of skin biopsies (figure 4), we used back-lit digital photographs and quantified the lightness channel, L*, (Svensson et al., 2005). This method is also good at detecting pigmentation changes caused by regulation of melanophores. In relatively small-bodies fish species, the same method can be used to quantify the transparency of live animals (figure 5).

Biopsies were placed on a light table, ideally still submerged in their respective treatment reagent. If necessary, the biopsies were flattened with a glass slide. When quantifying transparency of whole (live) animals, the fish were quickly transferred and placed either ventrally of laterally on the light table. The picture was taken with the camera affixed directly above the sample, with an opaque object placed next to it for calibration purposes (a zero-light reference). It is important that photography takes place in a dark room, or that the whole setup is covered by dark fabric, so that the light table is the only light source. Care should be taken that all biopsies are placed on the same area of the light table. One should also verify that the light levels do not change over time (e.g. from ageing fluorescent lights).

The image analysis was carried out in Adobe Photoshop, and photographs converted from RGB colour to Lab colour space. We further standardized the tonal range in the image by setting the centre of the opaque area to $L^* = 0$ and the background to $L^* = 255$. In Photoshop this is done with the pipettes in the curve or levels tool. The area of interest was selected with the polygon lasso tool with zero feathering. After the selection was made, the mean value of L* in the selected area was noted (in Photoshop this is given in the 'histogram/all channels view' dialogue). Lightness was converted to a measurement of transparency by calculating the percentage of L* in the selected area relative to the L* of the background ($\text{transparency} = 100 \times L^*_{\text{biopsy}} / 255$).

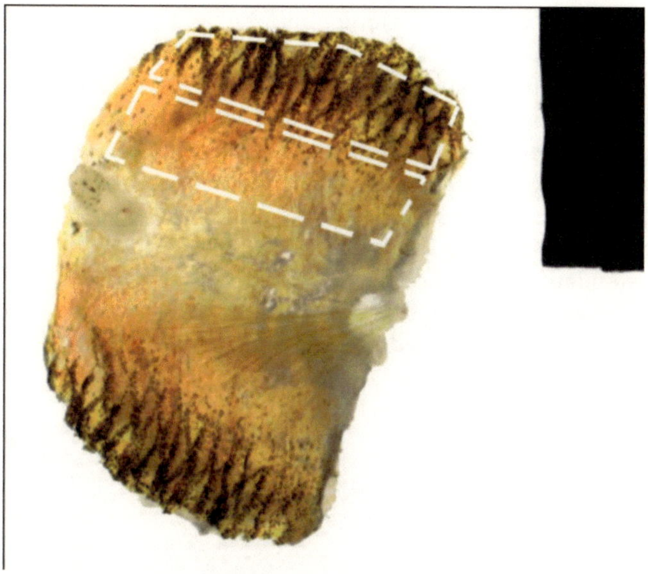

Fig. 4. Examples of photograph used to quantify abdominal skin coloration and transparency in *G. flavescens*. After excising the biopsy, it was placed next to a black piece of plastic (zero-light reference). It was placed on a light table and photographed with the light shining through the skin. The dashed line indicates the two areas selected for analysis (Sköld et al., 2008).

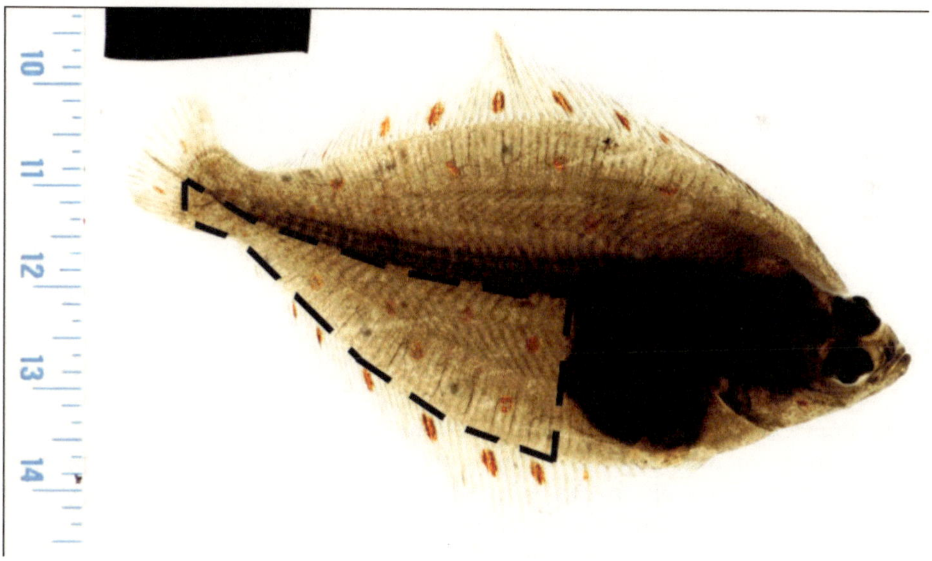

Fig. 5. Example photograph of whole-body transparency in juvenile plaice *P. platessa*. The live fish was placed on a light table and photographed with the light shining through the skin and body. The dashed line indicates a pre-defined area selected for analysis (Nilsson Sköld et al., 2010).

2.2.5 Method to quantify biopsy coloration

The coloration of a biopsy may be measured with the light passing through the biopsy. In this case the same method as described above (2.2.4) was used (figure 4). Alternatively, the biopsy may be lit from above (figure 6). For illumination our choice fell on photographic flashes, which are consistent, broad-spectrum light sources. We used two flash heads, fired at obtuse angles to avoid glare. Having the biopsy submerged and using diffusing flash filters may reduce glare further. It is important that the settings and position of the flash is kept constant, and that it is allowed to recharge fully between photographs. Apart from a matte black object as a zero-light reference one can use cut-outs of colour standards (e.g. Kodak™ Q13 colour separation guide) to assist in calibration. After converting the RGB image file to Lab and selecting the area of interest, the mean a* and b* values were noted. These values were used to calculate chroma and hue as described above.

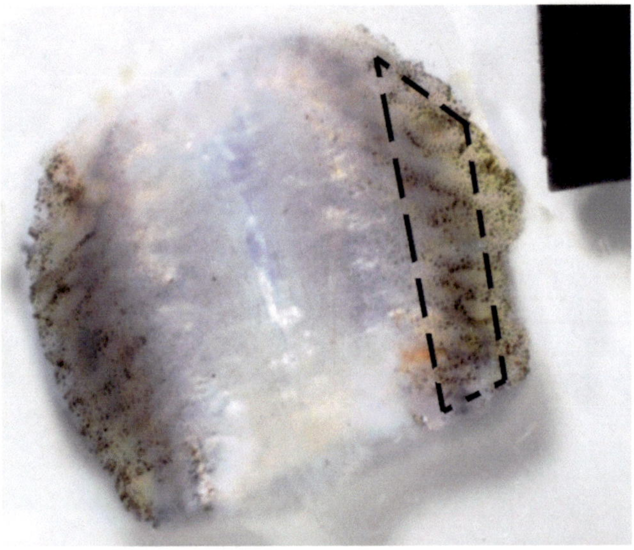

Fig. 6. Examples of photograph used to quantify abdominal skin coloration in *G. flavescens* after exposure to norepinephrine. In this case, the biopsy was lit from above with dual flash heads. The dashed line indicates the anatomically predefined area analysed.

3. Some notes on statistics

A major benefit of using scales or excised biopsies is the ability to apply treatments that would be impractical or unethical to administer to live animals. A major limitation is the inevitable, and non-randomizable, effect of time passing from the moment of euthanasia/excision. Time effects can be addressed with appropriate controls, for example by comparing "time only" with "time + reagent". A statistically powerful method is to collect several scales or to divide biopsies and to then expose the sub-samples from the same individual to different treatments. Such within-subject designs, also called block designs, can be analysed by using the identity of the animal as a random factor in a mixed model. In an experiment with only one factor (treatment) at only two levels, this will be equivalent to a paired t-test.

MI-scores and data describing the shapes of the CPM's are subjective by nature. It is therefore advisable that the same person do all such scoring within a study. Ideally, the person that scores shall also be blind with respect to treatments.

Percentages, and many colour parameters, such as L*, a* and b*, will always be bounded by a maximum and a minimum value. This may cause data to be non-normally distributed, especially if many values are close to the upper, or lower, limit. An arcsine square root transformation may improve normality in these cases (Crawley, 2007). The following formula is used will return a transformed value in degrees (i.e. ranging from 0 to 90):

$$\textit{transformed value} = \frac{180}{\pi} \times \text{asin}\left(\sqrt{p}\right) \qquad (3)$$

where p is the parameter converted into a proportion (i.e. ranging from 0 to 1).

For the determination of differences in amounts of spherical shapes of CMPs as well as for differences in of the rate of colour change reaction, we used factorial analysis of variance with treatment as fixed factor, individual fish as a random factor and percentage deformed CPMs or slope of MIs/minute during the linear phase of colour change reaction as response variables. MI score at a specific time point can be used to measure of the rate of a response, but as the data are discrete, non-parametric tests are typically more suitable.

4. Conclusions

We have described several different ways in which skin biopsies can be useful for studies of animal coloration and the mechanisms for colour change. Manipulations and observations of skin biopsies have given us an increased understanding of regulation of rapid colour change in general, and have been successfully applied to the study of colour signals in animals. Similarly, by using abdominal skin biopsies (containing both epidermis and the peritoneum) we have acquired novel insights into the functions of internal pigment cells in transparent fishes. At a cellular level, fish biopsies has been successfully used to isolate melanophores for immunocytechemistry, to trace the movements of individual melanosomes, for microinjections and other more direct manipulations. This cell-based approach has been instrumental in the construction of the current physiological model for rapid colour change in fishes. This model includes the function of the cytoskeleton and the coordinated actions of various molecular motors, and has increased the understanding intracellular organelle transport and positioning in all cell types.

However, many things remain to be discovered, and current methods have important limitations. In fish, the type of kinesin used in pigment dispersal during rapid colour change is still unidentified. We are yet to understand how the pigment organelles at an intracellular level are maintained in an evenly dispersed state. Although the important roles of cAMP and its downstream protein kinase A in pigment movement are clear, the possible roles of other second messengers, including the exact functions of calcium, are far from understood. From image analysis of skin biopsies, changes in a* and b* channels are thought to reflect changes in erythrophores and xanthophores, respectively, but this needs to be verified though measurements of isolated pigment cells. Many fishes perform rapid and complicated colour modifications during specific behaviours (such as courtship displays). Our photographic/microscopic techniques are not well suited for quantification of such ephemeral signals. Likewise, the quantification of other types of coloration, such as iridescent and UV colours will require a refined methodology. The use of skin biopsies as a tool to address questions from cell physiology to animal behaviour does hold a lot of promise. We strongly believe that future studies will lead to many exciting discoveries.

5. Acknowledgement

This work was possible through grants from Wåhlströms and C. F. Lundströms foundations to H.N.S.

6. References

Amundsen, T. & Forsgren, E. (2001). Male mate choice selects for female coloration in a fish. *Proc. Natl. Acad. Sci. U. S. A.* Vol. 98, pp. 13155–13160.

Andersson, T. P. M., Nilsson Sköld, H. & Svensson, S. P. S. (2003). Phosphoinositide 3-kinase is involved in *Xenopus* and *Labrus* melanophore aggregation. *Cell Signal.* Vol. 15, pp. 119-127.

Aspengren, S., Nilsson Sköld, H. & Wallin, M. (2009). Different strategies for color change. *Cell Mol. Life Sci.* Vol. 66, pp. 187-191.

Aspengren, S., Hedberg, D., Nilsson Sköld, H. & Wallin, M. (2008). New insights into melanosome transport in vertebrate pigment cells. *Int. Rev. Cell Mol. Biol. Vol.* 272, pp. 245-302.

Aspengren, S., Nilsson Sköld, H., Quiroga, G., Mårtensson, L. & Wallin, M. (2003). Noradrenaline- and melatonin-mediated regulation of pigment aggregation in fish melanophores. *Pigment Cell Res,* Vol. 16, pp. 59-64.

Barber, I., Arnott, S. A., Braithwaite, V. A., Andrew, J., Mullen, W. & Huntingford, F. A. (2000). Carotenoid-based sexual coloration and body condition in nesting male sticklebacks. *J. Fish Biol.* Vol. 57, pp. 777-790.

Craig, J. K. & Foote, C. J. (2001). Countergradient variation and secondary sexual color: Phenotypic convergence promotes genetic divergence in carotenoid use between sympatric anadromous and nonanadromous morphs of sockeye salmon (*Oncorhynchus nerka*). *Evolution,* Vol. 55, pp. 380-391.

Crawley, M. J. (2007). *The R book.* John Wiley & Sons Ltd, Chichester.

Frischknecht, M. (1993). The breeding coloration of male 3-spined sticklebacks (Gasterosteus aculeatus) as an indicator of energy investment in vigor. *Evolutionary Ecology,* Vol. 7, pp. 439-450.

Fujii R. The regulation of motile activity in fish chromatophores. Pigment Cell Res 2000;13:300–319

Fujii, R., & Oshima, N. (1994). Factors influencing motile activities of fish chromatophores. *Adv. Comp. Environ. Physiol.* Vol. 20, pp. 1–54.

Grundström, N., Karlsson, J.O.G. & Andersson, R.G.G. (1985). The control of granule movement in fish melanophores. *Acta. Physiol. Scand.* Vol. 125, pp. 415–421.

Haimo, L. T. (1998). Reactivation of vesicle transport in lysed teleost melanophores. *Methods Enzymol.* Vol. 298, pp. 389-399.

Hatlen, B., Jobling, M. & Bjerkeng, B. (1998). Relationships between carotenoid concentration and colour of fillets of Arctic charr, *Salvelinus alpinus* (L.), fed astaxanthin. *Aquaculture Research,* Vol. 29, pp. 191-202.

Heflin, B., Young, L. & Londraville, R. L. (2009). Short-term cycling of skin colouration in the blackspotted rockskipper *Entomacrodus striatus. J. Fish Biol.* Vol.74, pp. 1635–1641.

Hogben, L.T. & Slome, D. (1931). The pigmentary effector system. VI. The dual character of endocrine coordination in amphibian colour change. *Proc. R. Soc. Lond. Ser. B*, Vol. 108, pp. 10–53.

Kasukawa, H., Oshima, N. & Fujii, R. (1987). Mechanism of light reflection in blue damselfish motile iridophore. *Zool. Sci.* Vol. 4, pp. 243-257.

Leclercq, E., Taylor, J. F. & Migaud, H. (2010). Morphological skin colour changes in teleosts. *Fish and Fisheries,* Vol. 11, pp. 159–193.

Margulis, D. (2006). *Photoshop LAB Color. The canyon conundrum and other adventures in the most powerful colorspace*. Peachpit Press, Berkeley.

Mills, M. G. & Patterson, L. B. (2009). Not just black and white: Pigment pattern development and evolution in vertebrates. *Seminars in Cell & Developmental Biology,* Vol. 20, pp. 72–81.

Mårtensson, L. G. & Andersson, R. G. (1997). Denervation of pigment cells lead to a receptor that is ultrasensitive to melatonin and noradrenaline. *Life Sci.*Vol. 60, pp.1575-1582.

Nilsson Sköld, H., Svensson, P. A. & Zejlon, C. (2010). The capacity for internal colour change is related to body transparency in fishes. *Pigment Cell and Melanoma Research,* Vol. 23, pp. 292-295.

Nilsson, H, Steffen, W. & Palazzo, R. E. (2001). In vitro reconstitution of fish melanophore pigment aggregation. *Cell Motil. Cytoskel.* Vol. 48, pp. 1-10.

Nilsson Sköld, H., Norström, E. & Wallin, M. (2002). Regulation of both actin- and microtubule- dependent fish melanosome movement. *Pigment Cell Res.* Vol.5, pp. 357-366.

Nilsson, H. (2000). Melanosome and erythrosome positioning regulates cAMP induced movement in chromatophores in Spotted Triplefin, *Grahamina capito. J. Exp. Zool.* Vol. 287, pp. 191-198.

Nilsson, H. & Wallin, M. (1997). Evidence for several roles of dynein in pigment transport in melanophores. *Cell Motil. Cytoskel.* Vol. 38, pp. 397-409.

Nilsson, H., Rutberg, M. & Wallin, M. (1996). Localization of kinesin and cytoplasmic dynein in cultured melanophores from Atlantic cod, *Gadus morhua. Cell Motil. Cytoskel.* Vol. 33, pp. 183-196.

Nordeide, J. T. (2002). Do male sticklebacks prefer females with red ornamentation? *Can. J. Zool.* Vol. 80, pp. 1344-1349.

Palazzo, R. E., Brawley, J. B. & Rebhun, L. I. (1988). Spontaneous aster formation in the cytoplasmic extracts from eggs of the surf clam. *Zool Sci.* Vol. 5, pp. 603- 611.

Pelabon, C., Borg, A. A., Bjelvenmark, J., Forsgren, E., Barber, I. & Amundsen, T. (2003). Do male two-spotted gobies prefer large fecund females? *Behavioral Ecology,* Vol. 14, pp. 787-792.

Rogers, S. L., Tint, I. S. & Gelfand, V. I. (1998). In vitro motility assay for melanophore pigment organelles. *Methods Enzymol.* Vol. 298, pp. 361–372.

Siebeck, U. E. (2004). Communication in coral reef fish: the role of ultraviolet colour patterns in damselfish territorial behavior. *Animal Behaviour,* Vol. 68, pp. 273-282.

Siebeck, U. E., Parker, A. N., Sprenger,D., Mäthger L. M. & Wallis, G. (2010). A species of reef fish that uses ultraviolet patterns for covert face recognition. *Curr. Biol.* Vol. 20, pp. 407–410.

Skrede, G. & Storebakken, T. (1986). Instrumental color analysis of farmed and wild atlantic salmon when raw, baked and smoked. *Aquaculture,* Vol. 53, pp. 279-286.

Sköld, H. N., Amundsen, T., Svensson, P. A., Mayer, I., Bjelvenmark, J. & Forsgren, E. (2008). Hormonal regulation of female nuptial coloration in a fish. *Hormones and Behaviour*, Vol. 54, pp. 549-556.

Smith, B. E., Hardy, R. W. & Torrissen, O. J. (1992). Synthetic astaxanthin deposition in pan-size coho salmon (Oncorhynchus kisutch). *Aquaculture*, Vol. 104, pp. 105-119.

Stevens, M., Parraga, C. A., Cuthill, I. C., Partridge, J. C. & Troscianko, T. S. (2007). Using digital photography to study animal coloration. *Biol. J. Linn. Soc. Lond.* Vol. 90, pp. 211-237.

Svensson, P. A., Blount, J. D., Forsgren, E. & Amundsen, T. (2009a). Female ornamentation and egg carotenoids of six sympatric gobies. *Journal of Fish Biology*, Vol. 75, pp. 2777–2787.

Svensson, P. A., Forsgren, E., Amundsen, T. & Nilsson Sköld, H. (2005). Chromatic interaction between egg pigmentation and skin chromatophores the nuptial coloration of female two-spotted gobies. *J. Exp. Biol.* Vol. 208, pp. 4391-4397.

Svensson, P. A., Pélabon, C., Blount, J. D., Forsgren, E., Bjerkeng, B. & Amundsen, T. (2009b). Temporal variability in a multicomponent trait: nuptial coloration of female two-spotted gobies. *Behavioral Ecology*, Vol. 20, pp. 346-353.

Svensson, P. A., Pélabon, C., Blount, J. D., Surai, P. F. & Amundsen, T. (2006). Does female nuptial coloration reflect egg carotenoids and clutch quality in the two-spotted goby (*Gobiusculus flavescens*, Gobiidae)? *Functional Ecology*, Vol. 20, pp. 689-698.

Townsley, P.M., Wight, H.G., & Scott, M.A. (1963). Marin fish tissue culture. *J. Fish. Res. Bd. Can*. Vol. 20, pp. 679-686.

Villafuerte, R. & Negro, J. J. (1998). Digital imaging for colour measurement in ecological research. *Ecology Letters*, Vol 1, pp.151-154.

16

Multi-Trial Ecotoxicological Diagnostic Tool in Cetacean Skin Biopsies

Maria Cristina Fossi and Letizia Marsili
*Department of Environmental Sciences,
University of Siena, Siena,
Italy*

1. Introduction

In the last 20 years there has been growing concern about potential hazard to cetaceans occasioned by multiple stress factors due to bioaccumulation of anthropogenic contaminants combined with infectious diseases, food depletion and climate change. In this context, the main aim of this chapter is to present the development and the application of a non-lethal multi trial biomarker tool applied to cetacean skin biopsies to diagnose "toxicological stress syndromes" related to multiple human pressures. Here we present a multidisciplinary approach to detect presence and effects of anthropogenic contaminants combined with general stressors using a wide range of diagnostic markers (molecular and gene expression biomarkers, immunological and nutritional status) with contaminant analysis, for a complete assessment of health status of cetaceans. The chapter is subdivided in three sections: in section one we describe the main threats faced by cetaceans focusing on the case study of Mediterranean Sea; in the second part we will describe the sensitivity of the multi trial biomarker diagnostic tool in skin biopsy cetacean samples; and in the third part we will describe the application of the proposed multidisciplinary approach to explore the effects of multiple human pressures on cetacean health status (field applications), comparing fin whale (*Balaenoptera physalus*) (mysticete) population of Mediterranean compared to the one of Sea of Cortez (Mexico). Final development of this interdisciplinary diagnostic methodology, embedded in a statistical Expert System, will provide exhaustive information about "toxicological status" of cetaceans as a powerful frontier approach for the conservation of relevant species of sea biodiversity.

2. Section one - Threats faced by cetaceans: The case study of Mediterranean sea

Threats facing cetaceans have changed through time. While overkill from hunting was the most obvious and immediate threat to some species and populations during much of the 20th century, the relative importance of other threats, particularly bycatch in fisheries and contamination, has increased dramatically during the last few decades. It is difficult to distinguish the effects of one threat from those of another when multiple threats are acting simultaneously; this is particularly evident in the Mediterranean area. Exposure to contaminants combined with other human impacts can affect survivorship, recruitment, reproductive success, mutation rates and migration and may play a significant role in the partitioning of genetic variation among high stress exposed and less stress exposed populations (Whitehead et al., 2003). Taking into account this complex pattern, international institutions like IWC and ACCOBAMS have recently encouraged research for development of suites of sensitive non-lethal tools in skin biopsies of free-ranging animals, to define the "health status" of threatened cetacean species (Pollution 2000+, IWC Project). Threats faced by cetaceans can be schematized below.

2.1 Pollution: Bioaccumulation and effects of anthropogenic contaminants

Mediterranean top predators, and particularly cetacean odontocetes, accumulate high concentrations of anthropogenic contaminants such as organochlorine compounds (OCs), polycyclic aromatic hydrocarbons (PAHs) and trace elements. The pollutant burden is lower at the lowest levels of the food chain and becomes higher as the position in the food web increases. Important factors for bioaccumulation are also metabolic rates, gender, age and adipose tissue concentration. The ecotoxicological risk of some species is also related to their "biochemical vulnerability" to lipophilic xenobiotics due to the low capacity of their detoxifying enzymatic systems (Tanabe & Tatsukawa, 1992; Fossi et al., 1997). Since the incidence of pathology in these species is closely related to the level of pollution in their environments, bacterial and viral infections and contaminants must be considered from a holistic point of view. Mass mortalities of dolphins and seals have occurred in particularly polluted areas (such as the Mediterranean Sea), when levels of OCs, PAHs and heavy metals reached very high levels. It is reported that lipophilic contaminants cause immune and reproductive dysfunctions (Hammond et al., 2005). Some contaminants, such as OCs are also known as endocrine disrupting chemicals (EDCs) (Fossi et al., 2003). In fact several examples suggest that exposure to levels of OC insecticides and PCBs commonly detected in Mediterranean odontocetes has affected endocrine function and reproduction in other marine mammal species (Fossi & Marsili, 2003). Moreover there is growing concern about accumulation and effects of emerging contaminants and polybrominated diphenyl ethers (PBDEs, a major family of flame retardants) in the food chain. PBDEs are lipophilic, persistent and toxic to fauna and humans (Alaee et al., 2003). The highest levels of PBDEs have been found in top marine predators, including Mediterranean odontocetes. Also phthalates (found in numerous commercial products as additives and used primarily to soften polyvinyl chloride - PVC) are a relevant and emerging cause of concern for these species, considered as potential EDCs. Some phthalates have been linked to reproductive effects and altered hormone levels, however the effects and concentrations of these compounds have not been assessed yet. Another important class of contaminants for cetaceans is PAHs, derived from both natural (e.g., oil spill, forest fires, natural petroleum seeps) and anthropogenic sources (e.g., combustion of fossil fuels, use of oil for cooking and heating, coal burning). Studies have shown that PAHs with four or more rings can induce dioxin-like activity and weak estrogenic responses (Villeneuve et al., 2002). As pointed out by the 2010 scientific expedition undertaken by the program Mediterranean Endangered, new priorities in marine environment contamination are the so-called microplastics (usually defined as plastic particles smaller than 5 mm) (Barnes et al., 2009). Micro debris floating on the Mediterranean Sea have reached 115,000 particles per km^2 with a maximum of 892,000 particles. Impacts of microplastics to organisms and the environment are largely unknown. More than 180 species have been documented to absorb plastic debris including planktophagous species. For example, laboratory study has shown that krill species *Euphasia pacifica* ingested 20µm polyethylene fragments. Clearly, considerably reducing microplastic inputs must be a priority of this decade for the biodiversity conservation in the EU strategy.

2.2 Diseases: Immunosuppression and infectious diseases

Cetaceans are normally susceptible to a large plethora of pathogenic organisms. For example, the family *Cyamidae* comprises 28 species of parasitic crustaceans, all of which live exclusively on the cetaceans skin (Haney et al., 2004). The majority of these infective organisms are repelled by innate host defences that include nonimmunological anatomical and physiological barriers (e.g. mucociliary blanket), antimicrobial factors (e.g. lactoferrin, defensins, immuno-lysozyme) and immunological effector cells (e.g. neutrophils, eosinophyls, macrophages and natural killer cells). Several studies have suggested that contaminants could have immunosuppressive effects on marine mammals (Beckmen et al., 2003). Since 1987, at least 8 epidemics of *Morbillivirus* infection (MI) have caused mass mortality of various free-living pinniped and cetacean populations worldwide. Along the coast of Spain and Italy new cases of MI were reported in 2007 and 2008. Another intriguing issue regards the synergic effects, associated with chronic exposure to a number of environmental pollutants, such as OCs and trace elements, as previously mentioned. In fact, it is also unknown whether and how these chemicals contribute towards modulating the pathogenic and pathogenetic activity primarily displayed by sea mammal MI (Di Guardo et al., 2005).

2.3 Bycatch

Several species of marine mammals are at risk of extinction from being captured as bycatch in commercial fisheries. In the Mediterranean Sea sperm whales (*Physter macrocephalus*), striped dolphins (*Stenella coeruleoalba*), and short-beaked common dolphins (*Delphinus delphis*) are affected by pelagic driftnets and gillnets. The only mitigation measure applied today is the ban of swordfish driftnet fishery (Young & Iudicello, 2007). Other approaches that have been developed and implemented to address this problem, include devices and gear changes, time and area closures and moratoria. The scientific committee of ACCOBAMS and the IWC indicate the bycatch as one of the major threats to marine mammals. Between 1999 and 2004, SOS Grand Bleu counted 50,000 deaths due to sword fish "spadare".

2.4 Shipping, collision and noise pollution

All cetacean species, from fin whales to bottlenose dolphins (*Tursiops truncatus*) and from pelagic to coastal species are potentially subjected to collisions with boats, even if most collisions go unreported. Several cases of collisions between fin whales and large ships are reported from stranding cetaceans and from photo-identification data (Panigada et al., 2006). Cetaceans need acoustic signals to navigate, find and capture prey, and to locate mates, social partners and predators. Heavy vessel traffic, seismic testing, dredging, and drilling for oil and gas cause noise travelling thousands of km underwater. There is no doubt that cetaceans react to noise, but it is extremely difficult to quantify the effects and establish thresholds of disturbance. It is reported that use of mid-frequency long-range active sonar by navy caused the stranding of 11 Cuvier's beaked whales (*Ziphius cavirostris*) on the coastline of Greece (Frantzis, 1998).

2.5 Food depletion

Fisheries can have a major impact upon the status and distribution of various cetaceans. In the Mediterranean Sea, the decline in high-order marine predators feeding on epipelagic prey (cetaceans, large pelagic fish) is consistent with the hypothesis of prey depletion, presumably due to intensive exploitation of fish stocks (over-fishing). In fact the combination of some 50,000–100,000 small gillnet fishing boats, plus large bottom trawlers, has depleted numerous fish, crustacean, and mollusc populations. In eastern Ionian Sea, the short-beaked common dolphin shows evidence of decline correlated with food depletion (Bearzi et al., 2006).

2.6 Climate change

It is generally agreed that the Mediterranean region is an area sensitive to global climate change, due to its position on the edge of the climatologically determined Hadley cell, which makes it a transition area between two very different climate regimes to the North and the South (Li et al., 2006). Many global and regional models simulate several degrees of warming (from 3 to 7°C) in the Mediterranean by the end of the 21st century. The potential impacts of climate change include drought, decline of water quality, floods, and change in seawater temperature/salinity, the rising of sea levels and reduction of biodiversity. This would pose several threats to cetaceans, mainly linked to changes in the distribution of sufficient quality and quantity prey of marine mammals (Simmonds & Nunny, 2002). Climate-related effects may combine with other factors such as pollution and disease to have significant impacts on cetacean populations.

2.7 Genetic erosion

Studies to date have indicated a complex pattern of population genetic structure for most cetacean species investigated. Seasonal patterns of movement and the possibility of extremely large scale dispersal, or local isolation (sympatric or parapratic) between populations, generate a mosaic of genetic diversity that cannot easily be determined by an intuitive assessment of geography. Although the Mediterranean basin is closed and has the heavily industrialized coasts, it hosts several cetacean species biologically differentiated between pelagic (*Stenella coeruleoalba*) and coastal (*Tursiops truncatus*) odontocetes and the resident mysticete (*Balaenoptera physalus*). Previous studies showed evidence of clear genetic differentiation between Atlantic and Mediterranean populations of striped dolphin and found much lower genetic variation of Mediterranean specimens (Garcia-Martinez et al., 1999). Gene flow through the Gibraltar Strait appears to be limited and easily prevents the genetic exchange between the Atlantic and Mediterranean cetacean populations. For the determination of population structure of wild species, genetic information about population subdivision has practical applications for short- and long-term strategies for animal management, conservation and protection (Hoelzel, 1998) and genetic diversity appears to be a major factor determining the success of a species in harsh environments. High genetic diversity within a population increases the chance for survival of at least some individuals, and possible changes in the environment, due to natural causes or anthropogenic pressures, can be better tolerated. Exposure to contaminants combined with other human impacts can affect survivorship, recruitment, reproductive success, mutation rates and migration, and may play a significant role in partitioning genetic variation among high stress exposed and less stress exposed populations (Whitehead et al., 2003). This is particularly true for populations inhabiting a closed basin characterized by considerable concentrations of environmental contaminants (OCs), orders of magnitude higher than those detected in oceanic environments. Bioaccumulation of pollutants, combined with other factors, such as immunosuppression, infectious diseases, climate change, and food depletion could soon lead to a further additional decrease in total genetic variability of Mediterranean cetacean populations, posing alarming threat to these species.

3. Section two - Skin biopsy for diagnosis of anthropogenic threats

Cetacean skin biopsies are biological material suitable for the hazard assessment of free-ranging cetaceans (Fossi et al., 2010). Our research team firmly believe that the use of cetacean skin biopsies, as non-lethal biological material for the hazard assessment, is a powerful procedure to screen a large number of samples, with a minimal disturb to animals. In this chapter integument biopsy will be described as diagnostic tool for the comprehensive diagnosis of multiple stress factors, health status and genetic population variability. The diagnostic set developed in our lab and described in this chapter will enable to detect: i) presence of contaminants, ii) exposure to contaminants, iii) reproductive alteration, iv) genotoxicity, v) immunosuppression, vi) general stress, vii) feeding ecology (Fig.1).

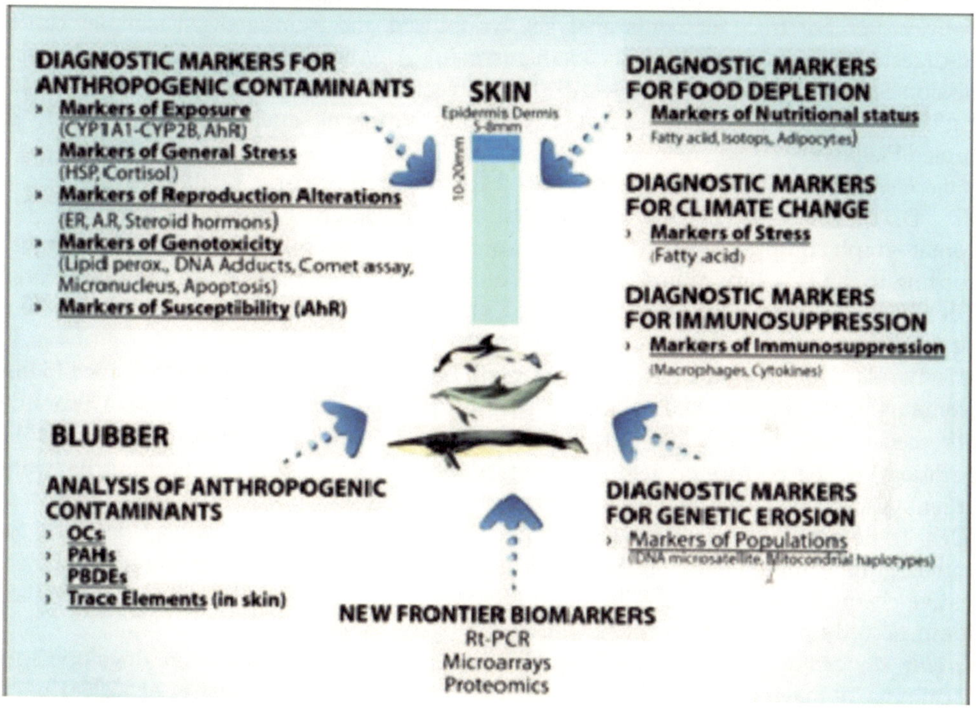

Fig. 1. Skin biopsy for diagnosis of anthropogenic threats

3.1 Sampling of integument biopsies

Samples of skin biopsy or integument biopsy (epidermis, dermis and blubber) can be obtained from free-ranging dolphin (es. *Tursiops truncatus, Stenella coeruleoalba)* from different study areas using an aluminium pole armed with biopsy tips (0.7 cm ø, 3.0 cm length) or with a crossbow and darts. Integument biopsies from large odontocete (es. *Physeter macrocephalus*) or mysticete *(Balaenoptera physalus)* can be obtained using a crossbow and darts armed with tips (0.9 cm ø, 4.0 cm length). A Barnett Wildcat II crossbow with a 150-pound test bow, using a biopsy dart with modified stainless steel collecting tip and floater, can be used to collect biopsies. To avoid the possibility of infection, the bolt tip need to be sterilised before shooting. Biopsy samples can be taken between the dorsal fin and the upper part of the caudal peduncle. The procedure consists in approaching the specimen at low-to-moderate speed and shooting the dart at a range of 20-50 m. The skin biopsy will be immediately placed in liquid nitrogen or stored in cell medium (CITES Nat. IT025IS, Int. CITES IT 007).

3.2 Detection of anthropogenic contaminants

Analysis of contaminant levels provide important data about exposure of cetaceans, that can be correlated with the biomarker data for a complete evaluation of their toxicological stress. The blubber layer of cetacean integument biopsy is the target tissue for the analysis of lipophilic and non-lipophilic contaminants in free-ranging populations (Fossi et al., 2000). A set of major POPs, trace elements and emerging contaminants can be analysed in skin biopsies of different cetacean species. The methods are reported below.

Trace elements: For trace elements analysis, lyophilised and homogenised samples can be acid-digested and analysed for trace elements using Atomic Absorption Spectrometry and Emission Spectrometry with FIMS-AAS (Flow Injection Mercury System) for determining Hg, THGF-AAS (Transversely Heated Graphite Furnace) and ICP-AES (Inductively Coupled Plasma).

Organochlorines: The analytical method used for quantitative and qualitative analysis of HCB, DDTs, PCDDs, PCDFs and PCBs will be High Resolution Capillary Gas chromatograph equipped with an electron capture detector (63Ni ECD)(AGILENT 6890/N), according to the U.S. Environmental Protection Agency (EPA) 8081/8082 modified (Marsili & Focardi, 1996). The GC has a SPB-5 bonded phase in a fused silica capillary column, 30 m long.

PAHs: Levels of PAHs and PAH fingerprint will be evaluated by High Performance Liquid Chromatography (Waters 600 HPLC) with Fluorescence Detector (Waters 474 Scanning Fluorescence Detector) and UV Detector (Waters 2487 Dual ë Absorbance Detector); PAH separation will be performed using a reversed phase column with an acetonitrile/water gradient (Marsili et al., 1997).

PBDEs: To detect PBDE, sample extracts will be analyzed on a GC/MS system (HP 6890 gas chromatograph coupled to an HP 5973 low-resolution mass spectrometer) using both EI and negative-chemical ionization (NCI) on an HP-5MS (5% phenyl methyl siloxane) capillary column, according to Pettersson et al. (2004).

Emerging contaminants (Pthalates): Several analytical methods have been developed for determining phthalates by GC (Feng et al., 2005), and HPLC (De Orsi et al., 2006) using different preconcentration techniques (Li et al., 2008).

3.3 Markers of exposure

A set of biomarkers of exposure to anthropogenic contaminants can be investigated in cetaceans skin biopsies (Fig.1). Particular attention will be paid to:

Cytochrome P450 (CYP) - Cytochrome P450 is the most important metabolic/detoxifying enzyme system in mammals. It is substrate-inducible and substrate-specific. CYP1A and CYP2B have been detected in cetacean skin and the induction of these isoforms was found after exposure to lipophilic contaminants both *in vitro* and in field studies (Fossi et al., 2006;

Montie et al., 2008; Hooker et al., 2008). Induction of CYP isoforms can thus be considered as a powerful biomarker of exposure. The induction of different CYP enzymes can be investigated by western blot (WB), immunohistochemistry and quantitative real-time PCR (qRT-PCR) (Spinsanti et al., 2006, 2008).

Nuclear receptors (AhR) - The cytosolic aryl hydrocarbon receptor (AhR) is a ligand inducible nuclear transcription factor which can induces the transcription of xenobiotic metabolizing enzymes such as CYP1A. AhR gene expression was found to be significantly induced in skin of chloracne patients subject to long-term exposure to dioxins and dibenzofuranes (Tang et al., 2008). Presence and modulation of AhR in cetacean skin samples will be here investigated by qRT-PCR.

3.4 Markers of reproductive alterations

Endocrine Disrupting Chemicals (EDCs) are a structurally diverse group of compounds that may adversely affect the health of humans and wildlife, or their progenies, by interaction with the endocrine system (Colborn, 1998). Many of the known EDCs are estrogenic, affecting particularly reproductive functions. A main mechanism of endocrine disruption occurs through receptor-mediated mechanisms or the cross-talk of these receptors with the AHR. In skin biopsy we can investigate the gene expression of steroid hormone receptors and any possible alterations due to contaminants.

Steroid hormone receptors. Estrogen receptor(s) (*ER),* androgen receptor(s) (*AR*) and progesteron receptor(s) (*PR*) presence can be investigated in biopsy samples of cetaceans by using WB and immunohistochemistry techniques. Gene expression will also be investigated by qRT-PCR. Steroid hormone receptors are known to be induced in various species and tissues by specific contaminants.

Steroid hormones and steroidogenic enzymes. A set of key genes (Hilscherova et al., 2004) involved in steroid hormone synthesis in humans can be investigated in cell cultures and skin biopsy samples by qRT-PCR and WB, to explore the expression and its potential alterations due to toxicants. We will explore the up/down-regulation of some genes including: CYP11A (cholesterol side-chain cleavage), CYP11B1 (steroid 11β-hydroxylase), CYP11B2 (aldosterone synthetase), CYP17 (steroid 17αHSD1-hydroxylase), CYP19 (aromatase) and CYP21B2 (steroid 21-hydroxylase).

3.5 Markers of genotoxicity

DNA integrity is essential for the correct transmission of genetic information to the next generation. Chemicals and/or physical agents that have the potential to cause loss of the DNA's structural and functional integrity are defined genotoxics (Shugart, 2000). Following failing of the repair mechanism, structural changes in DNA become irreversible (apoptosis, chromosome aberrations) and the cells may exhibit altered functions, from uncontrolled proliferation cells to carcinogenesis (Lee & Steinert, 2003). Finally the damage caused by genotoxic compounds leads to DNA mutations and possible alterations in subsequent generations (Gil & Pla, 2001). In this chapter we will present how to evaluate the presence of DNA damage and the efficiency of cells repair mechanism by comet assay. Diffusion assay will be used to evaluate apoptosis in cells.

The Comet Assay or single cell gel electrophoresis (SCGE) is a sensitive, rapid and inexpensive method for measuring DNA damage in individual cells. As reported by Frenzilli et al. (1999) the single cells are embedded in agarose on microscope slides, lysed to remove the majority of the proteins, electrophoresed, then stained with Sybr Safe in order to visualize the DNA. As result, the DNA of undamaged cells appears as a spherical mass occupying the cavity formed by the lysed cell. On the contrary, cells with DNA damage form a comet image, due to the amount of DNA fragments: smaller is the fragment size, greater is their number and the percentage of DNA that migrates in an electric field. The assay can be performed to examine DNA single strand breaks or to measure double strand breaks in individual cells.

Markers associated with apoptosis: to detect the apoptotic cells, a comet assay modified protocol will be used (Singh et al., 1988). This test, as the comet assay, is relatively easy to apply to most eukaryotic cell types, it is sensitive for detecting low levels of DNA damage or multiple classes of DNA damage and require a small cells number (Dhawan et al., 2009).

Lipid peroxidation: it involves a set of chain reactions by ROS because of their double bonds. Lipid peroxidation is the result of interactions of lipidic radicals and/or formation of non radical species by lipid proxy radicals. The resulting LOOH (lipid hydroperoxide) can easily decomposes into several reactive species, including lipid alkoxyl radicals (LO), aldehydes, lipid epoxides and alcohols. Most of these products are toxic and active mutagens. Peroxidised membranes become rigid and lose permeability and integrity (Valavanidis et al., 2006). Lipid peroxidation will be investigated in skin biopsies by measuring levels of MDA using a spectrophotometric test.

3.6 Diagnostic markers of immunosuppression

Mammal skin is an important immune organ, displaying various defence mechanisms which can be divided into three major functional compartments: epithelial defence, innate-inflammatory immunity and adaptive immunity (Meyer et al., 2007). IIn this biological material we will develop and validate a set of biomarkers in cultured fibroblasts and skin biopsies to monitor the immunological status of cetaceans. The Major Histocompatibility Complex (MHC) is a set of molecules displayed on cell surfaces that are responsible for lymphocyte recognition and "antigen presentation". These molecules control the immune response through recognition of "self" and "non-self" and are of two types: Class I and Class II molecules. In the Class I molecules there is a family of polymorphic genes, named MIC genes, where MICA and MICB are functional. MIC genes are mainly expressed in endothelial cells and fibroblasts. MIC molecules are considered to be stress-induced antigens that are recognized by cytotoxic T cells and natural killer (NK) cells. The evaluation of MICA protein expression in cetaceans can be used to evaluate the status of the immune system of the different species and will be investigated by WB, immunohistochemistry, qRT-PCR and indirect immunofluorescence (Marsili et al., 2008).

3.7 Diagnostic markers of general stress

Cetaceans are exposed to a diverse array of multiple stressors and here we propose a suite of skin biomarkers to assess general stress.

Heat-shock proteins (HSPs): A number of environmentally and chemical agents are known to induce a set of cellular stress proteins, the heat-shock proteins (HSPs) (Nover, 1991; Nover & Scharf, 1991). Their amount increases rapidly when cells are subjected or exposed to a wide variety of stresses such as heat, xenobiotics or drugs; pathological stimuli such as viral, bacterial and parasitic infections, inflammation and autoimmunity (Wu & Tanguay, 2006). In skin biopsy we can explore the expression of HSPs by WB and qRT-PCR (Cao et al., 1999; Rossner et al., 2003).

Cortisol alteration: Cortisol is mainly involved in carbohydrate, lipid, and protein metabolism and serves as an indicator of an animal's state of well-being, as its levels increase during times of distress ("stress hormone"). We can measure levels of cortisol in the blubber biopsies of cetaceans by enzyme immuno-assays. In fact adipocytes are equipped with a functional G6PT-hexose-6-phosphate dehydrogenase-11ß-hydroxysteroid dehydrogenase type 1 system that is a potential target for modulating local glucocorticoid activation (Marcolongo et al., 2007).

3.8 Diagnostic markers of feeding ecology

Assessing the diet and trophic position of cetaceans is important for understanding the ecology of marine food webs. Decreased quantity and quality of prey, due mainly to over-fishing, have been cited as factors promoting population decline of Mediterranean cetaceans (Bearzi et al., 2006). Feeding ecology is a fundamental aspect in the understanding, management and conservation of free-ranging marine mammals. Nutritional status of marine mammals is a factor that can limit reproductive output and thus population growth. However, foraging of large cetaceans can be difficult to assess when direct observation is not possible, and the use of chemical feeding ecology (i.e., stable isotope and fatty acid analysis) has become increasingly important (Dehn et al., 2006). Stable isotopes of carbon and nitrogen, evaluated using Isotope Ratio Mass Spectrometer (Herman et al., 2005), have been established as powerful tools in animal ecology. They occur naturally, and nitrogen isotope ratios of prey are reflected in tissues of the consumer, with slight enrichment occurring at each trophic step (Kelly, 2000). Stable carbon isotopes are generally used to provide information on spatial habitat use and carbon sources rather than trophic relationships as they enrich in consumer tissues only to a minor degree (Burton & Koch, 1999). An increase of $\delta^{15}N$ values has been shown in specimens in particular conditions such as nutritional stress (Fuller et al., 2005) or disease (Katzenberg & Lovell 1999). Thus, measurements of the fatty acid composition of the blubber of marine mammals, evaluated using quadruple gas chromatography/mass spectrometry (Krahn, 2004), allow the identification of the diet of these animals. The differences either between individuals or between populations (Møller et al., 2003) or between species (Borobia et al., 1995), are a direct function of their prey fatty acid composition.

3.9 Diagnostic markers for genetic erosion and population studies

Accurate screening of current overall genetic variability of Mediterranean cetaceans and its constant monitoring over the years would identify potential environmental threats and interspecies differences in susceptibility to contaminants.

DNA microsatellites: DNA microsatellites are short (10-50 copies) tandem repeats of mono- to hexa-nucleotide units, assumed to be randomly distributed throughout nDNA, cpDNA and mtDNA. SSRs can appear as simple, interrupted and compound repeats, and are usually distributed across non-coding (and, less often, coding) regions of the genome. Irrespective of hypotheses about their evolutionary mechanisms (slipped-strand mispairing (slippage) error during DNA replication of a single DNA double helix or recombination), SSRs have been appliedas a highly variable and powerful genetic marker in areas ranging from ancient and forensic DNA studies to population and conservation genetics (Jarne and Lagoda, 1996). Nucleotide sequence analysis of the genes encoded in the mitochondrial genome (mtDNA) constitutes an additional powerful tool of modern phylogeography and molecular population genetics (Bickham et al., 2000; Gaspari et al., 2007). mtDNA is located outside the nucleus and it encodes for a subset of the proteins necessary for the mitochondrion itself. The number of copies of mitochondrial genes greatly outnumbers that of nuclear encoded genes. The mitochondrial genome is inherited solely through the maternal line in a clonal fashion and usually does not undergo recombination. Moreover, its rapid rate of base substitution makes the mtDNA genome an ideal marker for establishing levels of variability between and among populations or species (Natoli et al., 2004, 2005).

4. Section three - The case study of the multi-trial diagnostic tool in fin whale *(Balaenoptera physalus)* skin biopsies of the Pelagos Sanctuary (Mediterranean Sea) and the Gulf of California (Mexico)

In this section we describe the application of the proposed multidisciplinary approach to explore the effects of multiple human pressures on cetacean health status (field applications), comparing *Balaenoptera physalus* cetacean population of Mediterranean with the Sea of Cortez population. As previously mentioned (section one) over the past decades, there has been a growing concern regarding the potential threat to Mediterranean cetaceans from persistent organic pollutants such as organochlorine compounds (OCs) (Fossi et al., 2006) and polybrominated diphenyl ethers (PBDEs). Cetaceans of the Gulf of California (Sea of Cortez – Mexico) are reputed to be less exposed to anthropogenic pressure. To date, OC concentrations have been investigated in only three marine mammal species from the Gulf of California (Niño-Torres et al., 2009). The main objective of this case study (Fossi et al. 2010) was to develop and apply a set of sensitive non-lethal diagnostic biomarkers to skin biopsies of fin whales to evaluate the toxicological status of this mysticete in the Pelagos Sanctuary (Ligurian, Corsica and North Tyrrhenian Seas) and in the Gulf of California. We propose a "multi-trial diagnostic tool", combining molecular biomarkers and gene expression with the analysis of OCs, PAHs and PBDEs.
Mediterranean fin whale – The fin whale is the only mysticete that is regularly found in the Mediterranean Sea (Bérubé et al., 1998), facing a number of anthropogenic threats, such as chemical and acoustic pollution, entanglement in fishing gear and disturbance and collisions from commercial and pleasure boats.
Gulf of California fin whale – Fin whales are permanent residents of the Gulf of California. This population of approximately 610 animals (Urbán-Ramírez et al., 2005) is considered one of the most isolated in the world (Bérubé et al., 1998), and it constitutes a unique and separate conservation unit vulnerable to anthropogenic effects. Although the Gulf of California is considered one of the most pristine and bio-diverse areas of the world (hosting 36 species of marine mammals), increasing human activity is beginning to affect it.

4.1 Experimental design

4.1.1 Sampling

Integument biopsies were obtained from free-ranging fin whales in the Pelagos Sanctuary (n = 12, 6 males and 6 females) and the Gulf of California (n = 5, 3 males and 2 females) during the summer of 2008, using biopsy darts launched with a crossbow (CITES Nat. IT 025IS, Int. CITES IT 007). Sex was determined according to Bérubé and Palsbøll (1996).

4.1.2 Skin biopsy as diagnostic tool

To validate this "multi-trial diagnostic tool", a two-phase experimental protocol was followed (Fig. 2). In the first phase of the project (field studies), we applied a multidisciplinary methodology to explore the effects of the exposure of Mediterranean and Mexican fin whales to anthropogenic contaminants, using skin biopsies as a diagnostic tool and combining the analysis of molecular biomarkers (Western Blot (WB) of CYP1A1 and CYP2B) and gene expression (qRT-PCR of HSP70, ERa, AHR, E2F-1) with the analysis of OC, PAH and PBDE residues in subcutaneous blubber. In the second phase (in vitro experiments), whale biopsy slices were treated with mixtures of OCs, as an innovative tool for the study of intra-species sensitivity to various classes of environmental contaminants.

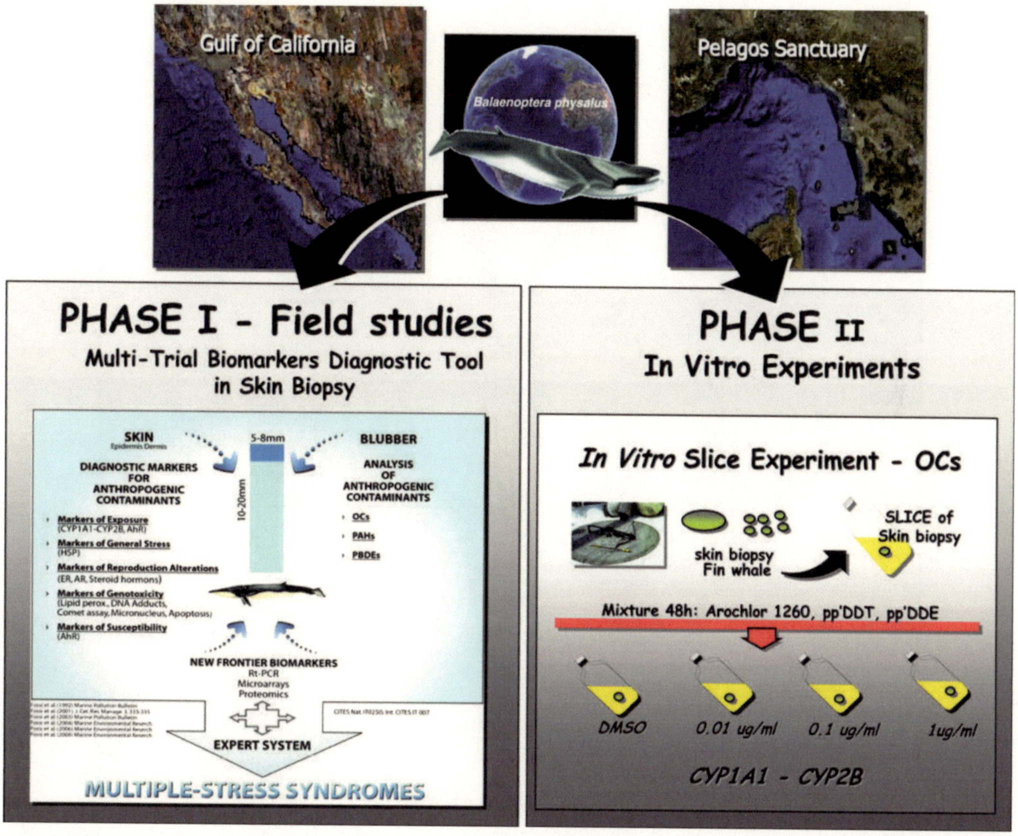

Fig. 2. Experimental design and sampling areas - validation of a "multi-trial diagnostic tool" to evaluate the toxicological status of fin whales in the Pelagos Sanctuary (Mediterranean Sea) and the Gulf of California (Sea of Cortez - Mexico). A two-phase experimental protocol was followed: first phase: field studies; second phase: in vitro experiments (Fossi et al, 2010).

4.1.3 Results

The two populations of fin whales (first phase results) showed differences in contaminant levels and biomarker responses.

Higher levels of PCBs, DDTs, OCs-EDCs and PAHs were found in both male and female (PAHs $p < 0.1$) Mediterranean fin whales in comparison to the Cortez specimens (Fig. 3a–d), confirming the high toxicological stress to which the fin whale population in the Pelagos Sanctuary is exposed.

Levels of low-brominated PBDEs were higher in samples from the Sea of Cortez (Fig. 3e), ranging from 282 to 30,506 ng/g dw, while samples from the Mediterranean sea showed lower average levels. The most abundant congener was PBDE 47. In general, samples from the Sea of Cortez had a major number of detected congeners, such as 47, 100, 99, 154 and 153.

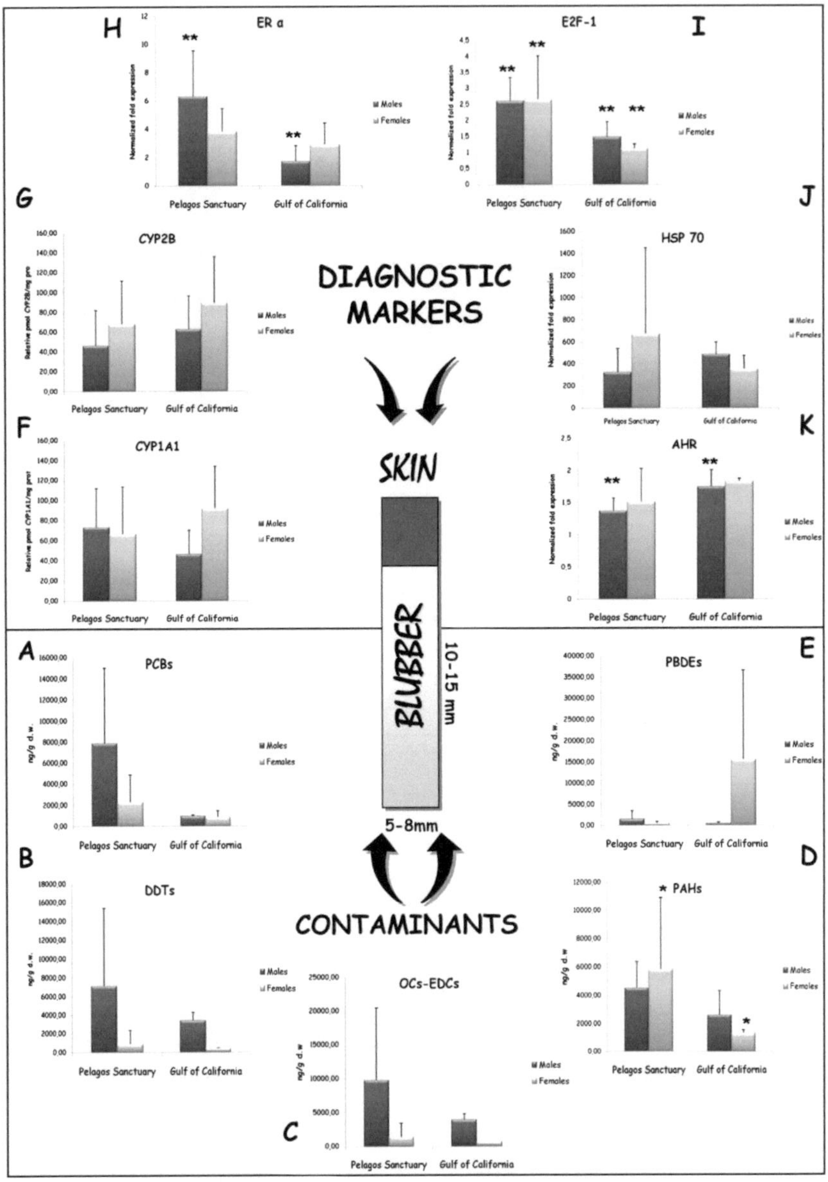

Fig. 3. First phase results - contaminant levels (PCBs (A), DDTs (B), OCs-EDCs (C), PAHs (D), PBDEs (E)) and biomarker responses WB of CYP1A1 (F), CYP2B (G), gene expression (qRT-PCR) of ERa (H), E2F-1 (I), HSP70 (J), AHR (K) in skin biopsies of specimens from the two populations of fin whales (*= $p < 0.1$; ** = $p < 0.05$). Pelagos Sanctuary (n = 12,males = 6; females = 6); Sea of Cortez (n = 5, males = 3; females = 2). (Fossi et al, 2010).

Exploring molecular biomarker responses, the induction of CYP1A1 in Mediterranean male whales, if compared to males from the Gulf of California (Fig. 3f), can be related to the presence of high levels of planar compounds, such as coplanar PCBs, and PAHs (Fig. 3a and 3d). A statistically significant positive correlation (rho Spearman = 0.73, $p = 0.003$) was found between total PAHs and CYP1A1 induction in male ($n = 11$) specimens.

A lack of CYP2B induction, despite high levels of lipophilic contaminants, was evident in both male and female Mediterranean whales, even though the differences between the Mediterranean and Mexican specimens are not statistically significant (Fig. 3g). On the other hand, a preliminary warning signal is represented by the high induction of CYP2B in the Mexican fin whales (Fig. 2g), but further investigations are needed.

Exploring gene expression biomarker responses (Fig. 2h–2k), the ERa and E2F-1 genes were up-regulated in the specimens from the Pelagos Sanctuary with respect to those from Mexico for both males (ERa: 3.6_-fold; E2F-1: 1.7_-fold) and females (ERa: 1.3_-fold; E2F-1: 2.4_-fold) ($p < 0.05$). These data suggest,in the first case (ERa), high exposure to EDC compounds such as OCs-EDCs and, in the second case (E2F-1), the presence of apoptosis processes as a sign of toxicological stress in the Mediterranean population. In contrast, the expression of HSP70 is higher in the Mexican male specimens than that of the Pelagos Sanctuary (1.5_-fold), whereas the Pelagos females exhibit an overexpression of the HSP70 gene with respect to the Mexican specimens (1.9_-fold). The AHR gene is slightly up-regulated in the Mexican specimens ($p < 0.05$ in males).

The results of the second phase (in vitro tests) show marked differences in CYP1A1 and CYP2B induction by OCs in the whale biopsy slices of the two populations (male specimens), with higher sensitivity responses in the Mexican mysticetes. A dose-dependent induction of CYP1A1 was detected only in biopsy slices from Cortez specimens (0.01 μg/ml = 2.6-fold, 0.1 μg/ml = 3.6-fold and 1 μg/ml = 4.4-fold with respect to the control). The in vitro tests showed no induction of CYP1A1 and CYP2B for the male Mediterranean whales (slices).

In conclusion, this "multi-trial diagnostic tool", applied to skin biopsies, underlined differences in OC, OC-EDC, PBDE and PAH levels and molecular and gene expression biomarker responses between the two populations. The presence of a higher "toxicological stress" in the Pelagos population is highlighted by warning signals such as CYP1A1 induction and the up-regulation of ERa and E2F-1 genes, combined with a lack of CYP2B induction in both field and in vitro experiments. Moreover, particular concern arises from the high levels of low-brominated PBDEs found in the Mexican whale specimens. Future development of this methodology could provide a statistical system for obtaining more complete information about the "toxicological stress syndrome" in cetaceans, providing a predictive model for hazards in susceptible areas targeted by increasing tourism, such as the Gulf of California (Fossi et al, 2010).

5. Conclusion

The data reported in this chapter confirm that cetacean skin biopsies are a biological material suitable for the hazard assessment of free-ranging cetaceans. This chapter shows that the use of cetacean skin biopsies, as non-lethal biological material for the hazard assessment, is a powerful procedure to screen a large number of samples, with a minimal disturb to animals. Here integument biopsy is proposed as diagnostic tool for the comprehensive diagnosis of multiple stress factors, health status and genetic population variability. The methods proposed could be used to:

- support in ranking the threatened levels for cetaceans populations/species;
- as an operative tool, suitable for both scientific and decision making purposes supporting in identification of proper mitigation measures;
- find application on two main EU areas of interest: Convention on Biological Diversity (CBD) (2010-2020) - EU Marine Strategy.

The final outcome of these studies will be the development of a prototype DSS - Decision Supporting System for ranking toxicological risk of cetacean populations/species based on integration and analysis of data from the above diagnostic approach. Such a scheme is currently not available to the scientific community nor to policy makers worldwide, neither in the terrestrial nor marine environment. In case of success these achievements are susceptible to be applied on a wider-scale to other marine threatened species.

6. Acknowledgements

The authors particularly thanks the precious collaborators Silvia Maltese, Cristina Panti, Giacomo Spinsanti, Silvia Casini, and Daniele Coppola. The projects described in this chapter were partially supported by the Italian and Mexican Ministry of Foreign Affair and the Italian Ministry of Environment.

7. References

Alaee, M., Arias, P., Sjodin, A. & Bergman, Å. (2003). An overview of commercially used brominated flame retardants, their applications, their use patterns in different countries/regions and possible modes of release. *Environment International*, Vol. 29, No. 6, pp. 683-689, ISSN 0160-4120.

Barnes, D.K.A., Galgani, F., Thompson, R.C. & Barlaz, M. (2009). Accumulation and fragmentation of plastic debris in global environments. *Philosophical Transactions of the Royal Society B (The Royal Society)*, Vol. 364, No. 1526, pp. 1985-1998, ISSN 0962-8436.

Bearzi, G., Politi, E., Agazzi, S. & Azzellino, A. (2006). Prey depletion caused by overfishing and the decline of marine megafauna in eastern Ionian Sea coastal waters (central Mediterranean). *Biological Conservation*, Vol. 127, No. 4, pp. 373-382, ISSN 0006-3207.

Beckmen, K.B., Blake, J.E., Ylitalo, G.M., Stott, J.L. & O'Hara, T.M. (2003). Organochlorine contaminant exposure and associations with hematological and humoral immune functional assays with dam age as a factor in free-ranging northern fur seal pups (*Callorhinus ursinus*). *Marine Pollution Bulletin*, Vol. 46, No. 5, pp. 594-606, ISSN 0025-326X.

Berubè, M. & Palsboll, P. (1996). Identification of sex in cetaceans by multiplexing wih three ZFX and ZFY specific primers. *Molecular Ecology*, Vol. 5, pp. 283-287, ISSN: 0962-1083.

Bérubé, M., Aguilar, A., Dendanto, D., Larsen, F., Notarbartolo di Sciara, G., Sears, R., Sigurjonsson, J., Urbàn, R. & Palsbøll, P. (1998). Population genetic structure of North Atlantic, Mediterranean Sea and Sea of Cortez fin whales, *Balaenoptera physalus* (Linnaeus, 1758); analysis of mitochondrial and nuclear loci. *Molecular Ecology*, Vol. 7, pp. 585-599, ISSN: 0962-1083.

Bickham, J.W., Sandhu, S., Hebert, P.D., Chikhi, L. & Athwal, R. (2000). Effects of chemical contaminants on genetic diversity in natural populations: implications for biomonitoring and ecotoxicology. *Mutation Research*, Vol. 463, No. 1, pp. 33-51, ISSN 0027-5107.

Borobia, M., Gearing, P.J., Simard, Y., Gearing, J.N.& Beland, P. (1995). Blubber fatty acids of finback and humpback whales from the Gulf of St. Lawrence. *Marine Biology*, Vol.122, pp. 341–353, ISSN: 0025-3162.

Burton, R.K. & Koch, P.L. (1999). Isotopic tracking of foraging and long-distance migration in northeastern Pacific pinnipeds. *Oecologia*, Vol.119, pp. 578-585, ISSN 0029-8549.

Cao, Y., Ohwatari, N., Matsumoto, T., Kosaka, M., Ohtsuru, A. & Yamashita, S. (1999). TGF-beta1 mediates 70-kDa heat shock protein induction due to ultraviolet irradiation in human skin fibroblasts. *Pflügers Archiv: European Journal of Physiology*, Vol. 438, No. 3, pp. 239–244, ISSN 0031-6768.

Colborn, T., Smolen, M.J. & Rolland, R. (1998). Enivironmental neurotoxic effects: the search for new protocols in functional teratology. *Toxicology and Industrial Health*, Vol.14, pp. 9-23, ISSN 1477-0393.

De Orsi, D., Gagliardi, L., Porrà, R., Berri, S., Chimenti, P., Granese, A. Carpani, I. & Tonelli, D. (2006). An environmentally friendly reversed-phase liquid chromatography method for phthalates determination in nail cosmetics. *Analytica Chimica Acta*, Vol. 555, pp. 238-241, ISSN 0003-2670

Dehn, L.A., Follmann, E. H., Rosa, C., Duffy, L. K., Thomas, D. L., Bratton, G. R., Taylor, R. J. & O'Hara, T. M. (2006). Stable isotope and trace element status of subsistence-hunted bowhead and beluga whales in Alaska and gray whales in Chukotka. *Marine Pollution Bulletin*,. Vol.52, pp. 301-319, ISSN 0025-326X.

Dhawan, A., Bajpayee, M. & Parmar, D. (2009). Comet assay: a reliable tool for the assessment of DNA damage in different models. *Cell Biology And Toxicology*, Vol. 25, No. 1, pp. 5-32, ISSN 0742-2091.

Di Guardo, G., Marruchella, G., Agrimi, U. & Kennedy, S. (2005). Morbillivirus infections in aquatic mammals: a brief overview. *Journal of Veterinary Medicine Series A-Physiology Pathology Clinical Medic*, Vol. 52, No. 2, pp. 88-93, ISSN 0931-184X.

Feng, Y.L., Zhua, J.P. & Robert, S. (2005). Development of a headspace solid-phase microextraction method combined with gas chromatography mass spectrometry for the determination of phthalate esters in cow milk. *Analytica Chimica Acta*, Vol.538, pp. 41-48, ISSN 0003-2670.

Fossi, M.C., Marsili, L., Junin, M., Castello, H., Lorenzani, J.A., Casini, S., Savelli, C. & Leonzio, C. (1997). Use of nondestructive biomarkers and residue analysis to assess the health status of endangered species of pinnipeds in the southwest Atlantic. *Marine Pollution Bulletin*, Vol. 34, No. 3, pp. 157-162, ISSN 0025-326X.

Fossi, M.C., Marsili, L., Neri, G., Casini, S., Bearzi, G., Politi, E., Zanardelli, M. & Panigada, S. (2000). Skin biopsy of Mediterranean cetaceans for the investigation of interspecies susceptibility to xenobiotic contaminants. *Marine Environmental Research*, Vol. 50, No. 1-5, pp. 517-521, ISSN 0141-1136.

Fossi, M.C. & Marsili, L. (2003). Endocrine disrupters in aquatic mammals. *Pure and Applied Chemistry*, Vol. 75, No. 11-12, pp. 2235-2247, ISSN 0033-4545.

Fossi, M.C., Marsili, L., Neri, G., Natoli, A., Politi, E. & Panigada, S. (2003). The use of non-lethal tool for evaluating toxicological hazard of organoclorine contaminants in Mediterranean cetaceans: new data ten years after the first paper published in MPB. *Marine Pollution Bulletin*, Vol. 46, pp. 964-971, ISSN 0025-326X.

Fossi, M.C., Marsili, L., Casini, S. & Bucalossi, D. (2006). Development of new-tools to investigate toxicological hazard due to endocrine disruptor organochlorines and emerging contaminants in Mediterranean cetaceans. *Marine Environmental Research*, Vol.62, pp. 200–204, ISSN 0141-1136.

Fossi, M. C., Urban, J., Casini, S., Maltese, S., Spinsanti, G., Panti, C., Porcelloni, S., Panigada, S., Lauriano, G., Nino-Torres, C., Rojas-Bracho, L., Jimenez, B., Munoz-Arnanz, J. & Marsili, L. (2010). A Multi-Trial diagnostic tool in fin whale (*Balaenoptera physalus*) skin biopsies of the Pelagos Sanctuary (Mediterranean Sea) and the Gulf of California (Mexico). *Marine Environmental Research*, Vol. 69, No. 1, pp.17-20, ISSN 0141-1136.

Frantzis, A. (1998). Does acoustic testing strand whales? *Nature*, Vol. 392, pp. 29, ISSN 0028-0836.

Frenzilli, G., Scarcelli, V., Taddei, F. & Nigro, M. (1999). Adaption of SCGE as a candidate for monitoring marine ecosystems. *Neoplasma*, Vol. 46, pp. 6–7, ISSN 0028-2685.

Fuller, B.T., Fuller, J.L., Sage, N.E., Harris, D.A., O'Connell, T.C. & Hedges, R.E.M. (2005). Nitrogen balance and δ^{15}N: why you're not what you eat during nutritional stress. *Rapid Communications in Mass Spectrometry*, Vol.19, pp.2481–2728, ISSN 0951-4198.

Garcia Martinez, J., Moya, A., Raga, J.A. & Latorre, A. (1999). Genetic differentiation in the striped dolphin *Stenella coeruleoalba* from European waters according to mitochondrial DNA (mtDNA) restriction analysis. *Molecular Ecology*, Vol. 8, pp. 1069-1073, ISSN 0962-1083.

Gaspari, S., Azzellino, A., Airoldi, S. & Hoelzel, A.R. (2007). Social kin associations and genetic structuring of striped dolphin populations (*Stenella coeruleoalba*) in the Mediterranean Sea. *Molecular Ecology*, Vol. 16, No. 14, pp. 2922-2933, ISSN 0962-1083.

Gil, F. & Pla, A. (2001). Biomarkers as biological indicators of xenobiotic exposure. *Journal of Applied Toxicology*, Vol. 21, pp. 245-255, ISSN 0260-437X.

Hammond, J.A., Hall, A.J. & Dyrynda, L. (2005). Comparison of polychlorinated biphenyl (PCB) induced effects on innate immune functions in harbour and grey seals. *Aquatic Toxicology*, Vol. 74, No. 2, pp. 126-138, ISSN 0166-445X.

Haney, T.A., De Almeida, A.O. & Reis, M.S.S. (2004). A new species of Cyamid (Crustacea: Amphipoda) from a stranded cetacean in Southern Bahia, Brazil. *Bulletin of Marine Science*, Vol. 75, No. 3, pp. 409-421, ISSN 0007-4977.

Herman, D.P., Burrows, D.G., Wade, P.R., Durban, J.W., LeDuc, R.G., Matkin, C.O. & Krahn, M.M. (2005). Feeding ecology of eastern North Pacific killer whales from fatty acid, stable isotope, and organochlorine analyses of blubber biopsies. *Marine Ecology. Progress Series*, Vol. 302, pp. 275–291, ISNN 0171-8630.

Hilscherová, K., Jones, P.D., Gracia, T., Newsted, J.L., Zhang, X., Sanderson, Yu, R.M.K., Wu, R.S.S. & Giesy, J.P. (2004). Assessment of the effects of chemicals on the expression of ten steroidogenic genes in the H295R cell line using real-time PCR. *Toxicological Sciences*, Vol.81, pp. 78-89, ISSN 1096-6080.

Hoelzel, A.R. (1998). Genetic structure of cetacean populations in sympatry, parapatry and mixed assemblages; implications for conservation policy. *Journal of Heredity*, Vol. 89, pp. 451-458, ISSN 0022-1503.

Hooker, S.K., Metcalfe, T.L., Metcalfe, C.D., Angell, C.M., Wilson, J.Y., Moore, M.J. & Whitehead, H. (2008). Changes in persistent contaminant concentration and CYP1A1 protein expression in biopsy samples from northern bottlenose whales, *Hyperoodon ampullatus*, following the onset of nearby oil and gas development. *Environmental Pollution*, Vol. 152, No. 1, pp. 205-216, ISSN 0269-7491.

Jarne, P. & Lagoda, P.J.L. (1996). Microsatellites, from molecules to populations and back. *Trends in Ecology and Evolution*, Vol. 11, pp. 424-429, ISSN 0169-5347.

Katzenberg, M.A. & Lovell, N.C. (1999). Stable isotope variation in pathological bone. International Journal of *Osteoarchaeology*, Vol.9, pp.316–324, ISSN 1047-482X.

Kelly, J.F. (2000). Stable isotopes of carbon and nitrogen in the study of avian and mammalian trophic ecology. *Canadian Journal of Zoology*, Vol.78, pp. 1–27, ISSN 0008-4301.

Krahn, M.M., Herman, D.P., Ylitalo, G.M., Sloan, C.A., Burrows, D.G., Hobbs, R.C., Mahoney, B.A., Yanagida, G.K., Calambokidis, J. & Moore, S.E. (2004). Stratification of lipids, fatty acids and organochlorine contaminants in blubber of white whales and killer whales. *Journal of Cetacean Research and Management*, Vol.6, pp. 175–189, ISSN 1561-0713.

Lee, R.F. & Steinert, S. (2003). Use of the single cell gel eletrophoresis/comet assay for detecting DNA damage in aquatic (marine and freshwater) animals. *Mutation Research*, Vol. 544, pp. 43-64, ISSN 0921-8262.

Li, L., Bozec, A., Somot, S., Beranger, K., Bouruet-Aubertot, P., Sevault, F. & Crepon, M. (2006). Chapter 7 Regional atmospheric, marine processes and climate modelling, In: P. Lionello, P. Malanotte-Rizzoli & R. Boscolo, (Eds), *Developments in Earth and Environmental Sciences*, Elsevier, Vol. 4, Mediterranean, pp. 373-397, ISSN 1571-9197, ISBN 9780444521705.

Li, J., Can, Y., Shia, Y., Moua, S. & Jiang, G. (2008). Analysis of phthalates via HPLC-UV in environmental water samples after concentration by solid-phase extraction using ionic liquid mixed hemimicelles. *Talanta*, Vol.74, No.4, pp. 498-504, ISSN 0039-9140.

Marcolongo, P., Piccirella, S., Senesi, S., Wunderlich, L., Gerin, I., Mandl, J., Fulceri, R., Bánhegyi, G. & Benedetti, A. (2007). The glucose-6-phosphate transporter-hexose-6-phosphate dehydrogenase-11ß-hydroxysteroid dehydrogenase type 1 system of the adipose tissue. *Endocrinology*, Vol. 148, No. 5, pp. 2487-2495.

Marsili, L. & Focardi, S. (1996). Organochlorine levels in subcutaneous blubber biopsies of fin whales (*Balaenoptera physalus*) and striped dolphins (*Stenella coeruleoalba*) from the Mediterranean Sea. *Environmental Pollution*, Vol. 91, No. 1, pp. 1-9.

Marsili, L., Fossi, M.C., Casini, S., Savelli, C., Jimenez, B., Junin, M. & Castello, H. (1997). Fingerprint of polycyclic aromatic hydrocarbons in two populations of southern sea lions (*Otaria flavescens*). *Chemosphere*, Vol. 34, No. 4, pp. 759-770, ISSN 0045-6535.

Marsili, L., Fossi, M.C., Bucalossi, D., Porcelloni, S., Maltese, S. & Casini, S. (2008). Use of immunofluorescence technique in cultured fibroblasts from Mediterranean cetaceans as new "in vitro" tool to investigate effects of environmental contaminants. *Marine Environmental Research*, Vol. 66, No. 1, pp. 151-153, ISSN 0141-1136.

Meyer, T., Stockfleth, E. & Christophers, E. (2007). Immune response profiles in human skin. *British Journal of Dermatology*, Vol. 157, No. 2, pp. 1-7, ISSN 1365-2133.

Møller, P., Born, E.W., Dietz, R., Ruzzante, D., Haug, T. & Øien, N. (2003). Differences in fatty acid composition of blubber in minke whales (*Balaenoptera acutorostrata*) from Greenland and the NE Atlantic. *Journal of Cetacean Research and Management*, Vol.5, n.2, pp.115-124, ISSN 1561-0713.

Montie, E.W., Fair, P.A., Bossart, G.D., Mitchum, G.B., Houde, M., Muir, D.C.G., Letcher, R.J., McFee, W.E., Starczak, V.R., Stegeman, J.J. & Hahn, M.E. (2008). Cytochrome P4501A1 expression, polychlorinated biphenyls and hydroxylated metabolites, and adipocyte size of bottlenose dolphins from Southeast United States. *Aquatic Toxicology*, Vol. 86, pp. 397-412, ISSN 0166-445X.

Natoli, A., Peddemors, V.M. & Hoelzel, A.R. (2004). Population structure and speciation in the genus Tursiops based on microsatellite and mitochondrial DNA analyses. *Journal of Evolutionary Biology*, Vol. 17, No. 2, pp. 363-375, ISSN 1420-9101.

Natoli, A., Birkun, A., Aguilar, A., Lopez, A. & Hoelzel, A.R. (2005). Habitat structure and the dispersal of male and female bottlenose dolphins (*Tursiops truncatus*). *Proceedings. Biological Sciences / The Royal Society*, Vol. 272, No. 1569, pp. 1217-1226, ISSN 0962-8452.

Nover, L. (1991). Inducers of hsp synthesis: heat shock and chemical stressors. In: *Heat Shock Response*, Nover L. (Ed.), CRC Press, Boca Raton, FL, pp. 5–40.

Nover, L. & Scharf, K.D. (1991). Heat shock proteins. In: *Heat Shock Response*, Nover L. (Ed.), CRC Press, Boca Raton, FL, pp. 41–128.

Panigada, S., Pesante, G., Zanardelli, M., Capoulade, F., Gannier, A. & Weinrich, M.T. (2006). Mediterranean fin whales at risk from fatal ship strikes. *Marine Pollution Bulletin*, Vol. 52, No. 10, pp. 1287-1298, ISSN 0025-326X.

Pettersson, A., van Bavel, B., Engwall, M. & Jimenez, B. (2004). Polybrominated diphenylethers and methoxylated tetrabromodiphenylethers in cetaceans from the Mediterranean Sea. *Archives of Environmental Contamination and Toxicology*, Vol. 47, No. 4, pp. 542-550, ISSN 0090-4341.

Rossner, P.Jr, Binkova, B. & Sram, R.J. (2003). Heat shock proteins hsp32 and hsp70 as biomarkers of an early response? *Mutation Research*, Vol. 542, pp. 105 --116, ISSN 0921-8262.

Shugart, L.R. (2000). DNA damage as a biomarker of exposure. *Ecotoxicology*, Vol. 9, pp. 329-340, ISSN 0963-9292.

Simmonds, M. & Nunny, L. (2002) Cetacean Habitat Loss and Degradation in the Mediterranean Sea. Accobams secretariat, Monaco, February 2002, section 7, 23 p.

Singh, N.P., McCoy, M.T., Tice, R.R. & Sch, E.L. (1988). A simple technique for quantitation of low levels of DNA damage in individual cells. *Experimental Cell Research*, Vol. 175, No.1, pp. 184-191, ISSN 0014-4827.

Spinsanti, G., Panti, C., Lazzeri, E., Marsili, L., Casini, S., Frati, F. & Fossi, M.C. (2006). Selection of reference genes for quantitative RT-PCR in striped dolphin (*Stenella coeruleoalba*) skin biopsies. *BMC Molecular Biology*, Vol. 7, No.32, ISSN 1471-2199.

Spinsanti, G., Panti, C., Bucalossi, D., Marsili, L., Casini, S., Frati, F. & Fossi, M.C. (2008). Selection of reliable reference genes for qRT-PCR studies on cetacean fibroblast cultures exposed to OCs, PBDEs, and 17β-estradiol. *Aquatic Toxicology*, Vol. 87, pp. 178-186, ISSN 0166-445X.

Tanabe, S. & Tatsukawa, R. (1992). Chemical modernization and vulnerability of cetaceans: increasing toxic threat of organochlorine contaminants. In: *Persistent Pollutants in Marine Ecosystems*, C.H. Walker & D.R. Livingstone, (Eds), 161-177, Pergamon Press Ltd, Oxford, ISBN 0-08-041874-0.

Tang, N.J., Liu, J., Coenraads, P.J., Dong, L., Zhao, L.J., Ma, S.W., Chen, X., Zhang, C.M., Ma, X.M., Wei, W,G., Zhang, P. & Bai, Z.P. (2008). Expression of AhR, CYP1A1, GSTA1, c-fos and TGF-alpha in skin lesions from dioxin-exposed humans with chloracne. *Toxicology Letters*, Vol. 177, No. 3, pp. 182-187, ISSN 0378-4274.

Urbán-Ramírez, J., Rojas-Bracho, L., Guerrero-Ruíz, M., Jaramillo-Legorreta, A. & Findley, L.T. (2005). Identification of sex in Cetaceans by multiplexing with ZFX and ZFY specific primer. In: Cartron, J.E., Ceballos, G., Felger, R.S. (Eds.), *Biodiversity Ecosystems and Conservation in Northern Mexico.* Oxford University Press, New York, pp. 276–297, ISBN 9780195348125.

Valavanidis, A., Vlahogianni, T., Dassenakis, M. & Scoullos, M. (2006). Molecular biomarkers of oxidative stress in aquatic organisms in relation to toxic environmental pollutants. *Ecotoxicology and Environmental Safety*, Vol. 64, pp. 178-189, ISSN 0147-6513.

Villeneuve, D.L., Khim, J.S., Kannan, K. & Giesy, J.P. (2002). Relative potencies of individual polycyclic aromatic hydrocarbons to induce dioxinlike and estrogenic responses in three cell lines. *Environmental Toxicology*, Vol. 17, pp. 128-137, ISSN 1520-4081.

Whitehead, A., Anderson, S.L., Kuivila, K.M., Roach, J.L. & May, B. (2003). Genetic variation among interconnected populations of *Catostomus occidentalis*: implications for distinguishing impacts of contaminants from biogeographical structuring. *Molecular Ecology*, Vol. 12, pp. 2817-2833, ISSN 0962-1083.

Wu, T. & Tanguay, R.M. (2006). Antibodies against heat shock proteins in environmental stresses and diseases: friend or foe? *Cell Stress Chaperones*, Vol. 11, No. 1, pp. 1–12, ISSN 1355-8145.

Young, N.M. & Iudicello, S. (2007). Worldwide Bycatch of Cetaceans. An evaluation of the most significant threats to cetaceans, the affected species and the geographic areas of high risk, and the recommended actions from various independent institutions. U.S. Dep. Commerce, *NOAA Technical Memorandum*, NMFS-OPR-36 July 2007, 236pp.